Orthodontic Diagnosis and Treatment of Malocclusion

Orthodontic Diagnosis and Treatment of Malocclusion

Editor: Philip Chiders

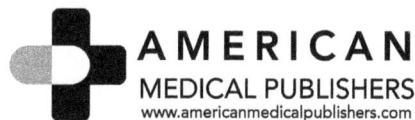

AMERICAN
MEDICAL PUBLISHERS
www.americanmedicalpublishers.com

AMERICAN
MEDICAL PUBLISHERS
www.americanmedicalpublishers.com

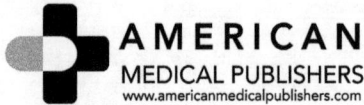

Cataloging-in-Publication Data

Orthodontic diagnosis and treatment of malocclusion / edited by Philip Chiders.
 p. cm.
Includes bibliographical references and index.
ISBN 978-1-63927-057-6
1. Malocclusion. 2. Orthodontics. 3. Occlusion (Dentistry). 4. Dentistry. I. Chiders, Philip.
RK523 .M35 2022
617.643--dc23

American Medical Publishers,
41 Flatbush Avenue,
1st Floor, New York,
NY 11217, USA

ISBN 978-1-63927-057-6 (Hardback)

Contents

Preface

Malocclusion is a condition that results in a misalignment between the teeth and the two dental arches when they approach each other when the jaw closes. Malocclusion can be divided into three types - class 1 is netrocclussion, class 2 is distocclussion and class 3 is mesiocclusion. Class 1 netrocclussion is a condition where the molar relationship of the occlusion is normal but the other teeth have problems like spacing, crowding and under eruption. Class 2 distocclussion is a condition where the mesiobuccal cusp of the upper first molar is anterior with the mesiobuccal groove of the lower first molar. Class 3 mesiocclusion is a condition where the upper molars are placed posteriorly to it and not in the mesiobuccal groove. Some common causes of malocclusion are extra teeth, impacted teeth, lost teeth and abnormally shaped teeth. It can be treated with the help of orthodontics which includes tooth extraction, dental braces and clear aligners. This book provides comprehensive insights into the field of malocclusion. It presents researches and studies performed by experts across the globe. This book is a resource guide for experts as well as students.

This book is a result of research of several months to collate the most relevant data in the field.

When I was approached with the idea of this book and the proposal to edit it, I was overwhelmed. It gave me an opportunity to reach out to all those who share a common interest with me in this field. I had 3 main parameters for editing this text:

1. Accuracy – The data and information provided in this book should be up-to-date and valuable to the readers.

2. Structure – The data must be presented in a structured format for easy understanding and better grasping of the readers.

3. Universal Approach – This book not only targets students but also experts and innovators in the field, thus my aim was to present topics which are of use to all.

Thus, it took me a couple of months to finish the editing of this book.

I would like to make a special mention of my publisher who considered me worthy of this opportunity and also supported me throughout the editing process. I would also like to thank the editing team at the back-end who extended their help whenever required.

Editor

Dental and skeletal components of Class II open bite treatment with a modified Thurow appliance

Helder Baldi Jacob[1], Ary dos Santos-Pinto[2], Peter H. Buschang[3]

Introduction: Due to the lack of studies that distinguish between dentoalveolar and basal changes caused by the Thurow appliance, this clinical study, carried out by the School of Dentistry — State University of São Paulo/Araraquara, aimed at assessing the dental and skeletal changes induced by modified Thurow appliance. **Methods:** The sample included an experimental group comprising 13 subjects aged between 7 and 10 years old, with Class II malocclusion and anterior open bite, and a control group comprising 22 subjects similar in age, sex and mandibular plane angle. Maxillary/mandibular, horizontal/vertical, dental/skeletal movements (ANS, PNS, U1, U6, Co, Go, Pog, L1, L6) were assessed, based on 14 landmarks, 8 angles (S-N-ANS, SNA, PPA, S-N-Pog, SNB, MPA, PP/MPA, ANB) and 3 linear measures (N-Me, ANS-Me, S-Go). **Results:** Treatment caused significantly greater angle decrease between the palatal and the mandibular plane of the experimental group, primarily due to an increase in the palatal plane angle. ANB, SNA and S-N-ANS angles significantly decreased more in patients from the experimental group. PNS was superiorly remodeled. Lower face height (ANS-Me) decreased in the experimental group and increased in the control group. **Conclusions:** The modified Thurow appliance controlled vertical and horizontal displacements of the maxilla, rotated the maxilla and improved open bite malocclusion, decreasing lower facial height.

Keywords: Angle Class II malocclusion. Open bite. Orthopedics.

[1] Post doc student in Orthodontics, Texas A&M Baylor College of Dentistry.
[2] Full professor in Orthodontics, School of Dentistry — State University of São Paulo/Araraquara.
[3] Professor, Department of Orthodontics, Texas A&M Baylor College of Dentistry.

» The authors report no commercial, proprietary or financial interest in the products or companies described in this article.

Helder Baldi Jacob
3302 Gaston Ave. - Texas A&M Baylor College of Dentistry
Department of Orthodontics - 75246 Dallas/TX – USA
E-mail: hjacob@bcd.tamhsc.edu

INTRODUCTION

Class II malocclusion can be due to skeletal or dental maxillary protrusion, mandibular retrusion or a combination of factors.[1,2,3] While Class II malocclusion can be addressed in a number of different ways (i.e. dentoalveolar changes, orthopedic forces to inhibit maxillary growth or stimulate mandibular growth, or surgical repositioning of the mandible in non-growing patients), maxillary protrusion is usually treated with orthopedic forces produced by headgear appliances.[3,4,5] Headgear appliances can be inserted into bands bonded onto the upper molars or into removable appliances. The issue of whether or not headgear therapy causes skeletal maxillary changes in humans remains controversial.[6-9]

When associated with hyperdivergence and anterior open bite, Class II malocclusions have proven to be a daunting challenge for orthodontists. The position of the tongue as well as thumb and finger sucking are perhaps the best known physical factors that cause open bite malocclusions.[10] Hyperdivergent open bite subjects have anterior and posterior dentoalveolar heights that tend to be excessive, palatal plane angles that are flatter, as well as increased mandibular plane and gonial angles.[11] To treat such malocclusion in growing patients, it is necessary to limit maxillary displacement and intrude the molars in order to rotate the mandible upwards and forward.[12,13]

The Thurow appliance was developed to apply distal and vertical forces while controlling molar rotation and tipping produced by forces directed through buccal molar tubes. The original appliance, which incorporates a high-pull headgear and a maxillary acrylic splint that serves as a bite block, has been shown to restrain maxillary growth, distally tip and displace the maxillary teeth, as well as restrain the eruption of posterior maxillary teeth.[14,15] Because the splint precisely covers the entire maxillary dentition, higher force levels dissipating over a larger surface area can be used. The acrylic smooth surface disoccludes the teeth and effectively eliminates occlusal interferences during force application, which facilitates maxillary tooth movement and allows the mandible to grow unimpeded by the maxilla. The Thurow appliance is thought to be particularly well suited for Class II patients with maxillary prognathism, steep mandibular plane angles and open bites.[16]

It has been reported that the Thurow appliance can be used to decrease the ANB angle, inhibit maxillary horizontal growth, control vertical growth of the maxilla, maintain the mandibular plane angle, move the upper first molars distally, and improve lip relationships.[12,13,16-19] However, these claims have been based on case reports which have not been compared to control groups. Existing case-control studies were not able to distinguish between dentoalveolar and basal changes produced by the appliance because mandibular and, especially, maxillary superimpositions were not performed.[14,20,21]

The ability to distinguish between skeletal/dental contributions and correction is important not only to ensure that treatment objectives were met, but also to further improve therapies performed with the appliance. Clinically, understanding the effects of Thurow high-pull headgear is vital to understand Class II correction in growing hyperdivergent patients. The aim of this retrospective study was to assess dental and skeletal changes produced by a Thurow high-pull headgear appliance for hyperdivergent patients with open bite and Class II division 1 malocclusion, by means of cephalometric radiographs.

MATERIAL AND METHODS
Sample

Fifteen children participated in this retrospective clinical study as a treated group. Recruitment was conducted at the orthodontic clinic of the School of Dentistry — State University of São Paulo/Araraquara. During treatment, two patients moved away from the city.

The final treated group included 13 children (1 male and 12 female) with Class II division 1 malocclusion as well as open bite. The children aged between 7 and 10 years old and were treated for 12 months before growth spurt (Table 1). The maxillary splint high-pull headgear comprised an acrylic plate, a vestibular arch, an extraoral arch fixed to the acrylic, a palatal crib, and an expansion screw at the level of the second deciduous molars (Fig 1); and it was based on the appliance introduced by Thurow[16] and modified by Santos-Pinto.[18] The acrylic plate extended laterally and occlusally, covering the cusps and approximately one-third of the molars buccal surfaces. Should expansion be necessary, the screw was activated once a week (0.25 mm) for as long as it was needed. The outer bow of the extraoral

Table 1 - Pre-treatment and follow-up ages of the treated (Thurow appliance) and untreated (control) groups.

	Group	Sample size	Mean ± SD	Prob.
Initial	Treated	13	8.85 ± 0.73	0.912
	Untreated	22	8.82 ± 0.73	
Final	Treated	13	9.84 ± 0.70	0.933
	Untreated	22	9.82 ± 0.73	

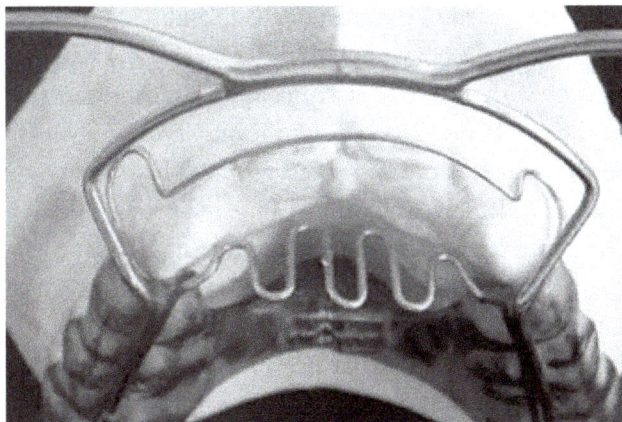

Figure 1 - Modified Thurow appliance.

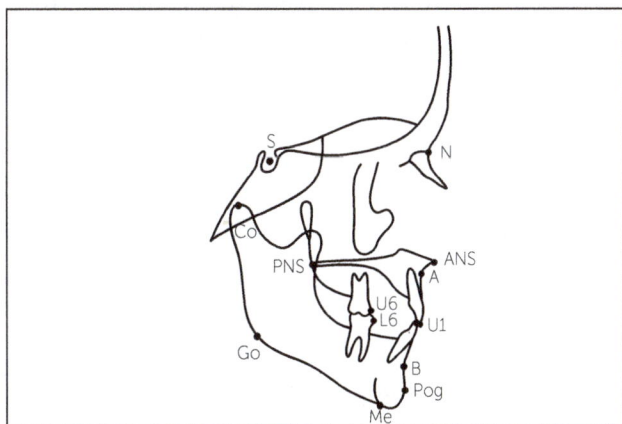

Figure 2 - Cephalometric landmarks digitized; (S) sella, (N) nasion, (PNS) posterior nasal spine, (ANS) anterior nasal spine, (A) A-point, (Co) condylion, (Go) gonion, (Me) menton, (Pog) pogonion, (B) B-point, (U6) maxillary mesial molar, (U1) maxillary incisor tip, (L6) mandibular mesial molar, (L1) mandibular incisor tip.

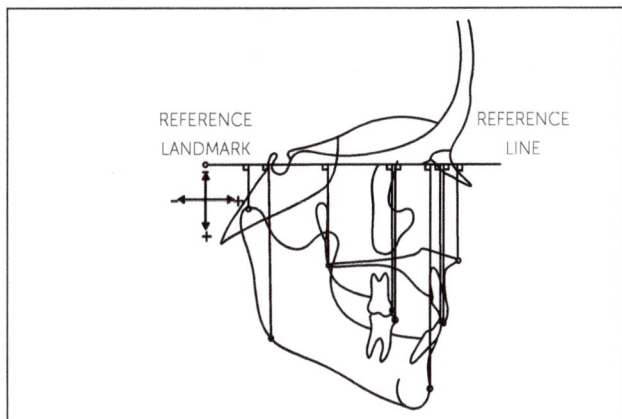

Figure 3 - Horizontal and vertical cephalometric landmarks position measured parallel and perpendicular to the reference line (SN = -7°).

arch was adjusted so that the line of force of the elastics slightly passed anteroposteriorly through the first and second deciduous molars and between the lower margin of the orbitale, and vertically through the apex of the first molar, which is slightly posterior to the maxilla center of resistance.[22,23] The high-pull headgear delivered approximately 400 g of force on each side and was worn 14 hours a day. After correction was achieved, the patients wore the headgear for 8 to 10 hours during sleep. They were seen monthly so that the splint could be adjusted, if necessary.

The untreated control group included children who were followed longitudinally at the Human Growth Research Center, University of Montreal, Canada. They were from three different school districts in Montreal and represented various socioeconomic strata.[24] The control group sample comprised 22 patients (2 males and 20 females) with Class II division 1 who were at the same age, with the same sex and mandibular plane angle when compared to the treated sample.

Cephalometric methods

Lateral cephalograms were obtained at the beginning of the treatment (T_1) and at the follow-up appointment (T_2) in the treated group. In the control group, the lateral cephalograms were obtained after one year, at least fifteen days before or after the initial day. The cephalograms were taken with the head positioned according to the Frankfort horizontal plane, and the lateral cephalometric tracings were performed on acetate paper. The tracings were digitized and analyzed with Viewbox 3.1-Cephalometric Software (Dhal Software, Athens, Greece) by one investigator. The linear measurements were adjusted to eliminate magnification. The analyses described growth and treatment changes of fourteen skeletal landmarks (Fig 2).

The horizontal and vertical movements of the selected landmarks were described on the basis of a horizontal reference line (RL), which was oriented in T_1 based on the sella-nasion plane with -7 degrees. For example, the horizontal change in the position of pogonion was measured parallel to the RL (distance between the pogonion projection to a reference point fixed 100 mm behind the sella), while the vertical change was measured perpendicular to the RL (Fig 3).

In general, tooth movements were calculated based on tracings superimposed to the stable cranial base structures, as described by Björk and Skieller.[25] To determine the actual movement of incisors and molars, maxillary and mandibular superimpositions were also performed, as described by Björk and Skieller.[25,26] After partial superimposition, tooth movements were subtracted from the overall tooth movements in order to estimate the movement of the skeletal bases. Horizontally, an anterior change was recorded as positive, whereas a posterior change was recorded as negative. Vertically, a superior change was recorded as negative, whereas an inferior change was recorded as positive (Fig 3).

Replicate analysis of 26 subjects showed small, but statistically significant systematic errors for the ANS horizontal (0.31 mm) and Go vertical (-0.21 mm). Random method errors ranged from 0.15 to 0.46 mm with PNS horizontal showing the largest random error.[27]

Statistical methods

The measurements were transferred to SPSS software (version 15.0, SPSS, Chicago, USA) for evaluation. Based on Skewness and Kurtosis, the variables were normally distributed. T-tests were used to compare the groups. A probability level of 0.05 was used to determine statistical significance.

RESULTS

T-tests showed significant (P < 0.05) differences between groups prior to treatment of five out of the 11 traditional variables measured (Table 2). In comparison to the control group, the treated group initially had greater ANB angles, smaller palatal plane angles and greater anterior and posterior facial heights. Analysis of covariance demonstrated that none of the traditional pretreatment variables were related to post-treatment changes.

Regardless of pretreatment measures, the treatment yielded significant differences. The palatal plane angle increased in the treated group and remained unchanged in the control. This difference, along with the greater, although not statistically significant decrease in the MPA, resulted in a significantly greater decrease in the PP/MPA of the treated group. The ANB angle significantly decreased more in treated patients than in the control group, primarily due to a significant treatment decrease in the SNA angle. While lower face height increased significantly in the control, it significantly decreased in the treated group.

In comparison to the treated group, which showed no statistically significant horizontal displacement, the maxilla and maxillary teeth of the control group were anteriorly displaced approximately 0.7 mm over the observation period (Table 4). Although the treated group showed anterior displacement of the mandible, the changes were not statistically significant. All mandibular landmarks of the control group showed significant anterior displacement, except for the condylion. None of the differences regarding horizontal displacement between groups were statistically significant.

Based on the maxillary superimpositions, the treated group demonstrated no statistically significant difference with regard to horizontal remodeling or tooth migration; the control group showed

Table 2 - Comparison of pretreatment values between treated and untreated groups.

Variable		Treated Mean ± SD		Untreated Mean ± SD		Prob. (difference)
S-N-ANS	Deg	87.45	5.88	86.38	2.62	0.548
SNA	Deg	82.37	5.93	81.27	3.19	0.550
PPA	Deg	3.99	3.40	6.91	2.79	0.016
SNPog	Deg	77.25	5.14	77.28	3.02	0.981
SNB	Deg	77.21	5.45	77.50	3.10	0.862
MPA	Deg	35.97	5.30	36.27	3.60	0.855
PP/MPA	Deg	31.96	4.62	29.19	3.41	0.076
ANB	Deg	5.16	1.90	3.72	2.00	0.046
N-Me	mm	96.58	4.58	92.03	4.02	0.007
ANS-Me	mm	58.23	3.99	53.02	2.66	0.001
S-Go	mm	60.82	5.25	57.27	3.90	0.047

Table 3 - Comparison of changes between treated and untreated groups.

Variable		Treated Mean ± SD		Untreated Mean ± SD		Prob. (difference)
S-N-ANS	Deg	-2.75	1.20	0.08	1.45	<0.001
SNA	Deg	-0.94	0.80	0.03	1.15	0.007
PPA	Deg	2.14	1.59	0.07	0.85	<0.001
S-N-Pog	Deg	0.27	1.12	0.33	0.66	0.871
SNB	Deg	0.16	0.95	0.22	0.59	0.846
MPA	Deg	-0.61	1.63	-0.17	0.99	0.392
PP/MPA	Deg	-2.73	1.92	-0.23	1.12	0.001
A-N-B	Deg	-1.10	0.88	-0.12	1.15	0.010
N-Me	mm	1.64	1.55	2.36	1.52	0.198
ANS-Me	mm	-0.92	1.44	1.14	1.26	<0.001
S-Go	mm	1.68	1.68	1.64	0.89	0.938

anterior and posterior remodeling of ANS and PNS, respectively, and mesial drift of the incisors molars. Except for the gonion of the control group, which drifted posteriorly, and for the lower molar of the treated group, which moved mesially, none of the mandibular measures showed statistically significant horizontal changes. While several of the group comparisons were at a significant level, none of the differences were statistically significant.

Both groups showed statistically significant inferior displacement, with no significant differences between groups (Table 5). The maxilla was inferiorly displaced for approximately 1 mm. The posterior and anterior aspects of the mandible were inferiorly displaced for approximately 2.9 to 3.4 mm and 1.5 to 2.3 mm, respectively. While ANS showed no significant remodeling changes, PNS showed slight superior drift in the treated group and inferior drift in the control group, with statistically significant differences.

The maxillary molars of the treated group showed no vertical changes, whereas the control molars erupted approximately 0.8 mm. There was little or no group difference in mandibular remodeling and tooth movements. Condylion showed the greatest growth (2.6 to 2.8 mm), gonion drifted superiorly, the incisors erupted 0.8 to 1.2 mm and the mandibular molars erupted 0.8 to 0.9 mm.

DISCUSSION

The modified Thurow appliance clearly restricted the forward growth of the maxilla. The treated subjects showed a decrease of 2.8° and 0.9° in S-N-ANS and SNA, respectively. The angles decreased in the treated group because the maxilla maintained its anteroposterior position while the nasion continued to drift anteriorly. The control group showed little or no change in SNA or S-N-ANS because the maxilla moved forward along with the nasion. This distinction is important

Table 4 - Horizontal skeletal and dental changes in treated and untreated patients (positive value = forward direction; negative value = backward direction).

| Variable | Horizontal values | | |
| | Displacement | | |
	Treated Mean ± SD	Untreated Mean ± SD	Prob. (difference)
ANS	0.01 ± 0.83	**0.72** ± 1.16	0.060
PNS	0.02 ± 0.84	**0.74** ± 1.21	0.068
U1	0.15 ± 1.62	**0.71** ± 1.56	0.315
U6	0.12 ± 1.35	**0.72** ± 1.41	0.229
Co	-0.42 ± 2.42	0.15 ± 1.73	0.418
Go	0.63 ± 2.12	**0.93** ± 1.37	0.618
Pog	1.32 ± 2.66	**1.44** ± 1.84	0.878
L1	0.59 ± 2.17	**0.86** ± 1.38	0.654
L6	0.55 ± 2.11	**0.86** ± 1.37	0.592

| Variable | Remodeling / tooth movement | | |
	Treated Mean ± SD	Untreated Mean ± SD	Prob. (difference)
ANS	0.35 ± 1.18	**0.78** ± 1.36	0.428
PNS	-1.14 ± 1.93	**-0.81** ± 1.14	0.699
U1	-0.02 ± 1.53	0.80 ± 1.14	0.091
U6	0.33 ± 1.15	0.56 ± 1.16	0.625
Co	0.25 ± 2.54	-0.54 ± 1.71	0.159
Go	-0.55 ± 1.64	**-1.45** ± 1.31	0.053
Pog	0.02 ± 0.13	-0.07 ± 0.25	0.271
L1	0.74 ± 1.44	0.34 ± 0.94	0.203
L6	**0.98** ± 1.28	0.36 ± 0.96	0.121

Bold = significant change between initial and final radiographs.

Table 5 - Vertical skeletal and dental changes in treated and untreated patients (positive value = inferior direction; negative value = superior direction).

| Variable | Vertical values | | |
| | Displacement | | |
	Treated Mean ± SD	Untreated Mean ± SD	Prob. (difference)
ANS	**0.80** ± 1.47	**0.98** ± 1.54	0.740
PNS	**1.02** ± 1.08	**1.00** ± 0.69	0.964
U1	**0.83** ± 1.42	**1.00** ± 1.48	0.749
U6	**0.96** ± 0.88	**0.96** ± 0.89	0.995
Co	**2.94** ± 2.30	**3.53** ± 2.13	0.448
Go	**2.86** ± 2.25	**3.40** ± 1.95	0.466
Pog	**1.51** ± 1.82	**2.31** ± 1.28	0.180
L1	**1.37** ± 1.97	**2.23** ± 1.36	0.181
L6	**1.89** ± 1.70	**2.59** ± 1.22	0.168

| Variable | Remodeling / eruption | | |
	Treated Mean ± SD	Untreated Mean ± SD	Prob. (difference)
ANS	0.22 ± 0.44	0.37 ± 1.75	0.775
PNS	**-0.50** ± 0.57	**0.21** ± 0.43	**0.001**
U1	**1.03** ± 0.91	**0.93** ± 1.45	0.243
U6	0.33 ± 1.15	**0.82** ± 0.95	0.073
Co	**-2.63** ± 2.69	**-2.82** ± 1.75	0.371
Go	**-1.25** ± 1.69	**-1.74** ± 1.85	0.489
Pog	**0.11** ± 0.14	0.04 ± 0.71	0.699
L1	**-1.24** ± 1.49	**-0.82** ± 1.14	0.319
L6	**-0.94** ± 0.86	**-0.84** ± 0.77	0.448

Bold = significant change between initial and final radiographs.

because previous studies have reported, based solely on decreases in SNA or S-N-ANS, that headgears used to correct Class II malocclusions are generally effective in posteriorly redirecting maxillary growth.[14,16,20,21,28-31]

Most studies have not assessed the actual antero-posterior movement of the maxilla. Baumrind et al,[8] who used the biologically defined "best fit" of palatal structures, showed small, but definite posterior movement of ANS. In the present study, ANS was not displaced posteriorly, perhaps due to the more superiorly oriented forces produced by the high-pull headgear.

The modified Thurow appliance produced 2.1° posteriorly, or a backward rotation of the palatal plane. In contrast with the control group, the treated group showed no statistically significant changes of the palatal plane angle, as expected for untreated subjects over a similar time period.[33-36] Other studies evaluating the effects of high-pull forces have all shown backward rotation of the palatal plane.[14,20,30,37,38]

In some situations, the orthodontist wants to prevent maxillary rotation, in which case the high-pull forces should be directed through the maxilla center of resistance.

In this study, the headgear forces were purposely directed behind the dental and maxillary centers of resistance in order to help correcting the open bite. Rotation of the palatal plane also explains the decrease observed in the lower anterior face height of the treated group.[20,31] Lower anterior face height of the control group increased, as expected during growth of untreated subjects.[33,34,36]

The modified Thurow appliance used in the present study had no real treatment effects on the antero-posterior mandibular position. The S-N-Pog and SNB angles did not significantly change in either treated or control group. Previous studies also show no changes in the anteroposterior position of the mandible.[14,20,21,32,39] Lahaye et al,[40] who evaluated methods commonly used to correct Class II skeletal malocclusions, including headgears and Herbst appliances, found no appreciable significant improvements in anteroposterior chin position. The authors stated that skeletal Class II correction in growing adolescents results primarily from maxillary growth restriction or inhibition.

The mandibular plane angle did not show statistically significant differences between groups either. Both groups showed forward rotation during the observation period. Most previous studies have shown that the mandibular plane angle changed or was maintained during treatment.[14,20,21,32,41] Except for Bhatia and Leighton,[36] who reported a slight increase for males and stable relations for females, previous longitudinal studies of untreated children have also shown decreases in the MPA between 10-15 years, ranging from 0.8 to 3.5°.[33,34,35]

CONCLUSION

1. The modified Thurow appliance held the maxilla and caused a slight backward rotation of the palatal plane.

2. The maxillary molars of the treated group showed neither horizontal nor vertical changes. The upper incisors were retroclined, but no significant change was observed over time.

3. Except for the lower molars, which moved mesially in the treated group, no treatment effect was observed in the mandible.

4. Lower facial height decreased in the treated group.

Acknowledgments

The authors would like to thank Dr. Demetrius Halazonetis for his intellectual expertise helping with the Viewbox 3.1-Cephalometric software.

REFERENCES

1. McNamara JA. Components of Class II malocclusion in children 8-10 years of age. Angle Orthod. 1981;51(3):177-202.

2. Proffit WR, Fields HW, Ackerman JL, Sinclair PM, Thomas PM, Tulloch JFC. Contemporary orthodontics. St. Louis: Mosby-Year Book; 1993.

3. Nanda R. Biomechanics in clinical orthodontics. Philadelphia: WB Saunders; 1997. 329 p.

4. Droschl H. The effect of heavy orthopedic forces on the maxilla in growing Saimiri sciureus (squirrel monkey). Am J Orthod. 1973;63(5):449-61.

5. Meldrum RJ. Alterations in the upper facial growth of Macaca mulatta resulting from high-pull headgear. Am J Orthod. 1975;67(4):393-411.

6. Klein PL. An evaluation of cervical traction on maxilla and the upper first permanent molar. Angle Orthod. 1957;27(1):61-8.

7. Bernstein L, Ulbrich WR, Gianelly A. Orthopedics versus orthodonticsin Class II treatment: an implant study. Am J Orthod. 1977;72(5):549-59.

8. Baumrind S, Korn EL, Isaacson RJ, West EE, Molthen R. Quantitative analysis of the orthodontic effects of maxillary traction. Am J Ortrhod. 1983;84:384-98.

9. Boecler PR, Riolo ML, Keeling SD, Tenhave TR. Skeletal changes associated with extraoral appliance therapy: an evaluation of 200 consecutively treated cases. Angle Orthod. 1989;59(4):263-70.

10. Graber TM, Swain BF. Orthodontics. Current principles and techniques. Saint Louis: Mosby; 1985.

11. Buschang PH, Sankey W, English JD. Early treatment of hyperdivergent open-bite malocclusions. Semin Orthod. 2002;8(3):130-40.

12. Henriques JFC, Martins DR, Almeida GA, Ursi WJS. Modified maxillary splint for Class II, division 1 treatment. J Clin Orthod. 1991;25(4):239-45.

13. Stuani MBS, Stuani AS, Stuani AS. Modified Thurow appliance: a clinical alternative for correcting skeletal open bite. Am J Orthod Dentofacial Orthop. 2005;128(1):118-25.

14. Caldwell SF, Hymas TA, Timm TA. Maxillary traction splint: a cephalometric evaluation. Am J Orthod. 1984;85(5):376-84.

15. Seckin O, Surucu R. Treatment of Class II, division 1, cases with a maxillary traction splint. Quintessence Int. 1990;21(3):209-15.

16. Thurow RC. Craniomaxillary orthopedic correction with en masse dental control. Am J Orthod. 1975;68(6):601-24.

17. Joffe L, Orth D, Jacobson A. The maxillary orthopedic splint. Am J Orthod. 1979;75(1):54-69.

18. Santos-Pinto A, Paulin RF, Martins LP, Melo ACM, Oshiro L. O splint maxilar de Thurow modificado no tratamento da Classe II com mordida aberta: caso clinico. Rev Dental Press Ortod Ortop Facial. 2001;6(1):57-62.

19. Souza MM, Freitas TM, Stuani AS, Stuani AS, Stuani MBS. Uso do aparelho de Thurow no tratamento da ma oclusao esqueletica de Classe II. Rev Dental Press Ortod Ortop Facial. 2005;10(4):76-87.

20. Orton HS, Slattery DA, Orton S. The treatment of severe "gummy" Class II division 1 malocclusion using the maxillary intrusion splint. Eur J Orthod. 1992;14(3):216-23.

21. Üner O, Yucel-Eroğlu E. Effects of a modified maxillary orthopaedic splint: a cephalometric evaluation. Eur J Orthod. 1996;18(3):269-86.

22. Miki M. An experimental research on the directional control of the nasomaxillary complex by means of external force: two dimensional analyses on the sagittal plane of the craniofacial skeleton. Shikwa Gakuho. 1979;79(8):1563-97.

23. Hirato R. An experimental study on the center of resistance of the nasomaxillary complex: 2-dimensional analysis of the coronal plane in the dry skull. Shikwa Gakuho. 1984;84(8):1225-62.

24. Demirjian A, Brault DM, Jenicek M. Etude comparative de la croissance de l'enfant canadien d'orige francais a Montreal. Can J Public Health. 1971;62:11-9.

25. Björk A, Skieller V. Normal and abnormal growth of the mandible: a synthesis of longitudinal Cephalometric implant studies over a period of 25 years. Eur J Orthod. 1983;5(1):1-46.

26. Björk A, Skieller V. Growth of the maxilla in three dimensions as revealed radiographically by the implant method. Br J Orthod. 1977;4(2):53-64.

27. Dahlberg G. Statistical methods for medical and biological students. New York: Interscience; 1940.

28. Ricketts RM. Cephalometric synthesis. Am J Orthod. 1960;46(9):647-73.

29. Wieslander L. The effect of force on craniofacial development. Am J Orthod 1974;65(5):531-8.

30. Brown P. A cephalometric evaluation of high-pull molar headgear and face-bow neck strap therapy. Am J Orthod. 1978;74(6):621-32.

31. Firouz M, Zernik J, Nanda R. Dental and orthopedic effects of high-pull headgear in treatment of Class II, division 1 malocclusion. Am J Orthod Dentofacial Orthop. 1992;102(3):197-205.

32. Martins RP, Martins JCR, Martins LP, Buschang PH. Skeletal and dental components of Class II correction with the bionator and removable headgear splint appliances. Am J Orthod Dentofacial Orthop. 2008;134(6):732-41.

33. Riolo ML, Moyers RE, McNamara JA, Hunter WS. An atlas of craniofacial growth: cephalometric standards from University School Growth Study. Ann Arbor: The University of Michigan, Center For Human Growth and Development; 1974. 380 p.

34. Saksena SS, Walker GF, Bixler D, Yu P. A clinical Atlas of Roentgenocephalometry in Norma Lateralis. New York: Alan R Liss; 1987. 208 p.

35. Nanda KS. Growth patterns in subjects with long and short faces. Am J Orthod Dentofacial Orthop. 1990;98(3):247-58.

36. Bhatia SN and Leighton BC. A manual of facial growth: a computer analysis of longitudinal cephalometric growth data. New York: Oxford University Press; 1993. 544 p.

37. Baumrind S, Molthen R, West EE, Miller DM. Mandibular plane changes during maxillary retraction. Am J Orthod. 1978;74(1):32-40.

38. Gautam P, Valiathan A, Adhikari R. Craniofacial displacement in response to varying headgear forces evaluated biomechanically with finite element analysis. Am J Orthod Dentofacial Orthop. 2009;135(4):507-15.

39. Fotis V, Melsen B, Williams S, Droschi H. Vertical control as an important ingredient in the treatment of severe sagittal discrepancies. Am J Orthod. 1984;86(3):224-32.

40. LaHaye MB, Buschang PH, Alexander RG, Boley JC. Orthodontic treatment changes of chin position in Class II Division 1 patients. Am J Orthod Dentofacial Orthop. 2006;130(6):732-41.

41. Malmgren O, Omblus J. Treatment with an orthopedic appliance system. Eur J Orthod. 1985;7(3):205-14.

2

Transdisciplinary treatment of Class III malocclusion using conventional implant-supported anchorage: 10-year posttreatment follow-up

Mariana Roennau Lemos Rinaldi[1], Susana Maria Deon Rizzatto[2], Luciane Macedo de Menezes[3], Waldemar Daudt Polido[3], Eduardo Martinelli Santayanna de Lima[4]

Introduction: Combined treatment offers advantages for partially edentulous patients. Conventional implants, used as orthodontic anchorage, enable previous orthodontic movement, which provides appropriate space gain for crown insertion. **Objective:** This case report describes the treatment of a 61-year and 10-month-old patient with negative overjet which made ideal prosthetic rehabilitation impossible, thereby hindering dental and facial esthetics. **Case report:** After a diagnostic setup, conventional implants were placed in the upper arch to anchor intrusion and retract anterior teeth. Space gain for lateral incisors was achieved in the lower arch by means of an orthodontic appliance. **Conclusions:** Integrated planning combining Orthodontics and Implantology provided successful treatment by means of conventional implant-supported anchorage. The resulting occlusal relationship proved stable after 10 years.

Keywords: Orthodontic anchorage procedures. Dental implants. Angle Class III malocclusion. Tooth loss.

[1] PhD resident in Orthodontics, Pontifícia Universidade Católica do Rio Grande do Sul (PUCRS), Porto Alegre, Rio Grande do Sul, Brazil.
[2] Professor of Orthodontics, Pontifícia Universidade Católica do Rio Grande do Sul (PUCRS), Porto Alegre, Rio Grande do Sul, Brazil.
[3] PhD in Oral and Maxillofacial Surgery, Pontifícia Universidade Católica do Rio Grande do Sul (PUCRS), Porto Alegre, Rio Grande do Sul, Brazil.
[4] Adjunct professor of Orthodontics, Pontifícia Universidade Católica do Rio Grande do Sul (PUCRS), Porto Alegre, Rio Grande do Sul, Brazil.

» The authors report no commercial, proprietary or financial interest in the products or companies described in this article.

Eduardo Martinelli S. de Lima
Av. Ipiranga, 6681 - Prédio 6 (Faculdade de Odontologia), Porto Alegre - RS, CEP 91530-000 - Brazil.
E-mail: elima@pucrs.br

INTRODUCTION

Transdisciplinarity is a trend in Dentistry as well as in other areas of the health sciences. This is because the interaction established among different specialties provides patients with a comprehensive treatment plan.[1,2,3] Osseointegration has opened up new possibilities not only for Prosthodontics, but also for Orthodontics. Proper anchorage has always been fundamental for orthodontic treatment efficiency, as it allows the desired orthodontic movements to be performed and reduces potential adverse effects. The use of conventional implants and temporary anchorage devices (TAD) has improved anchorage control and provided absolute resistance units against movement. Absolute anchorage allows space closure, intrusion, extrusion, protraction, retraction of teeth and stabilization of periodontally compromised teeth.[4-8]

Conventional implants for prosthetic restoration can also be used for orthodontic anchorage.[9] Implant selection and insertion site should be appropriate for the dual function of implants: rehabilitation and anchorage. The anatomical aspects of the case, the intended orthodontic movement and the ideal position for final rehabilitation should be planned ahead of time.[5,10,11] Combined treatment offers advantages for partially edentulous patients, and so does previous orthodontic movement, as it provides appropriate space gain for implant insertion.[12-15]

The aim of this case report is to demonstrate the transdisciplinary treatment of a Class III malocclusion patient with multiple missing teeth. Conventional implants were used as anchorage to retract lower teeth. This combined transdisciplinary plan intended to maximize patient's benefits, enhance dental esthetics and establish a balanced occlusion associated with healthy tissues. This report illustrates a case of successful 10-year posttreatment stability.

CASE REPORT

In 1998, a healthy female patient, aged 61 years and 10 months old, presented at the orthodontic service of the Brazilian Dental Association with anterior crossbite and multiple missing teeth. Her chief complaint was related to poor dental esthetics. Prosthetic rehabilitation was thought to be determined by the conditions of dental occlusion. There was premature contact between lower central incisors, and anterior crossbite was mostly caused by functional sliding resulting from contact.

In occlusion, the patient had Class I canine relationship on both sides (Figs 1 and 2).

Patient's face was symmetrical in frontal view, with a marked nasolabial fold. Facial profile was unbalanced, with mild maxillary deficiency and protrusion of the lower lip which was positioned ahead of the upper lip. The nasolabial angle denoted the incorrect anterior-posterior position of the maxilla, which was confirmed by cephalometric findings. The mentolabial sulcus was flat, most likely due to muscle adaptation to anterior crossbite.

Lower dentition was mutilated: molars and second premolars were absent on both sides. On the right side, there was a single-unit ceramic crown over the lower first premolar. In the upper arch, posterior teeth were extruded, left first molar was absent and right first premolar had a ceramic crown. A midline diastema of 5 mm was found in the upper arch and associated to the migration of central incisors and to the space of missing lateral incisors (Fig 3).

Periapical radiographs revealed generalized mild attachment loss, which suggested judicious periodontal control during orthodontic treatment. In spite of the edentulous regions, bone height was enough for conventional implant placement. Cephalometric evaluation revealed skeletal Class III malocclusion associated with retrusion of upper incisors and protrusion of lower incisors (Fig 4 and Table 1).

The objectives of treatment were: (1) correct anterior crossbite; (2) reestablish vertical dimensions in the posterior region, which would provide space gain for implant-retained prosthetic restorations in the region of lower premolars and molars; (3) close interincisal diastema; (4) gain space for implants and prosthetic crowns in the region of upper lateral incisors; and (5) improve the relationship established between upper and lower lips.

Delay in rehabilitation treatment after extraction of posterior teeth is expected to provoke alveolar bone atrophy; therefore, only basal bones of the maxilla and mandible remain intact. Lack of dental occlusion in the posterior region leads to a reduction in lower facial height and changes in the position of remaining teeth. The mandible rotates anticlockwise, remodeling the condyle process and the glenoid fossa.[16,17] Orthognathic surgery may be the first choice to correct anterior crossbite and provide the height necessary for prosthetic rehabilitation in the posterior region.

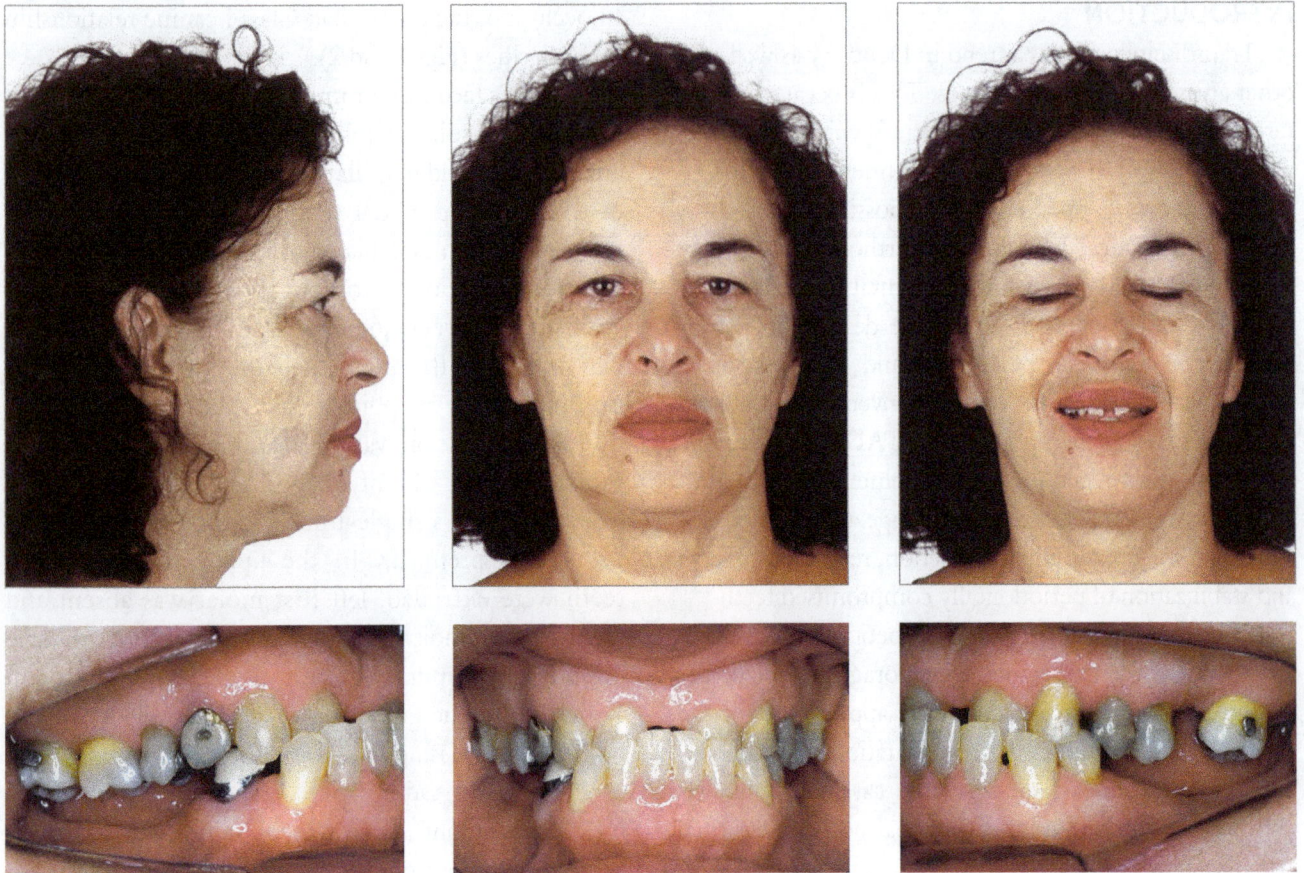

Figure 1 - Pre-treatment facial and intraoral photographs.

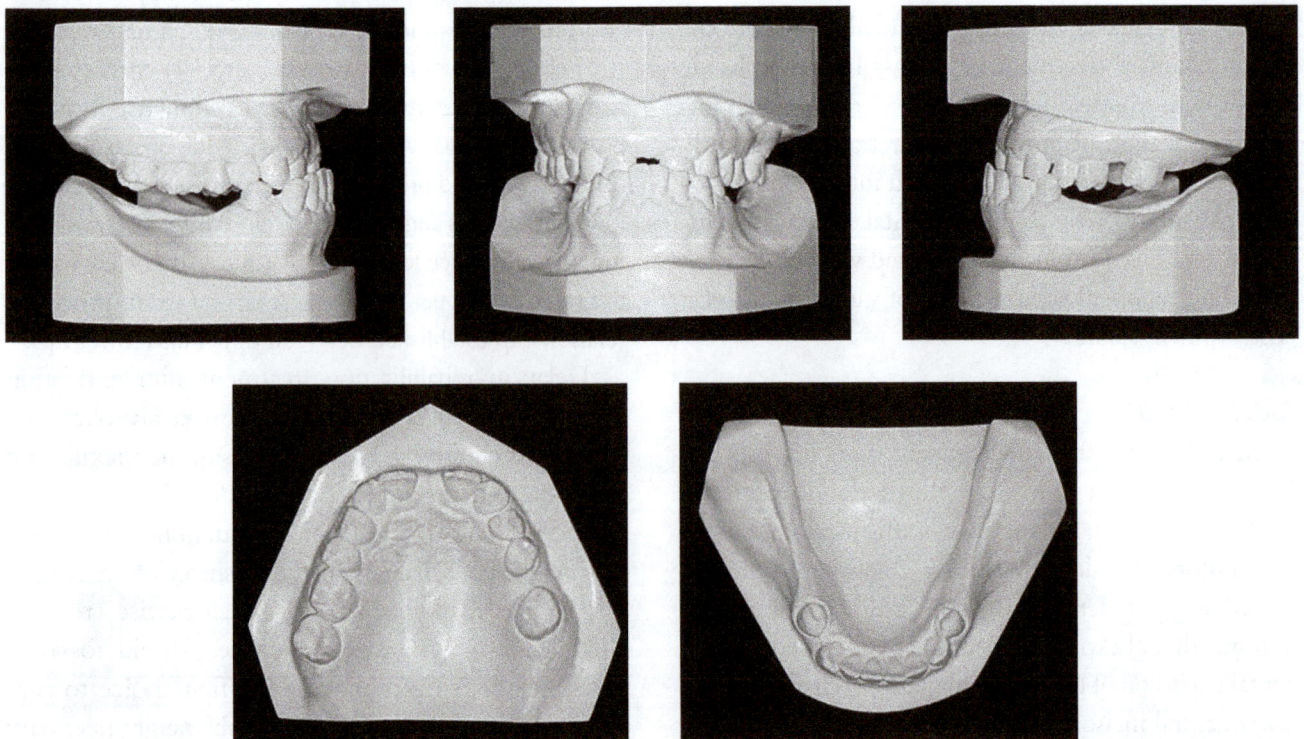

Figure 2 - Initial dental casts.

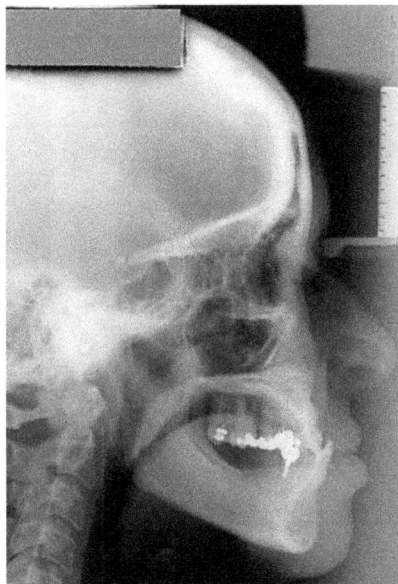

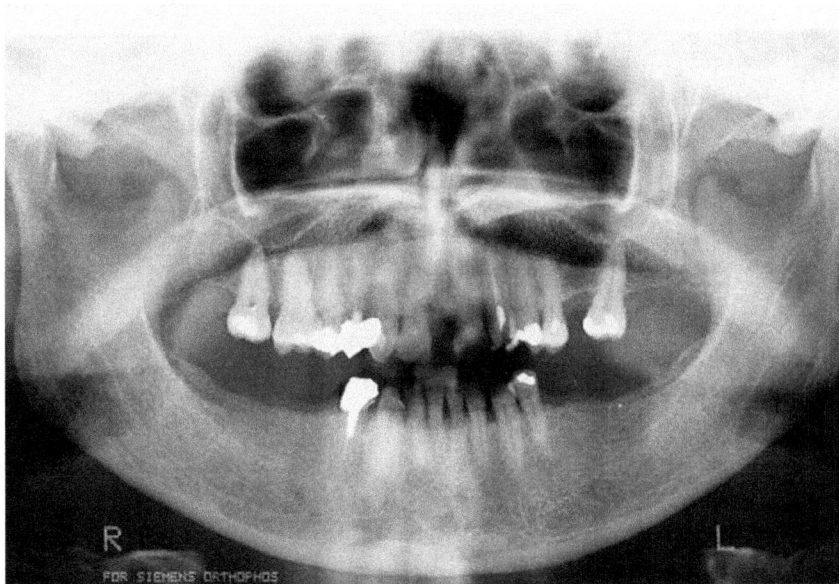

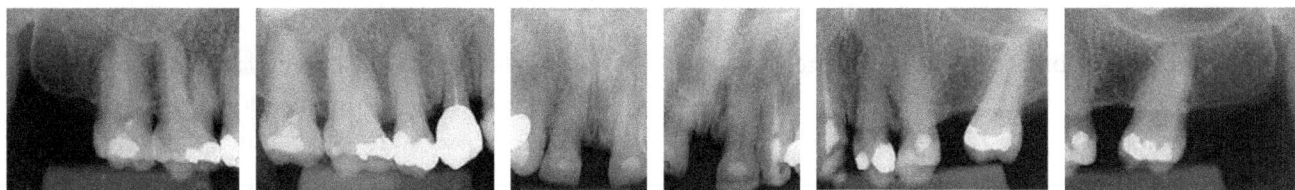

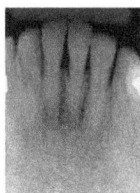

Figure 3 - Initial lateral cephalometric radiograph, panoramic and periapical radiographs.

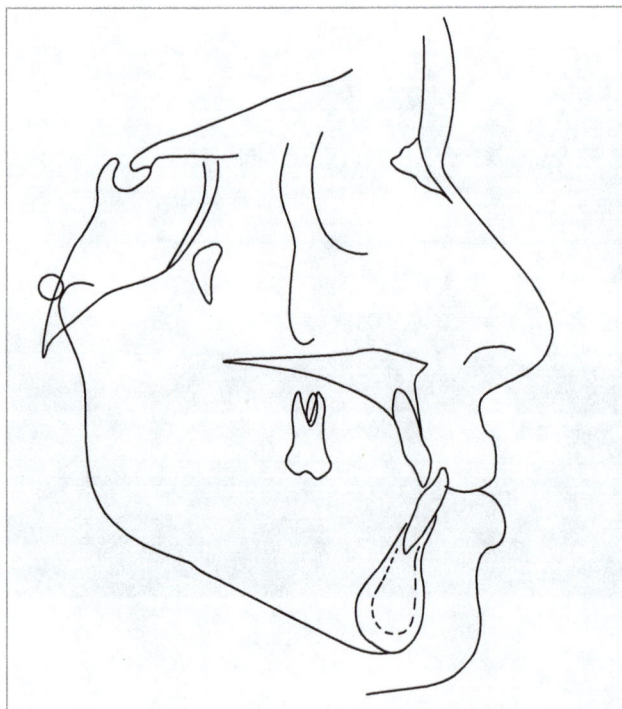

Figure 4 - Initial cephalometric tracing.

Table 1 - Cephalometric data.

	Pre-treatment	Post-treatment	10-year follow-up
SNA (degrees)	82	81	81
SNB (degrees)	83	81	81.5
ANB (degrees)	-1	0	-0.5
1.NA (degrees)	14	25	25.5
1-NA (mm)	4.0	9	9
1.NB (degrees)	24.5	23	23
1-NB (mm)	8.0	5.5	5.5
Pog-NB (mm)	1.5	0.5	0.6
1:1 (degrees)	142	132	
SN:OP (degrees)	9	12	12.5
SN:GoGn (degrees)	31	32	32
S to upper lip (mm)	-1	1	1
S to lower lip (mm)	2	1	3
FMA (degrees)	28	29.5	29.5
FMIA (degrees)	61	62.5	61.5
IMPA (degrees)	91	88	89
Angle of convexity (degrees)	-4	-2	-2.5

Presurgical Orthodontics may create space for implants to replace missing lateral incisors.

Surgery was considered a risky procedure for a 61-year-old patient. She presented favorable conditions for camouflage, since adequate anchorage could be provided. Conventional dental implants can also be used for orthodontic anchorage. Upper incisors should be proclined so as to increase arch perimeter, which would help space gain for upper lateral incisors. Treatment plan was designed according to patient's needs and expectations.

A diagnostic setup was performed according to cephalometric findings. Lower central incisors underwent retrusion of 4 mm and intrusion of 1.5 mm (Fig 5). Upper central incisors were subsequently positioned in contact, with an increase in buccal inclination so as to achieve a 2-mm overjet. Bilateral spaces of 6 mm were created to replace missing upper lateral incisors.

Implants should be inserted 2 mm distal to the lower right first premolar and 3 mm distal to the lower left first premolar. Temporary acrylic crowns were adapted over conventional dental implants (Brånemark System, Nobel Biocare, Kloten, Switzerland: 11.5 x 5 mm in the region of molars and 4 x 11.5 mm in the region of premolars) on both sides of the lower arch. Orthodontic brackets were bonded after six months. Absolute anchorage unit allowed distal movement of

lower right canine and left premolar; in addition, it provided retraction and intrusion of lower incisors.

Upper molars were banded and a full fixed orthodontic appliance was placed (Standard Edgewise 0.022 x 0.028-in, 3M-Unitek, Monrovia, USA). Leveling and alignment followed the sequence of stainless steel archwires in increasing stiffness (3M-Unitek, Monrovia, USA). Upper diastema closure and distal movement of lower teeth were performed by sliding mechanics with elastomeric chains.

Retraction of lower incisors and proclination of upper incisors occurred simultaneously. Tear drop loops were bent in 0.018 x 0.025-in stainless steel archwires halfway between lateral incisors and canines. Ideal 0.019 x 0.026-in stainless steel archwires allowed detailed angulation to be performed. Total treatment lasted 36 months.

Maxillary implants were inserted after orthodontic space opening (Brånemark System, Nobel Biocare, Kloten, Switerland: 3.3 x 13 mm on the right side and 3.3 x 15 mm on the left side).

RESULTS

By the end of orthodontic treatment, ideal overjet and overbite were achieved. In addition, the necessary space gain for implant-supported definite crowns, placed

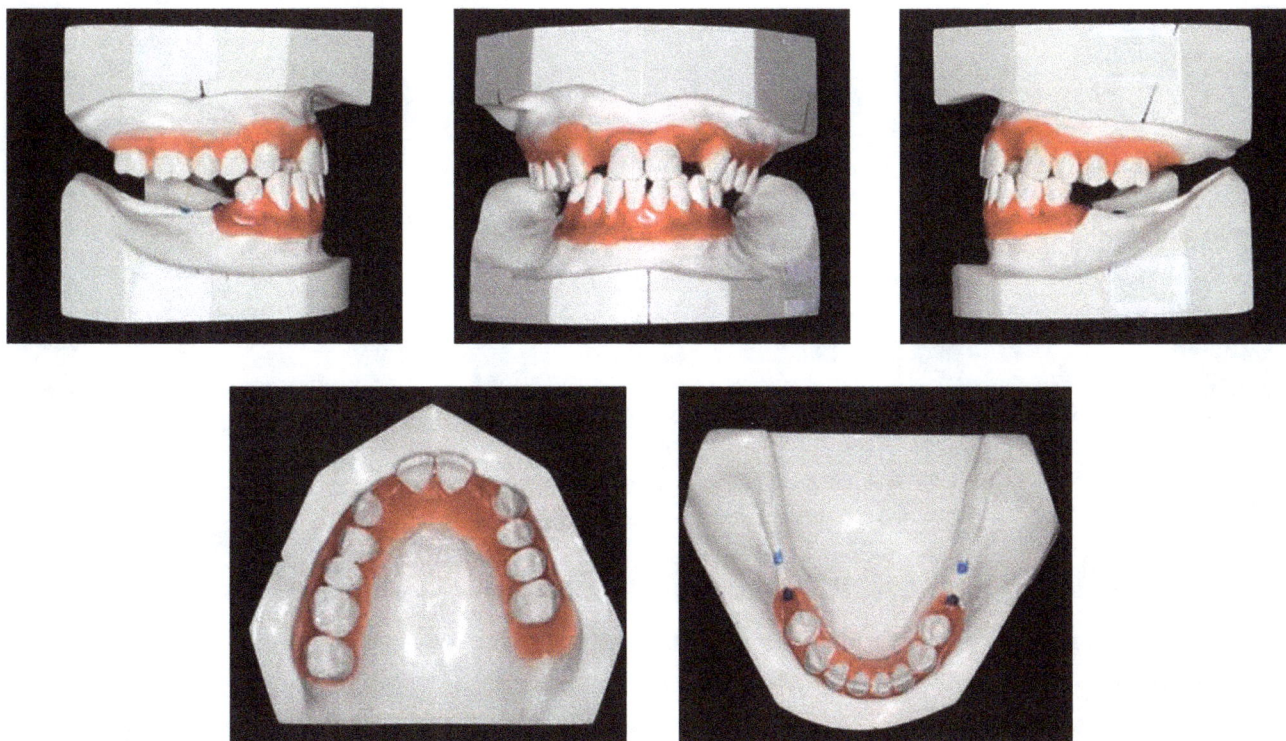

Figure 5 - Setup records.

in the posterior region of the lower arch, was achieved (Figs 6 and 7). Midline upper diastema was closed, which favored prosthetic rehabilitation of lateral incisors. After bracket debonding, definite crowns were placed over implants, central incisors were restored with resin veneers and other damaged restorations were replaced (Fig 8).

Superimposition of cephalometric tracings revealed that the mandible rotated clockwise (FMA from 28° to 29.5°). There was an increase in the occlusal plane angle (SN-OP from 9° to 12°) and a decrease in the incisor-mandible plane angle (IMPA from 91° to 88°), which reflects intrusion and retrusion, respectively, of lower incisors. Proclination of upper incisors was highlighted by an increase in the 1.NA angle (14° to 25°) (Figs 9 and 10, Table 1).

Regarding the facial profile, maxillary deficiency was camouflaged. Upper and lower lips were improved (upper lip to S-line, from -1 to 1 mm; lower lip to S-line, from 2 to 1 mm) with upper incisors support.

Ten years after the completion of the case, the patient showed occlusal stability, as well as integrity of dentition and prostheses. Resin veneers showed pigmentation and discoloration, as expected. Periodontal structures remained healthy (Figs 11 and 12).

DISCUSSION

Anterior-posterior and transversal Class III malocclusion relationships tend to worsen with aging.[18,19] Patient's Class III skeletal pattern associated with loss of lower posterior teeth were limiting factors in the planning of this case. Without orthognathic surgery, conventional mechanics would not solve the patient's problem. However, there are increased risks associated with surgery and, for this reason, the patient ultimately elected not to undergo surgery.

In this case, prognosis for camouflage was very favorable, considering mild maxillary deficiency and the possibility to procline upper central incisors. The need for oral rehabilitation led this case to be planned based on the use of implants and prostheses. Dentistry restored key features of patient's quality of life: proper mastication as well as smile and facial esthetics. In 1998, the life expectancy for women in Brazil was 72 years.[20] Thus, we offered a reliable treatment which promotes long-term oral health to our patient. Additionally, transdisciplinary treatment plan fulfilled patient's needs and expectations.

In the late 1990s, skeletal anchorage in Orthodontics was not as usual as it is today. Therefore, we considered

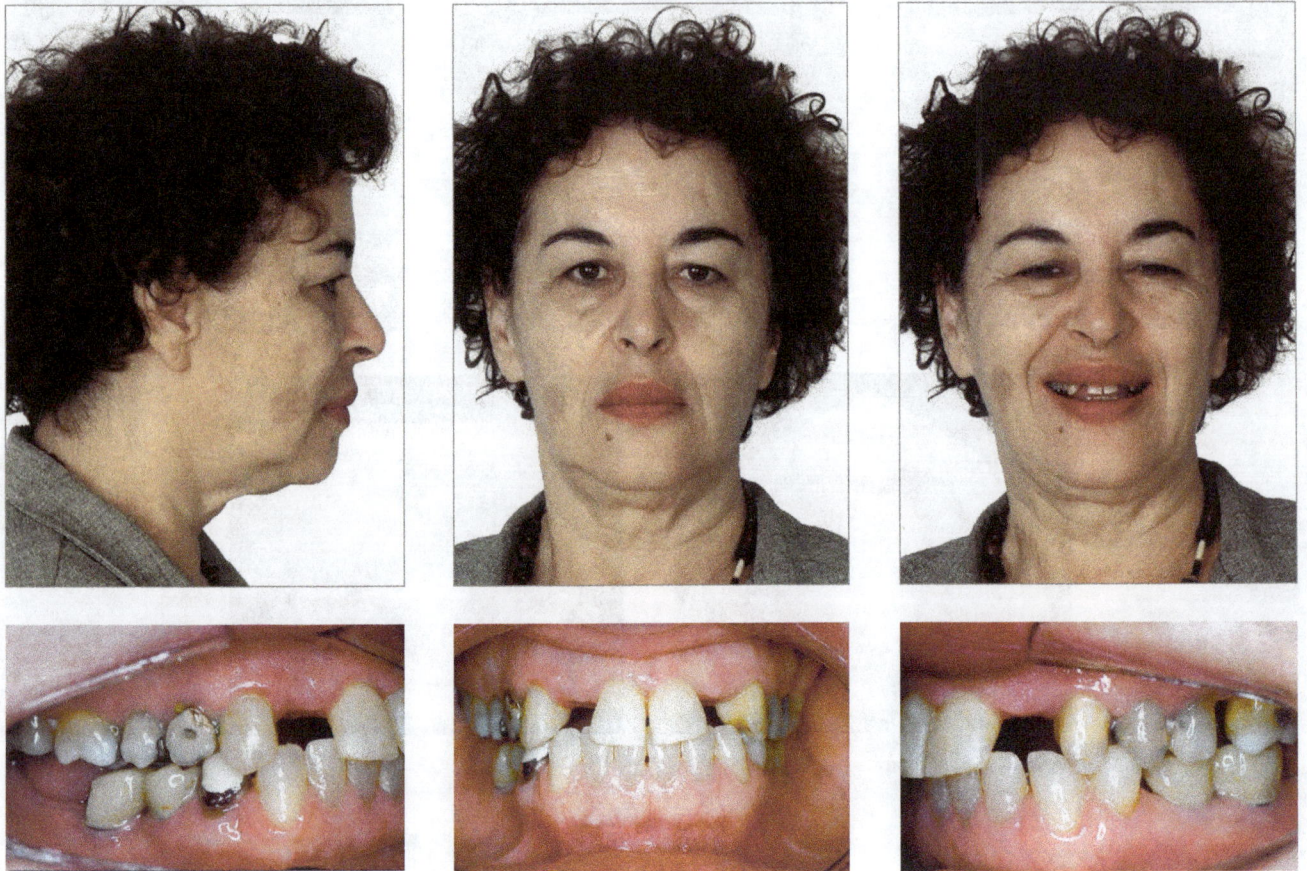

Figure 6 - Post-treatment facial and intraoral photographs.

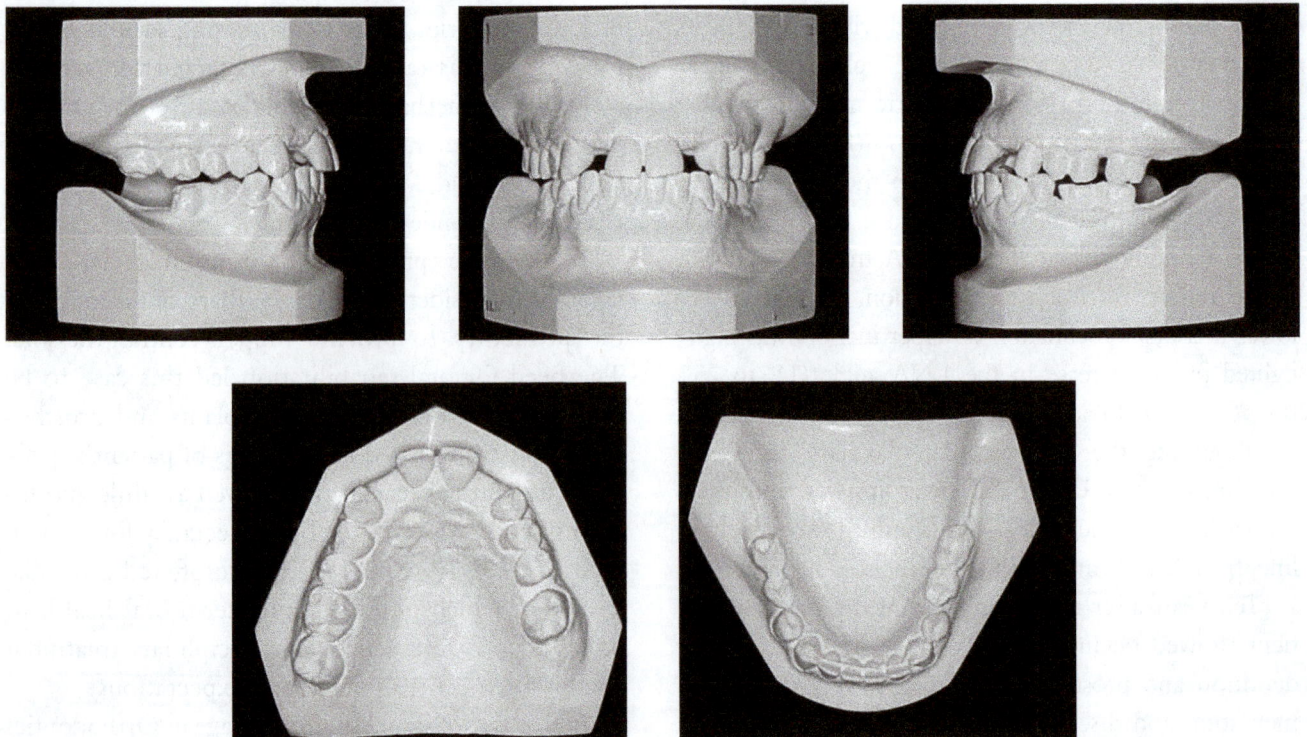

Figure 7 - Final dental casts.

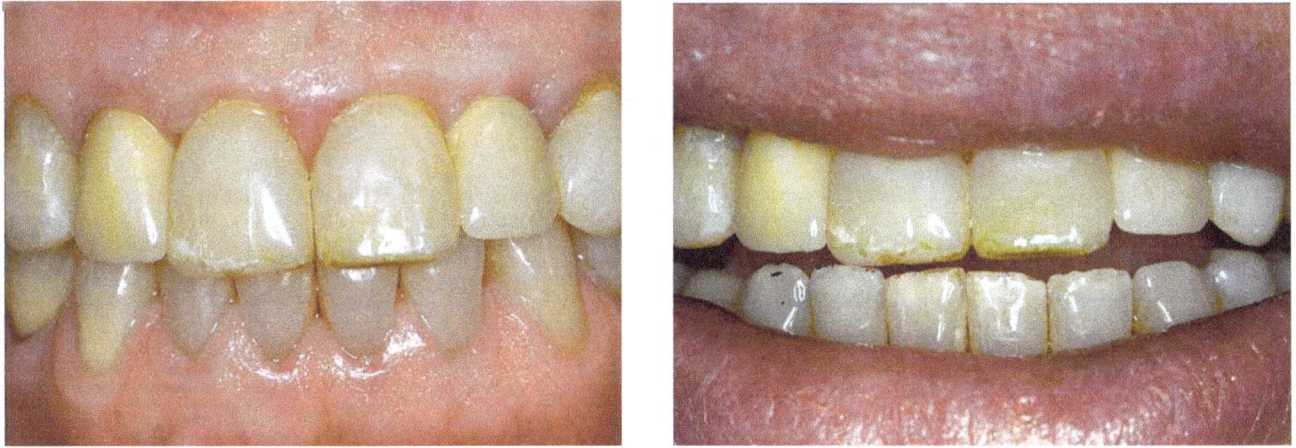

Figure 8 - Rehabilitation of the upper incisor region.

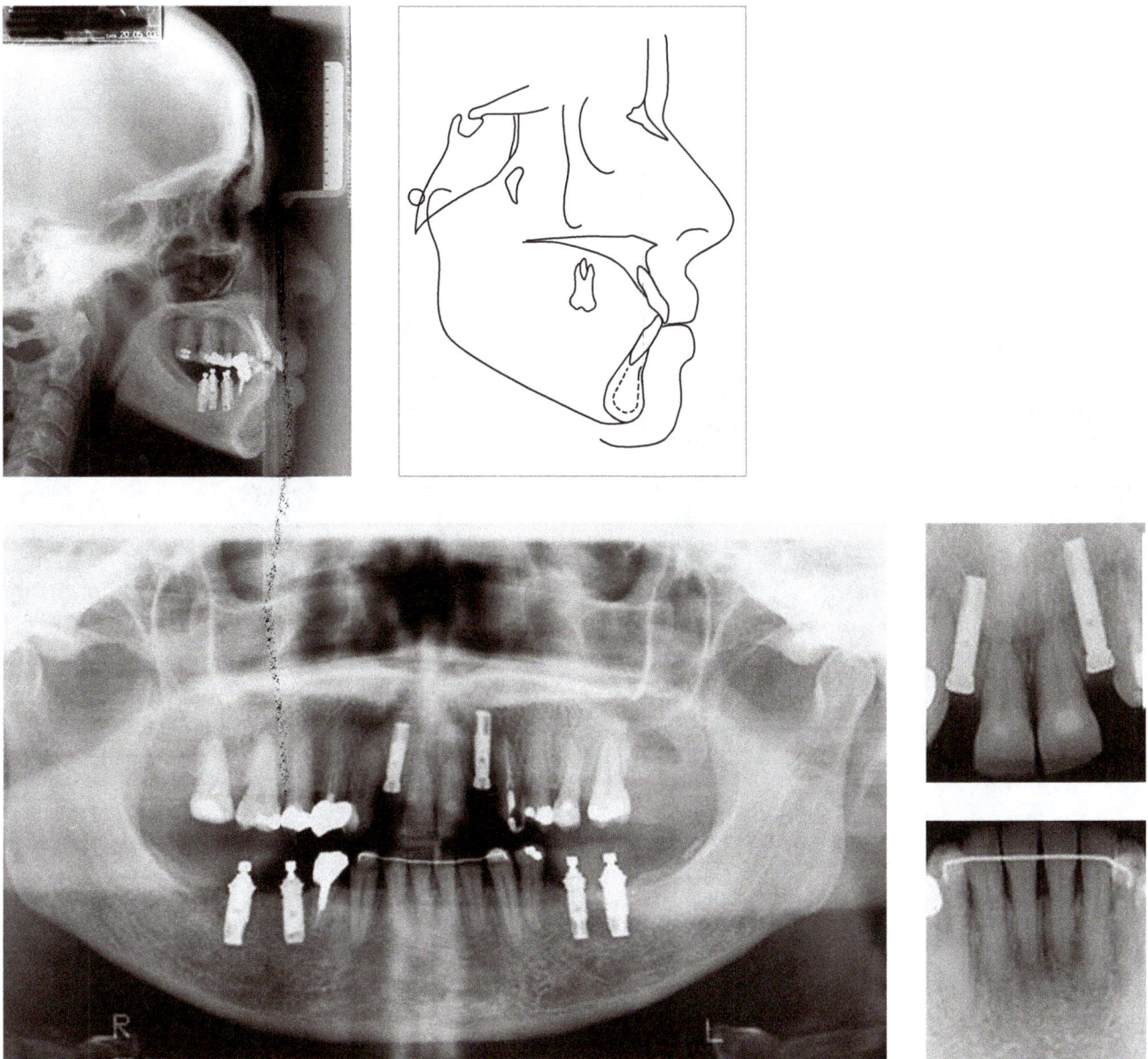

Figure 9 - Final lateral cephalometric radiograph, panoramic and periapical radiographs, and cephalometric tracing at treatment completion.

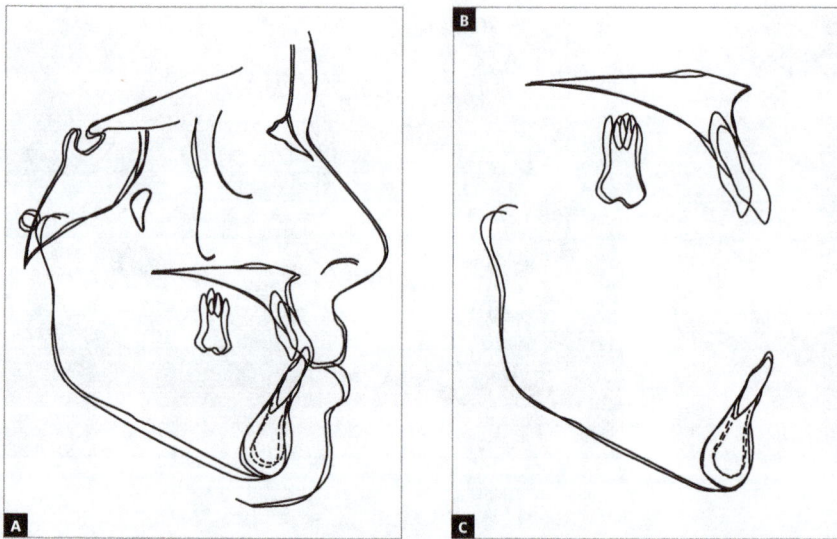

Figure 10 - Superimposition of cephalometric tracings at treatment onset (black) and after treatment completion (red): **A**) Sella-nasion plane at sella; **B**) Best-fit of the maxilla; **C**) Mandibular plane at the internal symphysis cortical plate to assess tooth movement, intrusion and incisor repositioning.

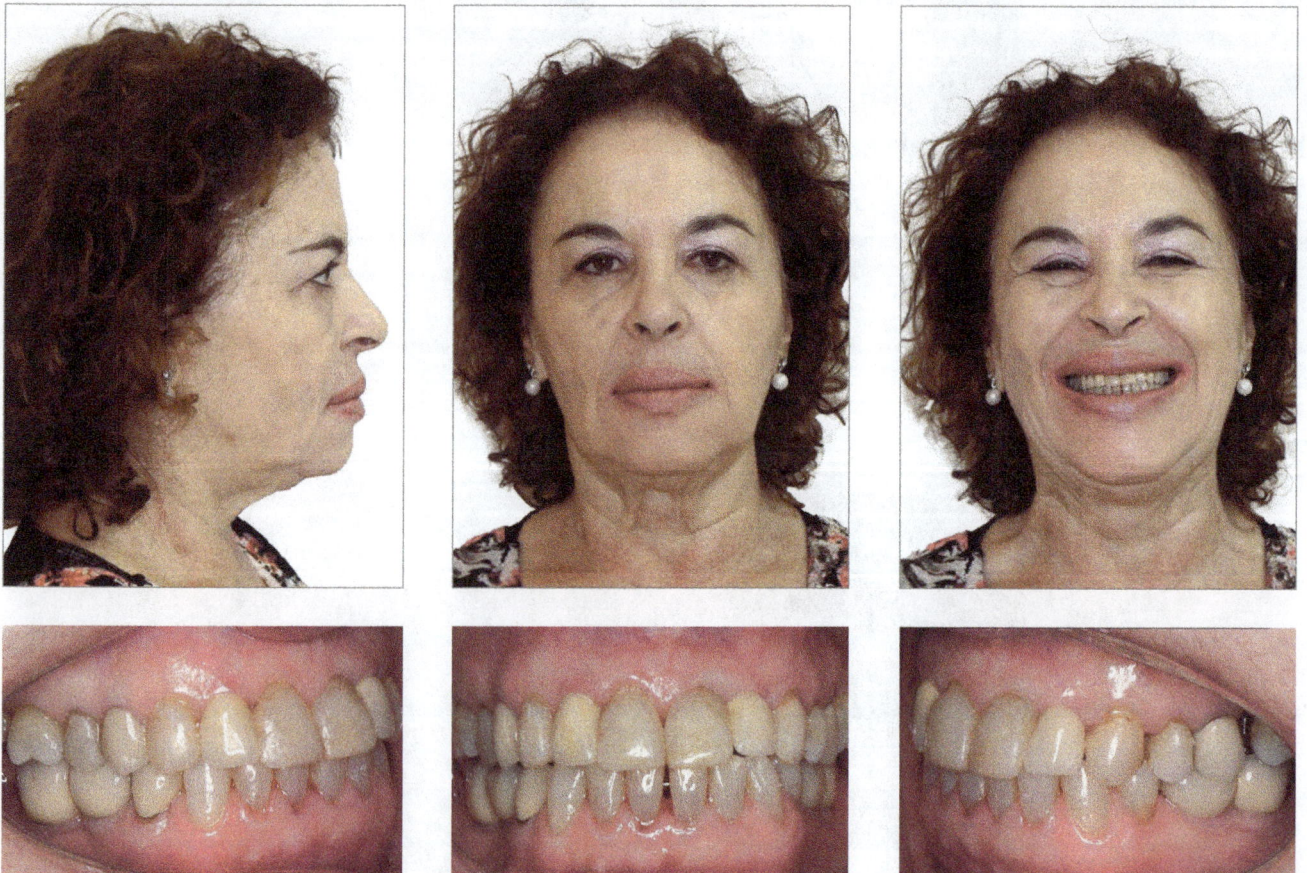

Figure 11 - Facial and intraoral photographs 10 years after treatment completion.

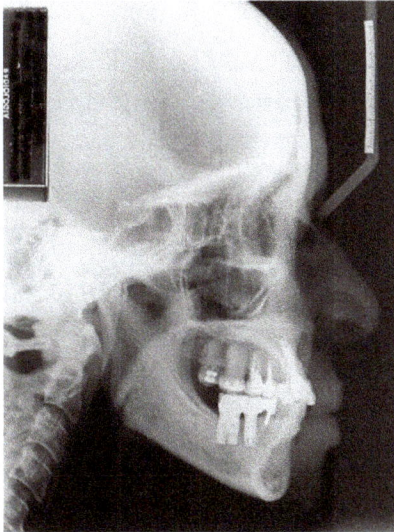

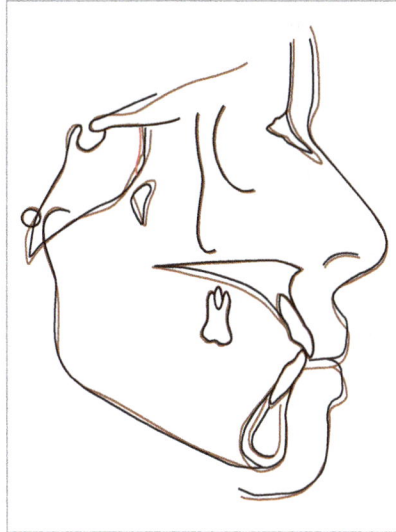

Figure 12 - Radiograph 10 years after treatment completion. Superimposition of cephalometric tracings at treatment completion (red) and 10 years after treatment (brown). Sella-nasion plane at sella.

the possibility of losing implants with the application of orthodontic movement and occlusal forces, leading to decreased alveolar width and height.

Orthodontic forces are small when compared to the complex system of intermittent and multidirectional forces acting on implants during mastication. Thus, biomechanical responses are within biological limits; for instance, an elastic chain used for canine retraction leads to a force of 1 N or less. The association between orthodontic forces and function stimulates responses of bone modeling and remodeling, which may lead to a new balance of forces.[10,16]

The approach presented herein took advantage of conventional implants which functioned as orthodontic anchorage before prosthetic procedures.[8,21] Therefore, implants placed in the region of lower molars provided anchorage necessary for intrusion and retraction of anterior lower teeth. This was considered a worthwhile strategy: previous orthodontic treatment improved occlusion and created space necessary for crown placement (Fig 6).[8,10,14,22] Implant selection and insertion site must consider patient's anatomical features, quality and quantity of bone available (alveolar width and height), gingival conditions, ideal position for teeth replacement and orthodontic movement.[4,14,23,24]

Whenever anterior teeth are missing, it is challenging to obtain a natural smile and achieve correct occlusion. Before implants were developed, alternative therapies for these cases included the use of adhesive crowns and preparation of healthy teeth to function as pillars. Both treatment options have esthetics limitations.[25,26]

The esthetic objectives of implant therapy include creating adequate gingival margins without abrupt changes in tissue height, maintaining the papilla intact and preserving alveolar crest convex contour. To this end, 1-mm space or more, between the implant and the adjacent tooth root, is required in addition to adequate space for crown placement.[14] Whenever it is impossible to gain the space required, space closure with mesial movement of posterior teeth is a reasonable option, especially if only one or two teeth are missing in the anterior region.[13]

No consensus has been reached regarding the best treatment option to replace missing lateral upper incisors.[27] It is important to consider various aspects of treatment, namely: patient's age, alveolar ridge and gingiva, type of malocclusion, other missing teeth and the possibility to restore space. Implant placement is the best choice for cases similar to that demonstrated in the present report: multiple missing teeth, interincisal diastema and mild Class III malocclusion. Space closure would have caused the collapse of the upper arch, thereby reducing arch perimeter. Mesial movement of central incisors produced the necessary space for implant placement. This was based on the margin of space required to the roots of adjacent natural teeth.[2,3,7]

In addition to absolute anchorage provided by implants, biomechanics was similar to the conventional technique. This treatment option requires the understanding of forces involved in the system and the ability to control the magnitude of forces on implants. Implants are structures fixed to bone and which transfer the load to the teeth which, in turn, are connected by the appliance. It is important to consider the functional characteristics of occlusion with implants, which assures stability and success (Figs 11 and 12).[17,28]

CONCLUSION

The goals of this transdisciplinary treatment were to create adequate space in vertical, transversal and horizontal planes for dental implant and prosthesis placement, with a view to establishing functional occlusion and attractive dentition. Treatment plan combining Implantology, Orthodontics and Prosthodontics proved to be effective in overcoming the challenges. Tissue stability and healthy conditions remain after a 10-year posttreatment follow-up, which confirms the usefulness of this approach.

REFERENCES

1. Agarwal S, Gupta S, Chugh VK, Jain E, Valiathan A, Nanda R. Interdisciplinary treatment of a periodontally compromised adult patient with multiple missing posterior teeth. Am J Orthod Dentofacial Orthop. 2014;145(2):238-48.

2. Pinho T, Neves M, Alves C. Multidisciplinary management including periodontics, orthodontics, implants, and prosthetics for an adult. Am J Orthod Dentofacial Orthop. 2012;142(2):235-45.

3. Uribe F, Janakiraman N, Nanda R. Interdisciplinary approach for increasing the vertical dimension of occlusion in an adult patient with several missing teeth. Am J Orthod Dentofacial Orthop. 2013;143(6):867-76.

4. Shapiro PA, Kokich VG. Uses of implants in orthodontics. Dent Clin North Am. 1988;32(3):539-50.

5. Nanda R. Biomechanics and esthetic strategies in clinical orthodontics. 1st ed. Philadelphia: WB Saunders; 2005. 385 p.

6. Uribe F, Nanda R. Intramaxillary and intermaxillary absolute anchorage with an endosseous dental implant and rare-earth magnets. Am J Orthod Dentofacial Orthop. 2009;136(1):124-33.

7. Barros LAB, Almeida Cardoso M, de Avila ÉD, Molon RS, Siqueira DF, Mollo-Junior FA, et al. Six-year follow-up of maxillary anterior rehabilitation with forced orthodontic extrusion: achieving esthetic excellence with a multidisciplinary approach. Am J Orthod Dentofacial Orthop. 2013;144(4):607-15.

8. Kuroda S, Iwata M, Tamamura N, Ganzorig K, Hichijo N, Tomita Y, et al. Interdisciplinary treatment of a nonsyndromic oligodontia patient with implant-anchored orthodontics. Am J Orthod Dentofacial Orthop. 2014;145(4 Suppl):S136-47.

9. Alani A, Bishop K, Renton T, Djemal S. Update on guidelines for selecting appropriate patients to receive treatment with dental implants: priorities for the NHS–the position after 15 years. Br Dent J. 2014;217(4):189-90.

10. Favero L, Brollo P, Bressan E. Orthodontic anchorage with specific fixtures: related study analysis. Am J Orthod Dentofacial Orthop. 2002;122(1):84-94.

11. Chang JZ-C, Liu P-H, Wang Y-T, Chen Y-J, Yao C-CJ, Lai EH-H. Orthodontic-prosthetic implant anchorage in a partially edentulous patient. J Dent Sci. 2011;6(3):176-80.

12. Farret MM, Benitez Farret MM. Skeletal Class III malocclusion treated using a non-surgical approach supplemented with mini-implants: a case report. J Orthod. 2013;40(3):256-63.

13. Bilodeau JE. A "midline dilemma" in an adult mutilated dentition. Am J Orthod Dentofacial Orthop. 2014;146(3):364-70.

14. Rose TP, Jivraj S, Chee W. The role of orthodontics in implant dentistry. Br Dent J. 2006;201(12):753-64.

15. Moslehifard E, Nikzad S, Geraminpanah F, Mahboub F. Full-mouth rehabilitation of a patient with severely worn dentition and uneven occlusal plane: a clinical report. J Prosthodont. 2012;21(1):56-64.

16. Higuchi KW. Orthodontic applications of osseointegrated implants. 1st ed. Hanover Park , IL: Quintessence; 2000. 218 p.

17. Melsen B, Lang NP. Biological reactions of alveolar bone to orthodontic loading of oral implants. Clin Oral Implants Res. 2001;12(2):144-52.

18. Berg RE, Espeland L, Stenvik A. A 57-year follow-up study of occlusion. Part 3: Oral health and attitudes to teeth among individuals with crossbite at the age of 8 years. J Orofac Orthop. 2008;69(6):463-83.

19. Miyajima K, McNamara JA, Sana M, Murata S. An estimation of craniofacial growth in the untreated Class III female with anterior crossbite. Am J Orthod Dentofacial Orthop. 1997;112(4):425-34.

20. IBGE. Coordenação de População e Indicadores Sociais. Gerência de estudos e análises da dinâmica demográfica projeção da população do Brasil por sexo e idade para o período 1980-2050 revisão 2008. Available from: http://www.ibge.gov.br/home/estatistica/populacao/tabuadevida/evolucao_da_mortalidade.shtm.

21. Martin W, Heffernan M, Ruskin J. Template fabrication for a midpalatal orthodontic implant: technical note. Int J Oral Maxillofac Implants. 2002;17(5):720-2.

22. Smalley WM. Implants for tooth movement: determining implant location and orientation. J Esthet Dent. 1995;7(2):62-72.

23. Odman J, Lekholm U, Jemt T, Branemark PI, Thilander B. Osseointegrated titanium implants—a new approach in orthodontic treatment. Eur J Orthod. 1988;10(2):98-105.

24. Thilander B, Odman J, Lekholm U. Orthodontic aspects of the use of oral implants in adolescents: a 10-year follow-up study. Eur J Orthod. 2001;23(6):715-31.

25. Zachrisson BU. Improving orthodontic results in cases with maxillary incisors missing. Am J Orthod. 1978;73(3):274-89.

26. Czochrowska EM, Skaare AB, Stenvik A, Zachrisson BU. Outcome of orthodontic space closure with a missing maxillary central incisor. Am J Orthod Dentofacial Orthop. 2003;123(6):597-603.

27. Andrade D, Loureiro C, Araújo V, Riera R, Atallah A. Treatment for agenesis of maxillary lateral incisors: a systematic review. Orthod Craniofac Res. 2013;16(3):129-36.

28. Southard TE, Buckley MJ, Spivey JD, Krizan KE, Casko JS. Intrusion anchorage potential of teeth versus rigid endosseous implants: a clinical and radiographic evaluation. Am J Orthod Dentofacial Orthop. 1995;107(2):115-20.

3

Class II malocclusion with accentuated occlusal plane inclination corrected with miniplate

Marcel Marchiori Farret[1], Milton M. Benitez Farret[2]

Introduction: A canted occlusal plane presents an unesthetic element of the smile. The correction of this asymmetry has been typically considered difficult by orthodontists, as it requires complex mechanics and may sometimes even require orthognathic surgery. **Objective:** This paper outlines the case of a 29-year-old woman with Class II malocclusion, pronounced midline deviation and accentuated occlusal plane inclination caused by mandibular deciduous molar ankylosis. **Methods:** The patient was treated with a miniplate used to provide anchorage in order to intrude maxillary teeth and extrude mandibular teeth on one side, thus eliminating asymmetry. Class II was corrected on the left side by means of distalization, anchored in the miniplate as well. On the right side, maxillary first premolar was extracted and molar relationship was kept in Class II, while canines were moved to Class I relationship. The patient received implant-prosthetic rehabilitation for maxillary left lateral incisor and mandibular left second premolar. **Results:** At the end of treatment, Class II was corrected, midlines were matched and the canted occlusal plane was totally corrected, thereby improving smile function and esthetics.

Keywords: Angle Class II malocclusion. Orthodontic anchorage procedures. Orthodontic appliance design.

[1] Professor, post-graduation courses, Specialization in Orthodontics, Centro de Estudos Odontológicos Meridional (CEOM), Passo Fundo, Rio Grande do Sul, Brazil; and Fundação para Reabilitação das Deformidades Crânio-Faciais (FUNDEF), Lajeado, Rio Grande do Sul, Brazil.
[2] Professor, Universidade Federal de Santa Maria (UFSM), Santa Maria, Rio Grande do Sul, Brazil.

Marcel Marchiori Farret
Rua Floriano Peixoto 100/113, Santa Maria/RS – CEP: 97.015-370 – Brazil
E-mail: marcelfarret@yahoo.com.br

» The authors report no commercial, proprietary or financial interest in the products or companies described in this article.

INTRODUCTION

Occlusal plane inclination has always represented a challenge for orthodontists.[1] The common options for treatment included asymmetric mechanics with high-pull headgears, asymmetric bite blocks,[2,3,4] or even orthognathic surgery in some cases.[5,6,7] In such cases, conventional mechanics require a long time to be performed, and adverse effects are often present, thus compromising and limiting treatment results.[2,8,9] Furthermore, patients frequently refuse orthognathic surgery and, as such, all treatment options for a canted occlusal plane have limitations.[10]

The introduction of skeletal anchorage has increased the number of treatment options for these cases.[2,8,11,12] Mini-implants or miniplates may aid intrusion of a group of teeth, either in the maxillary or mandibular arches, without adverse effects while greatly reducing total treatment time.[9,13] For large asymmetries, it is preferable to use miniplates, owing to the greater stability and success rate obtained with this device in comparison with mini-implants.[2,11,13,14,15]

In this paper, correction of occlusal plane inclination by means of skeletal anchorage is discussed. A case is presented in which significant asymmetry was corrected with a miniplate as the anchorage unit.

CASE REPORT
Diagnosis and etiology

A 29-year-old woman sought orthodontic treatment, complaining about an unesthetic smile due to occlusal plane inclination and midline deviation. This was caused by absence of maxillary left lateral incisor and mandibular left second premolar, with ankylosis of deciduous molar in this region. Facial analysis revealed good symmetry and vertical balance of the facial thirds, a convex profile, and accentuated occlusion plane inclination in a smiling photograph (Fig 1). Intraoral analysis revealed Angle Class II, Division 1 malocclusion, with absence of maxillary left lateral incisor, a peg-shaped maxillary right lateral incisor and the presence of mandibular left deciduous ankylosed second molar, which caused asymmetry on this side in both maxillary and mandibular arches (Figs 2 and 3). Maxillary midline was deviated 2 mm to the left while mandibular midline was deviated 2 mm to the right. Panoramic and periapical radiographs confirmed the absence of maxillary lateral incisor and mandibular second premolar and also revealed mandibular teeth greatly inclined towards the ankylosed deciduous molar. Initial lateral cephalogram and cephalometric tracing revealed skeletal Class II malocclusion, with upright maxillary incisors and well-positioned mandibular incisors (Fig 4 and Table 1).

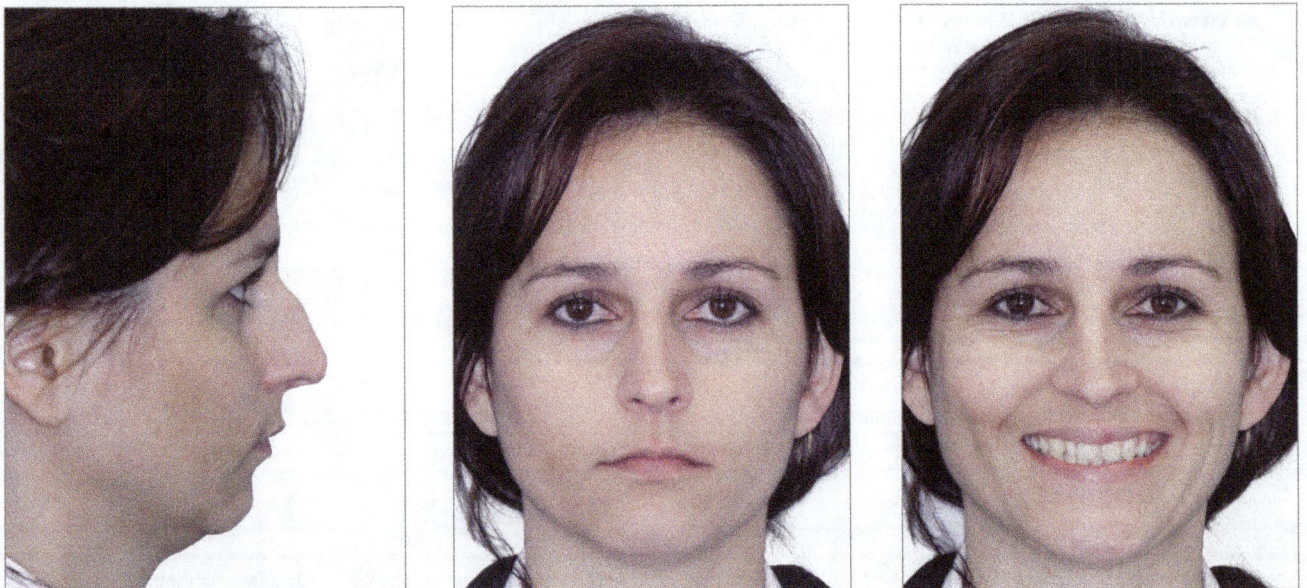

Figure 1 - Pretreatment facial photographs.

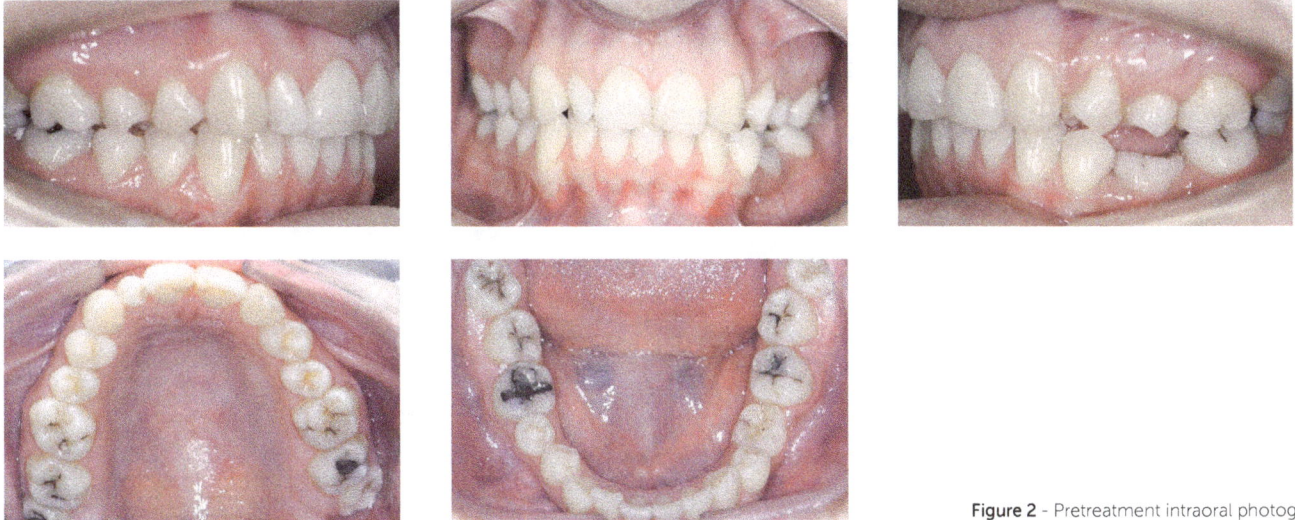

Figure 2 - Pretreatment intraoral photographs.

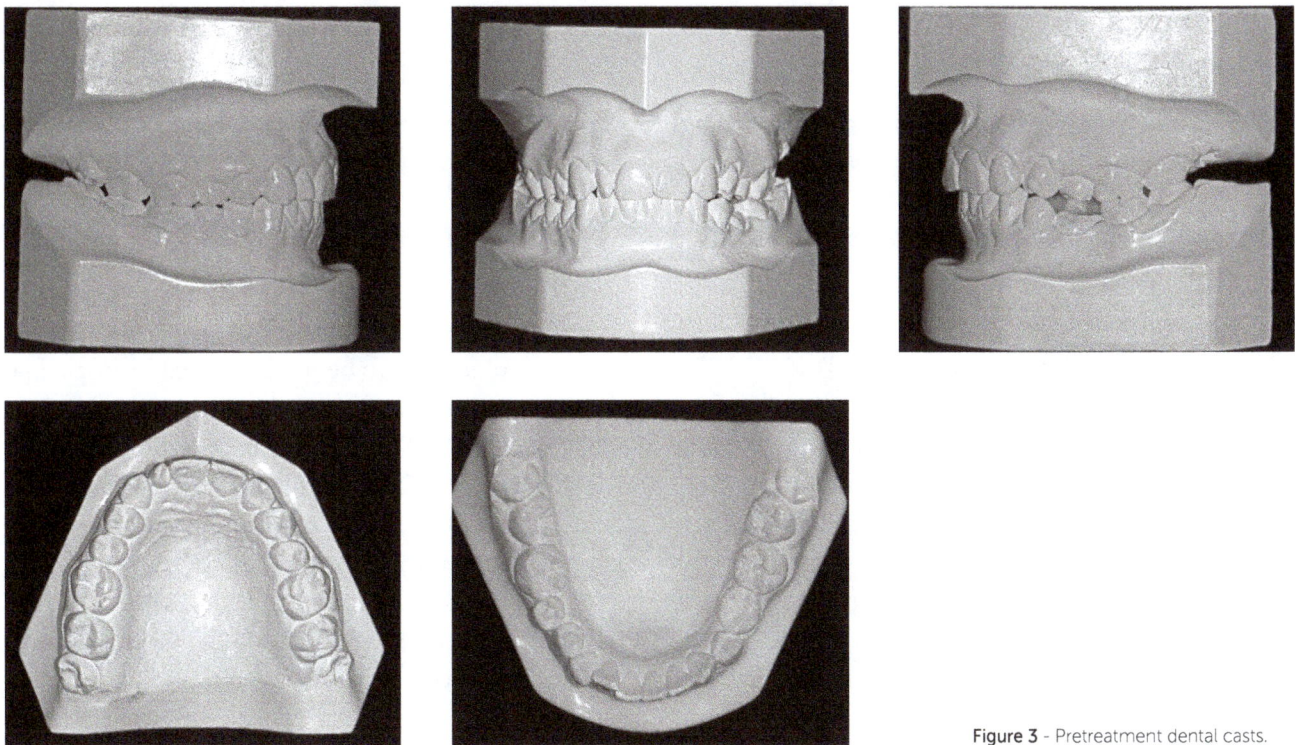

Figure 3 - Pretreatment dental casts.

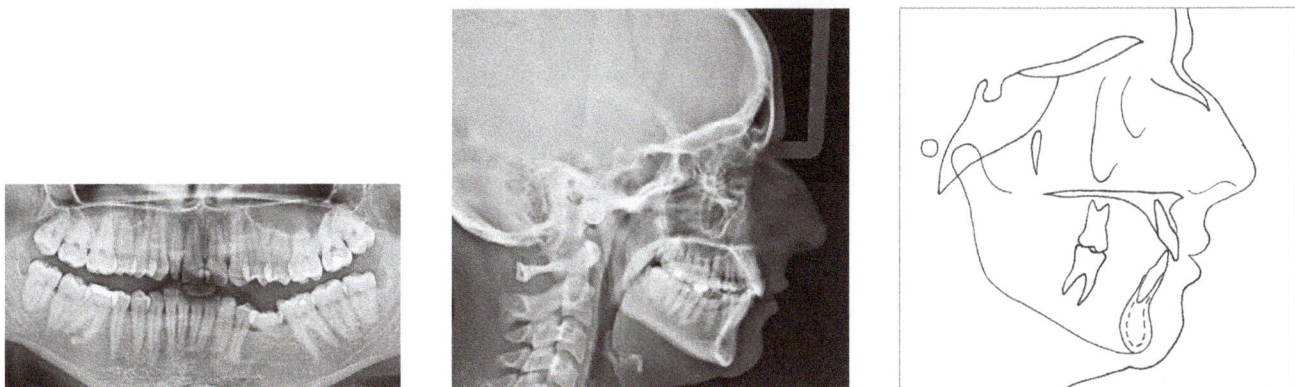

Figure 4 - Pretreatment panoramic radiograph, lateral cephalogram and cephalometric tracing.

Table 1 - Cephalometric measurements.

Measurements	Norms	Initial	Post-treatment
SNA	82°	81	80
SNB	80°	76	78
ANB	2°	5	2
Angle of convexity	0°	10	3
Facial angle	87°	85	87
Y-axis	59°	59	56
SN-GoGn	32°	33	29
1-NA (degrees)	22°	20	30
1-NA (mm)	4mm	3	5
1-NB (degrees)	25°	25	30
1-NB (mm)	4mm	5	6
$\frac{1}{1}$ - Interincisal angle	130°	129	116
Upper lip — S-line	0mm	1.5	1.5
Lower lip — S-line	0mm	0.5	1.5
IMPA	90°	97	102
FMA	25°	24	21
FMIA	65°	59	57

Treatment objectives

The objectives of treatment were as follows:

1. Correct occlusal plane inclination.
2. Obtain molar Class I relationship on the left side and Class II on the right side.
3. Establish canine Class I relationship on both sides.
4. Correct midlines.
5. Extract deciduous molar and replace the tooth with implant-prosthetic rehabilitation.
6. Open space in order to implant a prosthetic rehabilitation of the maxillary left lateral incisor.

Treatment alternatives

Orthognathic surgery was considered for occlusal plane correction, but the patient refused this option. Therefore, two other alternatives were considered to correct Class II malocclusion and tooth absences. The first option was to extract the maxillary right lateral incisor, replace lateral incisors with canines, and then replace canines with first premolars. This option was rejected in a meeting with the dentist responsible for the final rehabilitation. The dentist believed that the esthetic result would be better with implant-prosthetic rehabilitation of the maxillary lateral incisor, as

maxillary canines had large crowns and were too different in color, so as to be used as lateral incisors. The second option was to extract maxillary right first premolar and insert a mini-implant or miniplate on the left side to move the maxillary right dentition posteriorly. This option was rejected by the patient due to longer treatment time required in comparison to that for first premolar extraction to distalize all teeth. Thus, in agreement with the patient and the other dentist, it was decided to correct the occlusal plane by means of a miniplate on the maxillary left side, extract the maxillary right first premolar and open space for rehabilitation of the maxillary left lateral incisor.

Treatment progress

Treatment began with the bonding of 0.022×0.028-in standard Edgewise brackets on both arches, followed by alignment and leveling with 0.012 and 0.014-in Nickel-Titanium archwires and from 0.014-in to 0.020-in stainless steel archwires. Thereafter, maxillary right first premolar and mandibular left second deciduous molar were extracted and maxillary anterior teeth were moved to the right, tooth by tooth, with elastomeric chains, in order to correct maxillary midline and open space, thus allowing the insertion of an implant in the space left by the maxillary left lateral incisor. On the maxillary left side, after correction of premolars rotation, a 2-mm space was created and both premolar and canine were distalized with elastomeric chains to increase the space for implantation of the maxillary left lateral incisor prosthesis and to partially correct Class II. On the mandibular arch, an implant was inserted into the space of the missing premolar to aid mandibular midline correction. That implant was positioned above the proper position, considering that after occlusal plane correction with maxillary intrusion and mandibular extrusion on this side, the implant would be in adequate vertical position. Likewise, the implant was positioned closer to the mandibular left first molar and away from the left first premolar, thereby allowing distalization of mandibular left molars and distalization of mandibular anterior teeth, thus correcting the midline. After that, a miniplate in the shape of an Y was inserted in left zygomatic buttress and used to

intrude all maxillary left teeth, with elastics connected to 0.019×0.025-in wire segments inserted into a tube and connected to a miniplate, generating a force of 200 g/f each (Fig 5). Furthermore, the miniplate was used to distalize all teeth on the left side, with elastomeric chains connected to a hook welded between the lateral incisor and canine, so as to correct Class II relationship. After correction on the maxillary arch, the mandibular arch was extruded with intermaxillary 1/8-in elastics connected directly to the miniplate and on the mandibular teeth and archwire (Fig 6). In order to allow mandibular teeth extrusion, the mandibular arch was made bypassing the bracket of provisory crown over the implant. At that time, the space for maxillary left lateral incisor was already well defined and the implant was inserted. Maxillary right lateral incisor was provisionally restored with composite resin before appliance debonding, so as to precisely define the spaces on the anterior region. After 34 months of treatment, the appliance was removed.

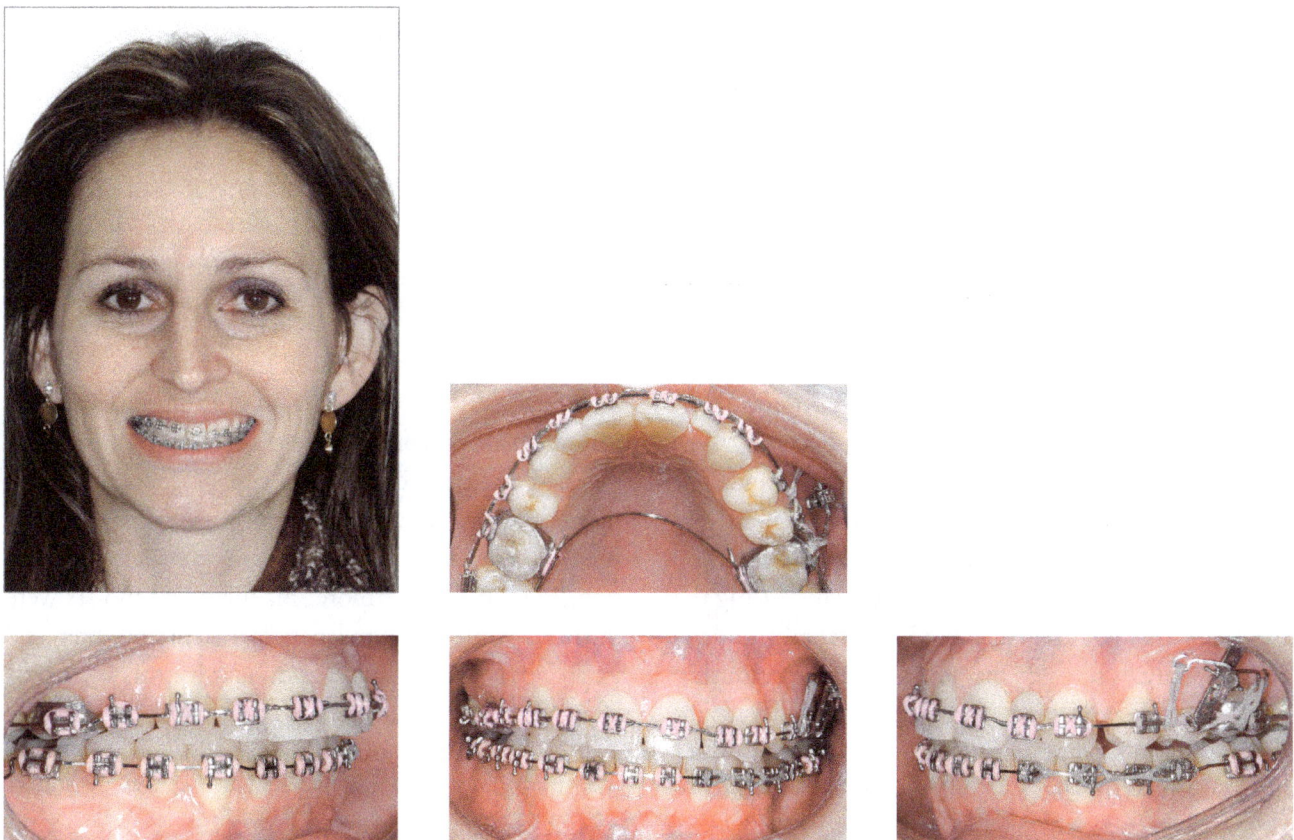

Figure 5 - Photographs after the insertion of miniplate and occlusal plane correction onset.

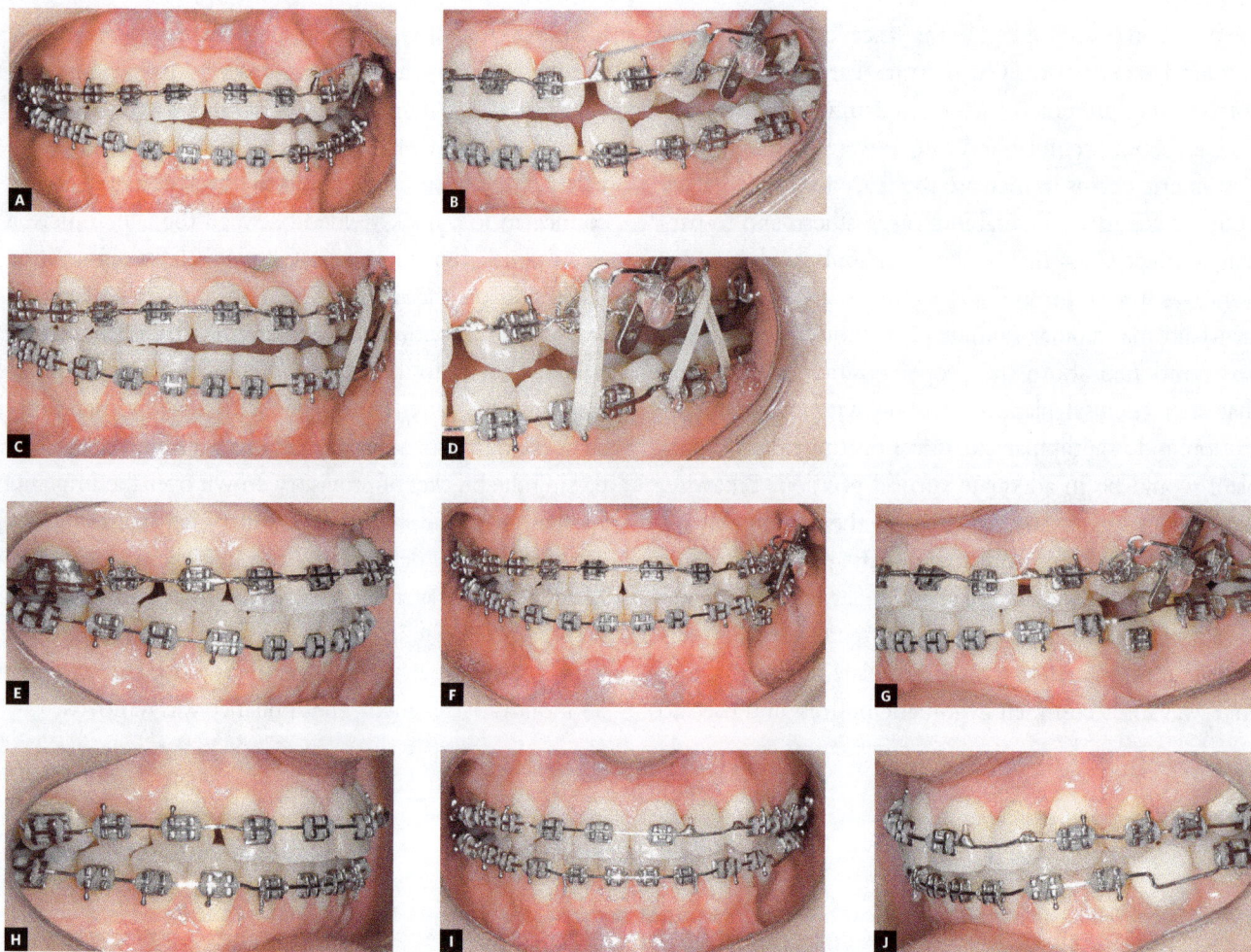

Figure 6 - Intraoral mechanic sequence. (**A** and **B**) After maxillary right teeth intrusion, (**C** and **D**) elastic mechanics employed to extruded mandibular left teeth, (**E** to **G**) after mandibular extrusion, (**H** to **J**) after miniplate removal and during the finishing procedures.

Treatment results

At the end of treatment, we noticed an improvement in smile esthetics due to correction of occlusal plane inclination and because the midlines were coincident with the facial midline (Fig 7). The profile remarkably improved as a result of counterclockwise rotation of the mandible, which reduced convexity, thus increasing the prominence of lips and chin (Fig 7). Intraoral and dental casts analyses revealed that Class I molar relationship on the left side, Class II molar relationship on the right side and Class I canine relationship on both sides were all obtained, with good intercuspation (Figs 8 and 9).

Panoramic radiograph showed good parallelism among roots, in addition to root resorption on maxillary left central incisor, which will be monitored after treatment. Post-treatment lateral cephalogram, cephalometric tracing and superimposition examinations confirmed accentuated mandibular counterclockwise rotation (Fig 10). Furthermore, maxillary left molars were intruded while mandibular molars were uprighted and extruded. Maxillary and mandibular incisors were proclined after treatment. The patient will be monitored every six months in order to have root resorption and treatment stability controlled.

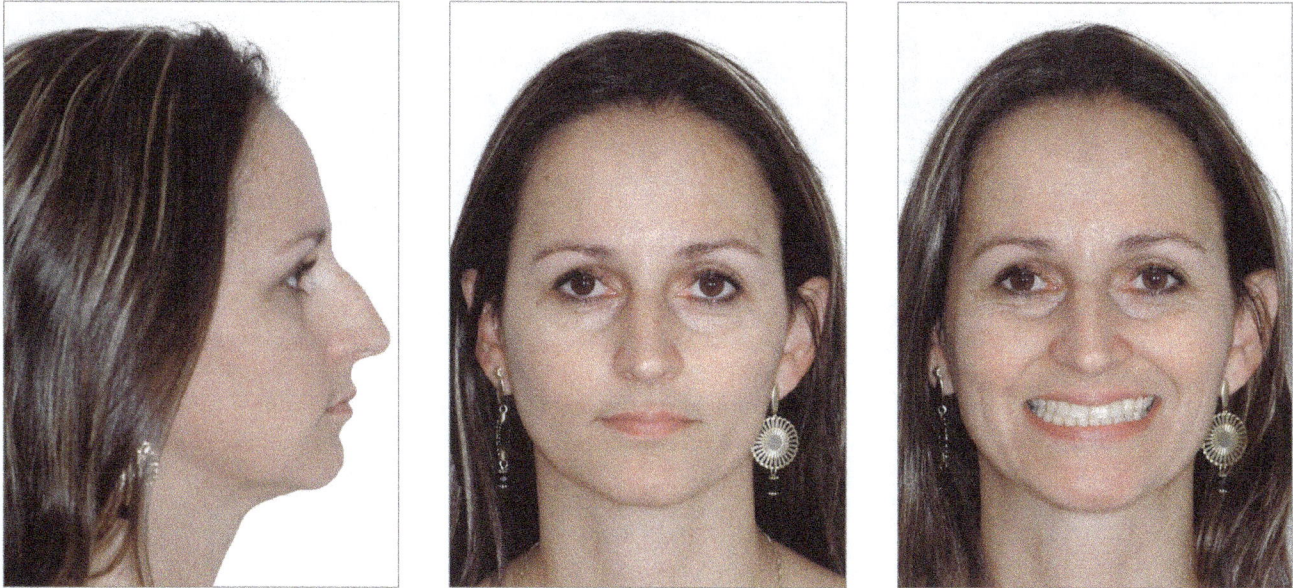

Figure 7 - Post-treatment facial photographs.

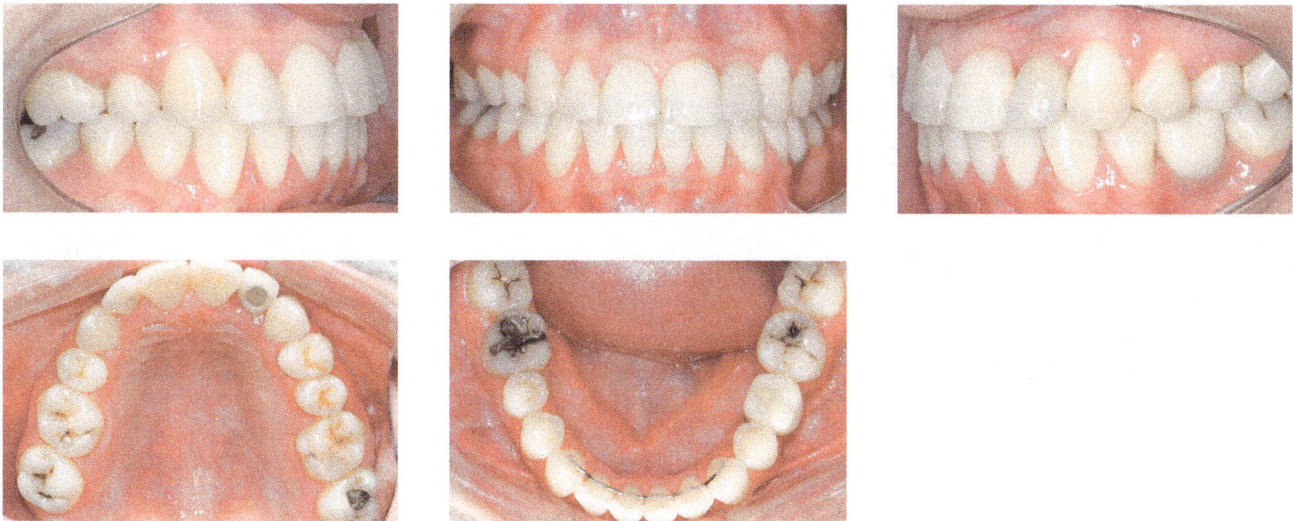

Figure 8 - Post-treatment intraoral photographs.

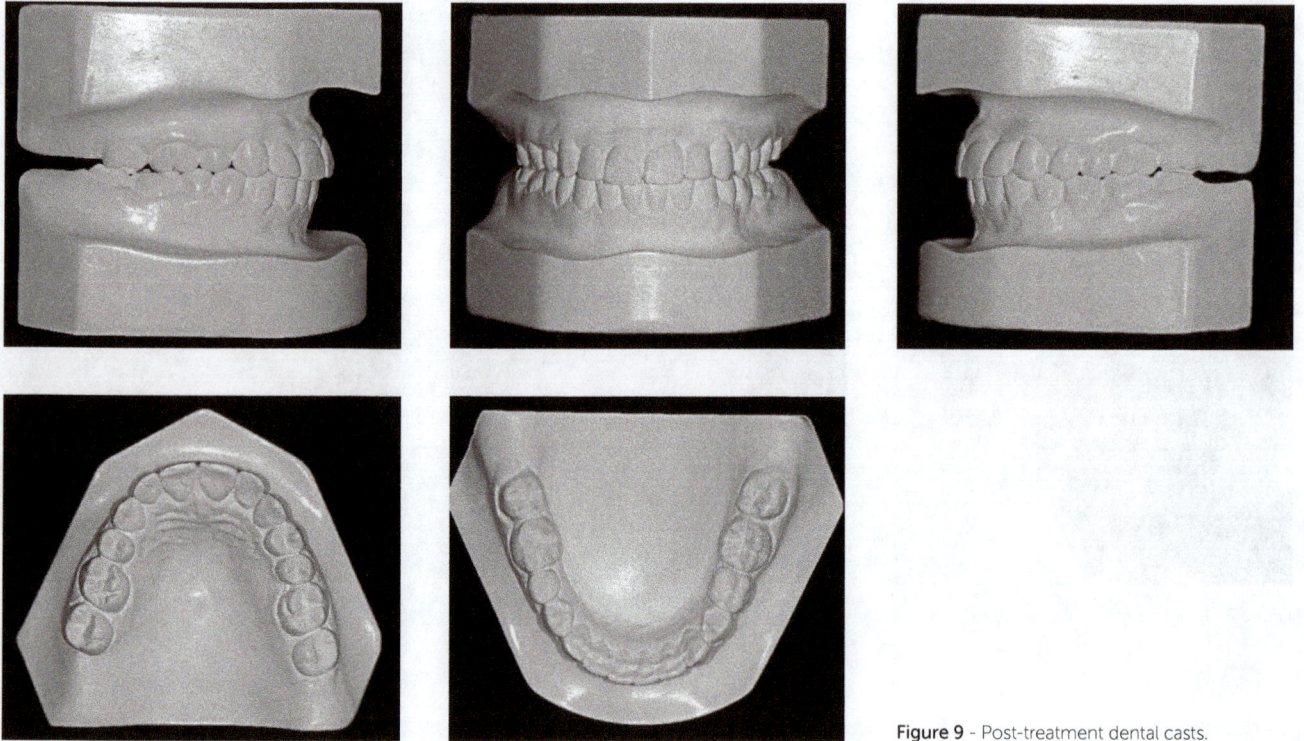

Figure 9 - Post-treatment dental casts.

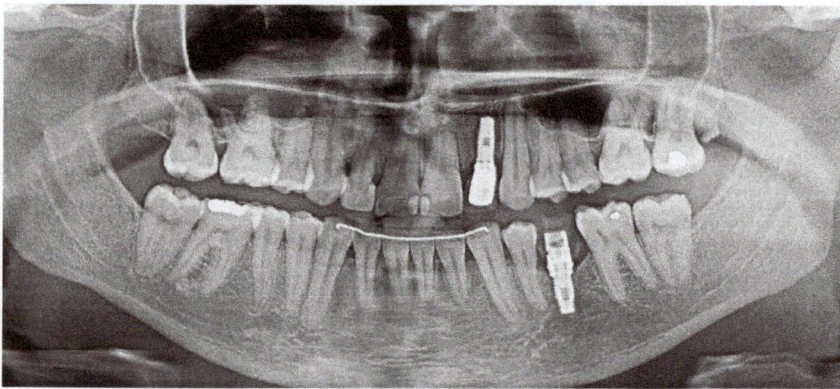

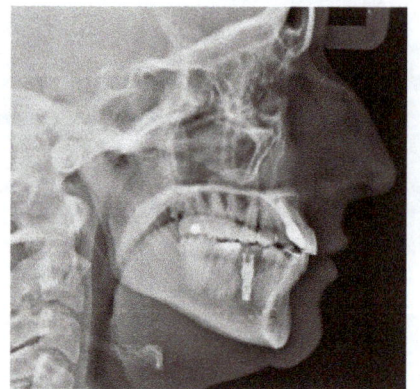

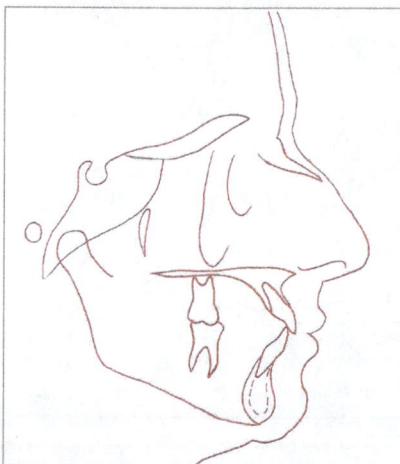

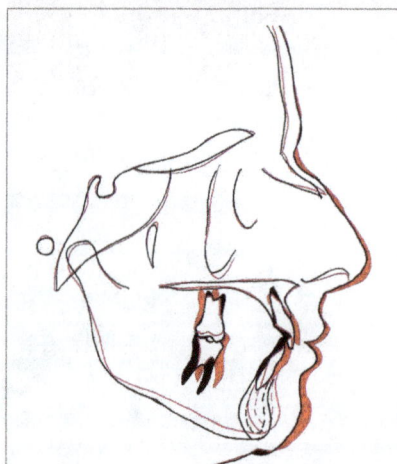

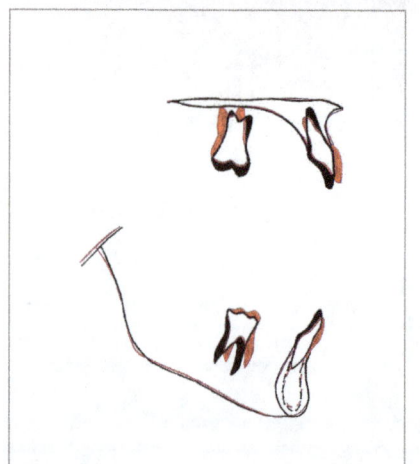

Figure 10 - Post-treatment panoramic radiograph, lateral cephalogram, cephalometric tracing, total superimposition, maxillary superimposition and mandibular superimposition.

DISCUSSION

Occlusal plane inclination is recognized as an asymmetry that impairs smile esthetics.[16,17] Padwa et al[17] and Pereira et al[18] studied some variations in occlusal plane inclination and found that as the degree of this asymmetry increases, the perceived attractiveness decreases. According to the authors, one of the reasons may be gingival exposure only on one side. This asymmetry should be corrected either by intrusion on one side, extrusion on the other side or a combination of both, depending on the diagnosis and treatment planning.[8] Intrusion is directed on the maxillary arch when gingival exposure is accentuated, followed by mandibular extrusion on the same side. Otherwise, when there is no gingival exposure associated with occlusal plane inclination, intrusion must be carried out on one side of the mandibular arch, followed by extrusion on the same side of the maxillary arch, considering that intrusion on the maxillary arch could extremely reduce maxillary teeth exposure, impairing smile esthetics. The combination of both procedures may be used in cases with moderate gingival exposure.[8] A precise esthetic diagnosis should be performed in these cases, including a series of smile photographs and thorough clinical examination. Frontal cephalograms are also an important tool for diagnosis and are essential, mainly when orthognathic surgery is being considered.[6,17]

Traditionally, the treatment options for asymmetries in the occlusal plane have been considered to be major challenges for orthodontists.[1] Despite the complexity of procedures, surgical approaches have always been considered to be a good option, as they have a reduced treatment time and avoid some adverse effects of conventional orthodontic mechanics.[5,6,8] However, the majority of patients refuse orthognathic surgery and treatment must therefore focus on orthodontic camouflage. One option is to use a unilateral bite block, which is another alternative for treatment and may provoke a minor intrusion on the side where it is located and a more significant extrusion on the other side. The limitation of this treatment modality is that it is not possible to attain moderate to high intrusion movements with these devices, in addition to the possibility of developing temporomandibular disorders after long periods of use. Other option consists in using an asymmetric high-pull headgear; however, it depends on patient's compliance and has limited results even after long periods of use.

The main reason for that is because the force between both sides cannot be very different in order to prevent displacement of occipital strap.

Skeletal anchorage appeared a few years ago as an excellent alternative for the treatment of asymmetries. It has no adverse effects on mechanics and does not rely on patient's compliance, meaning that treatment is more predictable and reliable.[11,19] Specifically for occlusal plane inclination, mini-implants may be the favored option for cases of minor discrepancies and two mini-implants should be preferably used in order to increase retention. Other problems related to mini-implants is the risk of root contact during treatment, as the intrusion movement is performed towards the mini-implant.[20] For these reasons, miniplates may be a better option for the treatment of vertical asymmetries on the occlusal plane, delivering an excellent capacity to intrude a group of teeth without the risk of coming into contact with any of the roots during treatment.[3,4,11,15] However, the disadvantage of miniplates is the need for two invasive surgical procedures to insert and remove the device, the reason why patients sometimes refuse miniplates.[15]

Root resorption may be a consequence of orthodontic treatment. Constant forces usually provoke higher root resorption in comparison with interrupt forces. Other authors agree with it and according to them it happens because the pause in force allows the resorbed cementum to heal and prevents further resorption.[21,22,23] Furthermore, intrusion movement is one of the main causes of resorption as well.[24] In the case described herein, the maxillary arch was intruded on the left side with constant forces delivered by elastics connected to the miniplate, which probably caused some root resorption on maxillary anterior teeth, which was more accentuated on the left side. After the end of active orthodontic treatment, root resorption tends to stop;[25,26] therefore, the patient will be monitored every six months to check whether resorption has indeed stopped.

Unfortunately, there are no studies in the literature that have analyzed the long-term stability of occlusal plane inclination correction by means of skeletal anchorage. The magnitude of orthodontic movement obtained with miniplates is remarkably higher than that obtained in the past with conventional mechanics. In order to avoid relapses, it is recommended that the appliance is stabilized for at least six months after correction, allowing for complete bone remodeling and reorganization of fibers. The retention protocol is the same as that usually used in other cases, with a 3 × 3 mandibular bonded retainer and a wraparound removable appliance on the maxillary arch. The patient must be monitored for a long period of time in order to identify any relapse and intercept or treat it.

CONCLUSION

The literature and case presented herein demonstrate that miniplates are a reliable device for the correction of occlusal plane inclination, eliminating the need for orthognatic surgery in some cases and reducing the complexity of orthodontic mechanics.

REFERENCES

1. Burstone CJ. Diagnosis and treatment planning of patients with asymmetries. Semin Orthod. 1998;4(3):153-64.
2. Jeon YJ, Kim YH, Son WS, Hans MG. Correction of a canted occlusal plane with miniscrews in a patient with facial asymmetry. Am J Orthod Dentofacial Orthop. 2006 Aug;130(2):244-52.
3. Sherwood KH, Burch JG, Thompson WJ. Closing anterior open bites by intruding molars with titanium miniplate anchorage. Am J Orthod Dentofacial Orthop. 2002 Dec;122(6):593-600.
4. Sherwood KH, Burch J, Thompson W. Intrusion of supererupted molars with titanium miniplate anchorage. Angle Orthod. 2003 Oct;73(5):597-601.
5. Hashimoto T, Fukunaga T, Kuroda S, Sakai Y, Yamashiro T, Takano-Yamamoto T. Mandibular deviation and canted maxillary occlusal plane treated with miniscrews and intraoral vertical ramus osteotomy: functional and morphologic changes. Am J Orthod Dentofacial Orthop. 2009 Dec;136(6):868-77.
6. Ko EW, Huang CS, Chen YR. Characteristics and corrective outcome of face asymmetry by orthognathic surgery. J Oral Maxillofac Surg. 2009 Oct;67(10):2201-9.
7. Takano-Yamamoto T, Kuroda S. Titanium screw anchorage for correction of canted occlusal plane in patients with facial asymmetry. Am J Orthod Dentofacial Orthop. 2007 Aug;132(2):237-42.
8. Kang YG, Nam JH, Park YG. Use of rhythmic wire system with miniscrews to correct occlusal-plane canting. Am J Orthod Dentofacial Orthop. 2010 Apr;137(4):540-7.
9. Park YC, Lee SY, Kim DH, Jee SH. Intrusion of posterior teeth using mini-screw implants. Am J Orthod Dentofacial Orthop. 2003 Jun;123(6):690-4.
10. Kuroda S, Sakai Y, Tamamura N, Deguchi T, Takano-Yamamoto T. Treatment of severe anterior open bite with skeletal anchorage in adults: comparison with orthognathic surgery outcomes. Am J Orthod Dentofacial Orthop. 2007 Nov;132(5):599-605.
11. Cornelis MA, Scheffler NR, Nyssen-Behets C, De Clerck HJ, Tulloch JF. Patients' and orthodontists' perceptions of miniplates used for temporary skeletal anchorage: a prospective study. Am J Orthod Dentofacial Orthop. 2008 Jan;133(1):18-24.
12. Park HS, Kwon TG, Kwon OW. Treatment of open bite with microscrew implant anchorage. Am J Orthod Dentofacial Orthop. 2004 Nov;126(5):627-36.
13. Leung MT, Lee TC, Rabie AB, Wong RW. Use of miniscrews and miniplates in orthodontics. J Oral Maxillofac Surg. 2008 July;66(7):1461-6.
14. De Clerck EE, Swennen GR. Success rate of miniplate anchorage for bone anchored maxillary protraction. Angle Orthod. 2011 Nov;81(6):1010-3.
15. Faber, J, Morum, TFA, Leal S, Berto PM, Carvalho CKS. Miniplates allow efficient and effective treatment of anterior open bites. Dent Press J Orthod. 2008 Sept-Oct;13(5):144-57.
16. Benson KJ, Laskin DM. Upper lip asymmetry in adults during smiling. J Oral Maxillofac Surg. 2001 Apr;59(4):396-8.
17. Padwa BL, Kaiser MO, Kaban LB. Occlusal cant in the frontal plane as a reflection of facial asymmetry. J Oral Maxillofac Surg. 1997 Aug;55(8):811-6; discussion 817.
18. Pereira CB, Justus R, Pinzan A, Bastos SHV, Bastos V, Lopes SL. The importance of evaluating the transverse cant of the occlusal plane in intraoral photographs. J World Federation Orthod. 2014;3(1):19-25.
19. Umemori M, Sugawara J, Mitani H, Nagasaka H, Kawamura H. Skeletal anchorage system for open-bite correction. Am J Orthod Dentofacial Orthop. 1999 Feb;115(2):166-74.
20. Kravitz ND, Kusnoto B. Risks and complications of orthodontic miniscrews. Am J Orthod Dentofacial Orthop. 2007 Apr;131(4 Suppl):S43-51.
21. Weiland F. Constant versus dissipating forces in orthodontics: the effect on initial tooth movement and root resorption. Eur J Orthod. 2003 Aug;25(4):335-42.
22. Acar A, Canyürek U, Kocaaga M, Erverdi N. Continuous vs. discontinuous force application and root resorption. Angle Orthod. 1999 Apr;69(2):159-63; discussion 163-4.
23. Owman-Moll P, Kurol J, Lundgren D. Continuous versus interrupted continuous orthodontic force related to early tooth movement and root resorption. Angle Orthod. 1995;65(6):395-401; discussion 401-2.
24. Han G, Huang S, Von den Hoff JW, Zeng X, Kuijpers-Jagtman AM. Root resorption after orthodontic intrusion and extrusion: an intraindividual study. Angle Orthod. 2005 Nov;75(6):912-8.
25. Consolaro A, Furquim LZ. Extreme root resorption associated with induced tooth movement: a protocol for clinical management. Dental Press J Orthod. 2014 Sept-Oct;19(5):19-26.
26. Weltman B, Vig KW, Fields HW, Shanker S, Kaizar EE. Root resorption associated with orthodontic tooth movement: a systematic review. Am J Orthod Dentofacial Orthop. 2010 Apr;137(4):462-76; discussion 12A.

4

Relationship between facial morphology, anterior open bite and non-nutritive sucking habits during the primary dentition stage

Melissa Proença Nogueira Fialho[1], Célia Regina Maio Pinzan-Vercelino[2],
Rodrigo Proença Nogueira[3], Júlio de Araújo Gurgel[4]

Introduction: Non-nutritive sucking habits (NNSHs) can cause occlusal alterations, including anterior open bite (AOB). However, not all patients develop this malocclusion. Therefore, the emergence of AOB does not depend on deleterious habits, only. **Objective:** Investigate a potential association between non-nutritive sucking habits (NNSHs), anterior open bite (AOB) and facial morphology (FM). **Methods:** 176 children in the primary dentition stage were selected. Intra and extraoral clinical examinations were performed and the children's legal guardians were asked to respond to a questionnaire comprising issues related to non-nutritive sucking habits (NNSHs). **Results:** A statistically significant relationship was found between non-nutritive sucking habits (NNSHs) and anterior open bite (AOB). However, no association was found between these factors and children's facial morphology (FM). **Conclusions:** Non-nutritive sucking habits (NNSHs) during the primary dentition stage play a key role in determining anterior open bite (AOB) malocclusion regardless of patient's morphological facial pattern (FM).

Keywords: Open bite. Face. Primary dentition.

[1] Professor, School of Dentistry, CEUMA Univeristy, UNICEUMA.
[2] Assistant professor, Department of Orthodontics, School of Dentistry, CEUMA Univeristy, UNICEUMA.
[3] Assistant professor, Brazilian Dental Association/Maranhão.
[4] Assistant professor, Department of Orthodontics, CEUMA University, UNICEUMA.

» The authors report no commercial, proprietary or financial interest in the products or companies described in this article.

Célia Regina Maio Pinzan Vercelino
Alameda dos Sabiás, 58 – Portal dos Pássaros – Boituva/SP — Brazil
CEP: 18550-000 – E-mail: cepinzan@hotmail.com

INTRODUCTION AND LITERATURE REVIEW

Much has been published about facial morphology (FM) analysis.[1,2,3] Orthodontic diagnosis on children requires not only proper occlusal and model analyses, but also a thorough assessment of facial configuration for growth prediction. In most cases, growth assessment means advancing a prognosis and, as a consequence, reducing the need for a more complex treatment in future.[4]

Anterior open bite (AOB) is one of the most common malocclusions in the primary dentition, and non-nutritive sucking habits (NNSHs) are among its etiologic factors.[1,5-9] Continuous thumb and pacifier sucking habits hinder proper teeth and alveolar processes development, especially in the anterior region.[10]

Long-facial morphology (dolichofacial) is closely associated with the development of AOB due to counterclockwise rotation of the mandible and consequent lip incompetence.[10]

AOB is the most prevalent malocclusion in primary dentition.[2,10-13] It is very often associated with the presence of NNSHs,[6,7,8] however, it tends to self-correct when the habit is eliminated at an early stage.[14]

To this day, the effect of facial morphology (FM) on growing patients with complete primary dentition and NNSH is seldom found in the orthodontic literature.[15] Most studies focusing on the association between facial morphology and AOB — with or without NNSH — consider patients in the mixed dentition stage.[11,16,17]

In 2004, Katz et al[1] examined 4-year-old children in the primary dentition stage to assess the relationship between NNSHs, FM and malocclusions. The authors found no association between facial morphology and malocclusion.

Despite the strong correlation between NSSHs and AOB,[18-22] not all children develop this malocclusion of which determinant factors are NNSH-related (duration, frequency and intensity) as well as patient-related (alveolar resistance and growth pattern). In light of a notorious lack of studies focusing on patients in the primary dentition stage, the aim of this study was to test the null hypothesis that there is no relationship between facial morphology (FM), anterior open bite (AOB), and non-nutritive sucking habits (NNSH).

MATERIAL AND METHODS

This cross-sectional study was conducted with subjects randomly selected from a population of children attending elementary schools in the city of São Luís, Brazil. The sample comprised 176 children with primary dentition (96 females and 80 males) aged between 3 and 6 years old (mean age: 4.9 years, maximum age, 6.8 years and minimum age, 2.1 years). The sample was divided into two groups: Group 1 consisting of children with NNSHs, and group 2 comprising children without any history of NNSHs.

The following inclusion criteria were applied: Children in the primary dentition stage; presence of all primary teeth; absence of extensive caries; no significant anomalies of tooth shape or size; no history of previous orthodontic treatment; NNSH and non-NNSH patients. Additionally, children's legal guardians were required to sign an informed consent form. The exclusion criterion was the absence of the habit, only. This study was approved by the Institutional Review Board of CEUMA University under protocol nº 00785/10.

The study was conducted in three major phases. At first, school principals were presented with the permits issued by the City Health Department, the children were selected according to the inclusion criteria and a second meeting was scheduled with the guardians. Secondly, the children's legal guardians were provided with detailed information about the study, its purpose and how the children would be examined. Thereafter, an informed consent form was signed by those who agreed with the research. NNSH data were collected by means of a questionnaire answered by the children's legal guardians. The questionnaire was applied individually by the researcher herself. Thirdly, the study was geared towards examining the children both intra and extraorally by means of an individual clinical assessment. Intraoral examination was performed under natural light with the child positioned in front of the examiner with their dental arches positioned in centric relation. The examiner was previously calibrated and during clinical examination, had no access to the questionnaire that provided information about the children's sucking habits (blinded).

A flexible ruler was used to assess overbite. Measurements were taken from the incisal edge of the maxillary right central incisor to the incisal edge of the lower right central incisor. Children with negative overbite and linear measurement greater than 1 mm were deemed to have anterior open bite (AOB).

Extraoral examination was conducted to determine the children's facial morphology (short face, balanced face or long face). The Facial Morphologic[23] index (FMI) was applied based on the ratio between morphological facial height (MFH) and bizygomatic distance (BD) established by means of the following formula: FMI = MFH/BD. Morphological facial height was determined based on the linear distance between the nasion and gnathion, and the bizygomatic distance between the zygomatic points (Fig 1).

A digital caliper (Mitutoyo Digimatic Caliper 200mm/.0005 "- 8"; cat. No. 500 - 147B; Battery: SR44, serial number: BH012006 - Suzano - São Paulo - Brazil) was used for extraoral measurements. Based on the values obtained, children's facial morphology was then classified into short face (< 83.9), balanced face (84.0 to 87.9) and long face (≥ 88.0).[1,23]

To ensure reliability, 36 children were randomly selected and re-assessed after 4 weeks. Numeric variables (bizygomatic distance, morphological facial height and overbite) were remeasured and the difference between the first and second measurements was determined. Dependent Student's t test was applied to assess the significance of differences observed between the two measurements, thereby revealing systematic error, according to Houston.[24] To assess random error, Dahlberg's formula[25] was employed ($Se^2 = \Sigma d^2/2n$).

Qualitative variables were described by absolute (n) and relative (%) frequencies. The *overbite* variable was described by mean and standard deviation.

To investigate the association between sucking habit and variable AOB, sucking habit and facial morphology, as well as the association between FM, AOB and NNSH, chi-square test was applied. Additionally, when the smallest expected frequency was less than or equal to 5, Fisher's Exact Test was applied.

Relationships were also expressed by odds ratio with confidence interval set at 95%.

One-way analysis of variance (ANOVA) was applied to compare AOB severity between the different facial types.

Level of significance was set at 5% ($p < 0.05$) for all tests. Statistical analyses were performed with Statistica version 5.1 software (StatSoft Inc., Tulsa, USA).

RESULTS

The error of the method results revealed reproducibility of measurements, since there were no systematic or random errors (Table 1).

A statistically significant association was found between NNSHs and the presence of AOB (Table 2). Nevertheless, there was no association between FM and AOB (Table 3).

Overall, children's FM showed no significant association with AOB malocclusion even in the presence of NNSHs. Children with balanced face and with NNSHs had the greatest percentages of AOB, followed by short-faced children (Table 4).

Among children with AOB, those with a short face had more severe anterior open bite, followed by those with a balanced face, and finally, a short face. No statistically significant difference was found between facial morphology and AOB severity (Table 5).

Finally, test power was applied, since no sample size calculation was performed at baseline to validate the results. Test power results showed that the study sample (n = 176) had 80% power to detect a difference of 22 percentage points in the association test between two variables.

DISCUSSION

This study was conducted with a sample of children in the complete primary dentition stage, given that AOB malocclusions often occur during this period. Moreover, only a few studies have focused on this phase of occlusion development, since most researches associating habits with malocclusions focus on the mixed dentition stage.[11,16,17] In addition, studies about facial morphology are scarce both in the mixed dentition and primary dentition stages,[4] particularly those seeking to correlate facial morphology with the presence of non-nutritive sucking habits and anterior open bite.[1]

In Dentistry and other healthcare areas, there is an ongoing concern about the radiation doses applied to patients. Recent studies have been conducted to assess the acceptable doses employed in the different imaging methods[26] with the purpose of reducing radiation in humans. Great emphasis has been given to facial analysis. Morphological facial index is a method used to classify facial patterns (facial morphology) without the need to expose the child to unnecessary radiation.

Table 1 - Error of the method – results of paired t test and Dahlberg's formula.[25]

Occlusal Indexes	1st Measurement Mean ± SD	2nd Measurement Mean ± SD	p	Dahlberg
Bizygomatic distance	100.17 ± 5.08	100.11 ± 5.14	0.10	0.13
Morphological facial height	84.32 ± 3.88	84.30 ± 3.87	0.26	0.08
Overbite	0.58 ± 2.65	0.57 ± 2.64	0.25	0.04

*Statistically significant: $p < 0.05$

Table 2 - Association between non-nutritive sucking habits and anterior open bite.

Groups	No AOB n	%	AOB n	%		Odds ratio (IC 95%)
NNSH	16	40.0	24	60.0	40	Reference
No NNSH	133	97.8	3	2.2	136	66.50 (17.99 – 245.80)
Total	149	84.7	27	15.3	176	
			$c2 = 79.49; p < 0.00*$			

*Statistically significant: $p < 0.05$

Table 3 - Association between facial morphology and anterior open bite.

Morphology	No AOB n	%	AOB n	%	Total	Odds ratio (IC 95%)
Short face	56	84.8	10	15.2	66	Reference
Balanced face	46	83.6	9	16.4	55	0.91 (0.34 – 2.44)
Long Face	47	85.4	8	14.6	55	0.87 (0.31 – 2.45)
Total	149	84.7	27	15.3	176	
			$c2 = 0.07; p = 0.96$			

*Statistically significant: $p < 0.05$

Table 4 - Association between NNSHs, AOB and facial morphology.

Deleterious habit and facial morphology	No AOB n	%	AOB n	%	Total	Odds ratio (IC 95%)
NNSH and short face	6	37.5	10	62.5	16	Reference
NNSH and balanced face	5	35.7	9	64.3	14	0.93 (0.21 – 4.11)
NNSH and long face	5	50.0	5	50.0	10	0.56 (0.11 – 2.90)
Total	16	40.0	24	60.0	40	
			$c2 = 0.57; p = 0.75$			

*Statistically significant: $p < 0.05$

Table 5 - Comparison among the three facial morphology patterns in terms of overbite in children with AOB, expressed in mm.

Facial morphology	Negative overbite Mean ± SD	p
Balanced face	-3.67 ± 2.00	
Short face	-4.80 ± 1.75	0.33
Long Face	-3.63 ± 2.00	
ANOVA: F = 1.15		

*Statistically significant: $p < 0.05$

For this reason, it was employed in the present study. It should be added that other studies[1,2] with similar methods were also conducted in the primary dentition stage and previously published in the literature using morphological facial index.

Results yielded with children with non-nutritive sucking habits reveal a 60% occurrence of AOB, which corroborates the values obtained by Sousa et al[2] (63.4%), but are nowhere near the values found by Katz et al[1] (35.5%). Other authors also found a positive relationship for the NNSH / AOB ratio.[6-8,19-21]

Results revealed no association between facial morphology, NNSHs and AOB. It is speculated that, although NNSHs act as etiological factors of malocclusions,[5-8] facial morphology does not interfere in this process as a facilitating factor in the emergence of this malocclusion during primary dentition.[1]

Katz et al[1] reported that the different types of facial morphology and NNSHs produce independent effects on malocclusions. Among these is AOB which should therefore be studied separately. These authors[1] endorse the idea that genetic factors seem to play a less important role than commonly believed, and that many types of malocclusions are actually acquired rather than inherited. However, Cozza et al[11] refute this idea, stating that chronic non-nutritive sucking habits and the characteristics of facial hyperdivergence (long face) pose significant risks for the development of AOB when occurring together. It should be emphasized, however, that in the aforesaid study[11] assessments were performed based on the cephalograms of children with a mean age of 9 years and 3 months, and in the mixed dentition stage, which differs from the sample used in the present study.

In this study, it was observed that among all children presenting with AOB, 14.6% had long face pattern, 15.2% short face, and 16.4% balanced face. Thus, the fact that patients with long face exhibited the lowest values in determining the onset of AOB shows an independent relationship between the presence of AOB and long face morphology, as well as other morphologies, in agreement with the results of Katz et al[1] and Sousa et al,[2] who applied a methodology that was similar to the one used in this study.

None of the types of facial morphology was prevalent, given that the values of 31.25%, 37.5% and 31.25% found for the balanced face, short face and long face, respectively, showed no statistically significant differences. This contrasts with the findings of Sousa et al[2] and Silva Filho et al[15] who argue that balanced face is the predominant pattern. It is believed that this difference in outcomes may be related to the fact that their investigation was carried out in different regions and in populations with different morphological characteristics.

With regard to the relationship between AOB severity and facial morphology, short-faced children exhibited the highest values of negative overbite, followed by balanced-faced, and long-faced children (Table 5). NNSH duration is of paramount importance in determining AOB emergence.[19] The literature shows that factors such as NNSH duration, frequency and intensity affect AOB severity.[17] This finding probably explains the higher values of negative overbite observed in short-faced children.

CONCLUSIONS

According to the methods applied in this study and after careful analysis of results, it seems reasonable to conclude that non-nutritive sucking habits (NNSHs) during the primary dentition stage play a key role in determining anterior open bite (AOB) malocclusion regardless of morphological facial pattern.

REFERENCES

1. Katz CRT, Rosenblatt A, Gondim PPC. Nonnutritive sucking habits in Brazilian children: Effects on deciduous dentition and relationship with facial morphology. Am J Orthod Dentofacial Orthop. 2004;126(1):53-7.
2. Sousa RLS, Lima RB, Florêncio Filho C, Lima KC, Diógenes AMN. Prevalência e fatores de risco da mordida aberta anterior na dentadura decídua completa em pré-escolares na cidade de Natal/RNR. Rev Dental Press Ortod Ortop Facial. 2007;12(2):129-38.
3. Cabrera CA, Cabrera MC. Ortodontia clínica. Curitiba: Interativas; 1997.
4. Proffit WR. Contemporany Orthodontics. 3nd ed. St Louis: Mosby; 2000.
5. Thomaz EBAF, Cangussu MCT, Assis AMO. Maternal breastfeeding, parafunctional oral habits and malocclusion in adolescents: a multivariate analysis. Int J Pediatr Otorhinolaryngol. 2012;76(4):500-6.
6. Furtado ANM, Vedovello Filho M. A influência do período de aleitamento materno na instalação dos hábitos de sucção não nutritivos e na ocorrência de maloclusão na dentição decídua. RGO: Rev Gaúch Odontol. 2007;55(4):335-41.
7. Leite-Cavalcanti A, Medeiros-Bezerra PK, Moura C. Aleitamento natural, aleitamento artificial, hábitos de sucção e maloclusões em pré-escolares brasileiros. Rev Salud Pública. 2007;9(2):194-204.
8. Oliveira AC, Pordeusb IA, Torresc CS, Martinsc MT, Paivab SM. Feeding and nonnutritive sucking habits and prevalence of open bite and crossbite in children/adolescents with Down syndrome. Angle Orthod. 2010;80(4):748-53.
9. Mercadante MMN. Hábitos em Ortodontia. In: Ferreira FV. Ortodontia: diagnóstico e planejamento clínico. São Paulo: Artes Médica; 2004. p. 253-79.
10. Forte FDS, Bosco VL. Prevalência de mordida aberta anterior e sua relação com hábitos de sucção não nutritiva. Pesq Bras Odonto Clin Integr. 2001;1(1):3-8.
11. Cozza P, Baccetti T, Franci L, Mucedero M, Polimeni A. Sucking habits and facial hyperdivergency as risk factors for anterior open bite in the mixed dentition. Am J Orthod Dentofacial Orthop. 2005;128(4):517-9.

12. Adair SM, Milano M, Dushku JC. Evaluation of the effects of orthodontic pacifiers on the primary dentitions of 24 to 59 month old children: preliminary study. Pediatric Dent. 1992;14(1):13-8.

13. Santana VC, Santos RM, Silva LAS, Novais SMA. Prevalência de Mordida Aberta Anterior e hábitos bucais indesejáveis em crianças de 3 a 6 anos de incompletos na cidade de Aracaju. J Bras Odontopediatr Odonto Bebe 2011;4(18):154-69.

14. Almeida RVD, Nogueira Filho JJ, Jardim MCAM. Prevalência de maloclusão e sua relação com hábitos bucais deletérios em escolares. Rev Pesq Bras Odontoped Clin Integr. 2002;2(1):43-5.

15. Silva Filho OG, Herkrath FJ, Queiroz APC, Aiello CA. Padrão facial na dentadura decídua: estudo epidemiológico. Rev Dental Press Ortod Ortop Facial. 2008;13(4):45-59.

16. Nisula KK, Lehto R, Lusa V, Nisula LK Varrela J. Occurrence of malocclusion and need of orthodontic treatment in early mixed dentition. Am J Orthod Dentofacial Orthop. 2003;124(6):631-8.

17. Tausche E, Luck L, Harzer W. Prevalence of malocclusions in the early mixed dentition and orthodontic treatment need. Eur J Orthod. 2004;26(3):237-44.

18. Moyers RE. Etiologia da má oclusão. In: Moyers RE. Ortodontia. 4ª ed. Rio de Janeiro: Guanabara Koogan; 1991. p. 212-37.

19. Warren JJ, Bishara SE. Duration of nutritive and nonnutritive sucking behaviors and their effects on the dental arches in the primary dentition. Am J Orthod Dentofacial Orthop. 2002;121(4):347-56.

20. Diouf JF, Ngom PI, Badiane A, Cisse B, Ndoye C, Diop-ba K, Diagne F. Influence of the mode of nutritive and nonnutritive sucking on the dimensions of primary dental arches. Int Orthod. 2010;8(4):372-85.

21. Thomaz EBAF, Valença AMG. Prevalência de má-oclusão e fatores relacionados à sua ocorrência em pré-escolares da cidade de São Luís – MA – Brasil. RPG Rev Pos Grad. 2005;12(2):212-21.

22. Tibolla C, Rigo L, Nijima LI, Estacia A, Frizzo EG, Lodi L. Associação entre mordida aberta anterior e hábito de sucção de chupeta em escolares de um município do sul do Brasil. Dental Press J Orthod. 2012;17(6):89-96.

23. Rakosi T, Jonas I, Grabe TM. Color atlas of dental medicine orthodontic-diagnosis. New York: Thieme; 1993. p. 108-9.

24. Houston WJB. Analysis of errors in orthodontics measurements. Am J Orthod. 1983;5(83):382-90.

25. Dahlberg G. Statistical methods for medical and biological students. New York: Intercience; 1940.

26. Grünheid T, Schieck JRK, Pliska BT, Ahmad M, Larsone BE. Dosimetry of a cone-beam computed tomography machine compared with a digital x-ray machine in orthodontic imaging. Am J Orthod Dentofacial Orthop. 2012;141(4):436-43.

5

Lateral cephalometric diagnosis of asymmetry in Angle Class II subdivision compared to Class I and II

Aparecida Fernanda Meloti[1], Renata de Cássia Gonçalves[1], Ertty Silva[2], Lídia Parsekian Martins[3], Ary dos Santos-Pinto[3]

Introduction: Lateral cephalometric radiographs are traditionally required for orthodontic treatment, yet rarely used to assess asymmetries. **Objective:** The objective of the present study was to use lateral cephalometric radiographs to identify existing skeletal and dentoalveolar morphological alterations in Class II subdivision and to compare them with the existing morphology in Class I and II relationship. **Material and Methods:** Ninety initial lateral cephalometric radiographs of male and female Brazilian children aged between 12 to 15 years old were randomly and proportionally divided into three groups: Group 1 (Class I), Group 2 (Class II) and Group 3 (Class II subdivision). Analysis of lateral cephalometric radiographs included angular measurements, horizontal linear measurements and two indexes of asymmetry that were prepared for this study. **Results:** In accordance with an Index of Dental Asymmetry (IDA), greater mandibular dental asymmetry was identified in Group 3. An Index of Mandibular Asymmetry (IMA) revealed less skeletal and dental mandibular asymmetry in Group 2, greater skeletal mandibular asymmetry in Group 1, and greater mandibular dental asymmetry in Group 3. **Conclusion:** Both IDA and IMA revealed greater mandibular dental asymmetry for Group 3 in comparison to Groups 1 and 2. These results are in accordance with those found by other diagnostic methods, showing that lateral cephalometric radiography is an acceptable method to identify existing skeletal and dentoalveolar morphological alterations in malocclusions.

Keywords: Facial asymmetry. Malocclusions. Radiography. Cephalometry.

[1] PhD in Orthodontics and Facial Orthopedics, School of Dentistry — State University of São Paulo (UNESP)/Araraquara.
[2] Specialist in Orthodontics and Facial Orthopedics, PUC-RJ.
[3] Adjunct professor, Department of Pediatric Dentistry and Orthodontics, School of Dentistry — State University of São Paulo (UNESP)/Araraquara.

» The authors report no commercial, proprietary or financial interest in the products or companies described in this article.

Aparecida Fernanda Meloti
Rua Carlos Antônio de Azevedo, 333 – Jardim São José – Urupês/SP — Brazil
CEP: 15.850-000 – E-mail: fermeloti@yahoo.com.br

INTRODUCTION

Class II subdivision is characterized by an asymmetrical posterior occlusal relationship in which the dental arches demonstrate a Class I relationship on one side and a Class II relationship on the other side. This asymmetrical occlusal relationship is of skeletal and/or dentoalveolar origin.[1] Knowing the origin of this asymmetry is extremely important to ensure correct treatment of individuals with Class II subdivision.

Slight degrees of facial asymmetry are common among the general population.[2] Individuals with Class II subdivision typically present an accentuated degree of asymmetry that involves the lower third of the face and the mandible.[3,4,5]

Alavi et al[6] reported the distal position of the first lower molar as the main cause of Class II subdivision asymmetry. Additionally, these authors stated that asymmetry could have dentoalveolar or skeletal etiology. Rose et al[7] also observed first lower molar in Class II subdivision asymmetry positioned more posteriorly on the Class II side; however, these authors stated that asymmetry resulted from dentoalveolar involvement without observable changes in the jaw. The position of dental midlines in relation to the facial midline was examined and revealed[8] that lower dental midline deviation was more common than upper midline deviation, suggesting the cause of this asymmetry to be mandibular in nature.

While observing maxillary and mandibular changes in Class II subdivision and Class I malocclusions, Janson et al[9] showed that dentoalveolar changes occurred in jaws without positional asymmetry. The main cause of Class II subdivision relationship was the distal position of lower molars on the Class II side. The position of upper mesial molars, also on the Class II side, was a secondary cause. The lower dental midline also presented more frequent deviations on the Class II side than the upper dental midline did. Therefore, this study[9] as well as others[4,7,8,10,11] demonstrated that asymmetries present in Class II subdivision patients are mainly of dentoalveolar origin.

Computed tomography is considered an optimal diagnostic method for asymmetry assessment,[12] but the cost of this method is higher and its radiation dose is greater in comparison to other methods. Photographs have been compared to posteroanterior radiographs, but no significant correlation has been found between methods.[13] Edler et al[14] argued that photographs should be used simultaneously with posteroanterior radiographs. When photographs were compared to submentovertex radiographs and posteroanterior radiographs,[15] a small correlation was found between methods. Posteroanterior radiographs allow observations of vertical and transversal changes; however, reports in the literature[6-9,11,12] have noted a greater change in the anteroposterior positioning of molars in Class II subdivision malocclusion.

Although anteroposterior changes can be observed with submentovertex radiographs, Lew and Tay[16] found a distortion in linear measurements taken with these radiographs. Additionally, Arnold et al[17] reported difficulties in using submentovertex radiographs. The use of 45° cephalometric radiographs offers another method that allows visualization of structures in the anteroposterior direction, but this method is not routinely applied because it requires two further radiographic images in addition to those required for basic orthodontic documentation. Study models may be used for observation of dental structures in the anteroposterior direction, but these models do not allow skeletal observations. In addition, panoramic radiographs do not enable anteroposterior morphological alterations to be visualized.[18,19]

Because they are traditionally required for orthodontic treatment, lateral cephalometric radiographs allow visualization of anteroposterior structures in a simple manner without additional costs to the orthodontist. Only one study[6] has used lateral cephalometric radiographs to observe the position of molars and the existence of an asymmetrical mandibular relationship in the anteroposterior direction.

Therefore, the objectives of our study were to use lateral cephalometric radiographs to identify skeletal and dentoalveolar morphological alterations in cases of Class II subdivision; to compare these changes with morphology of Class I and Class II; and to assess the incidences of dental and skeletal symmetry and asymmetry of the maxilla and mandible.

MATERIAL AND METHODS

This research was approved by the School of Dentistry — State University of São Paulo Institutional Review Board. The sample comprised 90 male and female Brazilian children aged between 12 and 15 years old, randomly selected in the archives of the School of Dentistry,

State University of São Paulo/Araraquara. The sample was divided into three equal groups of Class I, Class II or Class II subdivision patients. Malocclusion criteria were based on the occlusal relationship between upper and lower arches obtained on study models and photographic documentation. Molar and canine relationships in Group 1 (Class I) were bilateral and symmetrical, whereas those in Group 2 (Class II) were displaced in more than half the width of a cusp. In Group 3 (Class II subdivision), molar and canine exhibited a Class I relationship on one side and a Class II relationship on the other side. Additional inclusion criteria for all groups were as follows: normal lower arch or a lower arch with slight lower-anterior crowding, and the presence of all permanent teeth in the dental arches (from first molar to first molar) with eminent eruption or eruption of second molars. Subjects were excluded if they had occlusal interferences that might cause functional alterations (e.g., dental crossbite, open bite or history of facial trauma).

Standardized lateral cephalometric radiographs were taken with patients' teeth in maximum habitual intercuspation with relaxed lips and face positioned with Camper's plane parallel to the ground. Radiographs were taken with Rotograph plus model MR05, adjusted for 85 Kvp, 10 mA and 0.5 seconds of exposure time. The equipment had fixed and constant focus-object distance of 1.5 meters. The chassis with Kodak^{tm} - TMG/RA, 20.3cm x 25.4 cm film was positioned 15 cm away from the medial sagittal plan, giving an average magnification factor of 10%.

Cephalometric analysis was performed by digitizing twenty-one points identified in the lateral radiographs (Fig 1) by the same researcher using a Numonics Accu-Grid digitizer (TPL 1212 – Kurta, Seymour, Connecticut – USA) and Dentofacial Planner Plus, version 6.5, 1995 (Dentofacial software Inc. Toronto, Ontario – Canada). Radiographs were randomly digitized by means of simple random sampling without group identification.

For characterization of the sample, the following angular measurements were used: SNA, SNB, ANB, SNPP (angle formed by the SN line and the palatal plane [ANS – PNS]), SNOP (angle formed by the SN line and the occlusal plane [Op – Oa]), SN-GoMe, U1.SN, L1GoMe, U1.L1 and NAPog. Study analysis involved two indexes (i.e., the index of dental asymmetry and the index of mandibular asymmetry) as well as five linear measurements (RA-RP,

D7UA-D7UP, D6UA-D6UP, D7LA-D7LP and D6LA-D6LP) (Fig 2).

Index of dental asymmetry (IDA)

An IDA was developed based on the difference in distance between the most anterior and the most posterior molars in the upper and lower dental arches [IDA1 = (D6UA-D6UP) – (D6LA-D6LP)]. Similarly, this index was applied for second upper and lower molars [IDA2= (D7UA-D7UP) – (D7LA-D7LP)].

Mathematically, a difference of zero represents upper-lower dental symmetry. A variation from normality of ± 0.5 mm was used for the tolerance criterion; this value corresponds to the degree of magnification between the right and left sides in cephalometric measurements. Values greater than 0.5 mm represented a greater distance between upper molars than between lower molars, and thus indicated upper dental asymmetry. Values of less than -0.5 mm represented a greater distance between lower molars than between upper molars, and thus indicated lower dental asymmetry.

For example, the IDA using the first molars is described as follows:
» IDA1= (D6UA-D6UP) – (D6LA-D6LP), where
» (D6UA-D6UP) = distance between the most anterior image of the upper first molar (D6UA) and the most posterior molar (D6UP); and
» (D6LA-D6LP) = distance between the most anterior image of the lower first molar (D6LA) and the most posterior molar (D6LP).
If:
» IDA > 0.5 mm = upper dental asymmetry;
» IDA < -0.5 mm = lower dental asymmetry;
» -0.5 mm ≥ IDA ≤ 0.5 mm = upper and lower dental symmetry.

Index of mandibular asymmetry (IMA)

Following the same logic, an IMA was developed based on the difference in distance between the most anterior and the most posterior portions of the mandibular ramus, and the distance between the most anterior and the most posterior lower first molars [IMA1 = (RA-RP) – (D6LA-D6LP)]. Similarly, this index was applied for second molars [IMA2= (RA-RP) – (D7LA-D7LP)].

Mathematically, a difference of zero between skeletal and dental mandibular distances indicated dental

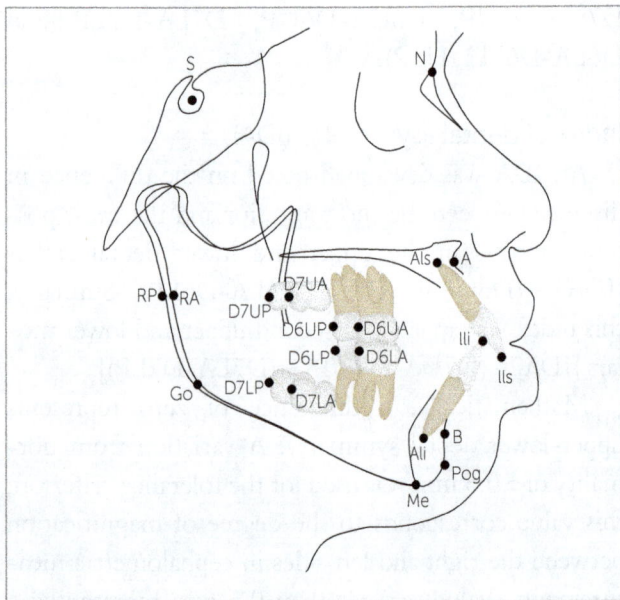

Figure 1 - Skeletal and dental cephalometric points. S (Sella), N (Nasion), A (Subspinal), B (Supramental), Go (Gonial), Me (Mentalis), Pog (Pogonion), IIs (Incisal edge of maxillary central incisor), AIs (Apex of upper incisor), IIi (Incisal edge of the lower central incisor), AIi (Apex of lower incisor), RA (Anterior ramus), RP (Posterior ramus), D7UA (Point in the distal face of the most anterior image of the second upper molar crown), D7UP (Point in the distal face of the most posterior image of the second upper molar crown), D6UA (Point in the distal face of the most anterior image of the first upper molar crown), D6UP (Point in the distal face of the most posterior image of the first upper molar crown), D7LA (Point in the distal face of the most anterior image of the second lower molar crown), D7LP (Point in the distal face of the most posterior image of the second lower molar crown), D6LA (Point in the distal face of the most anterior image of the first lower molar crown), D6LP (Point in the distal face of the most posterior image of first lower molar crown).

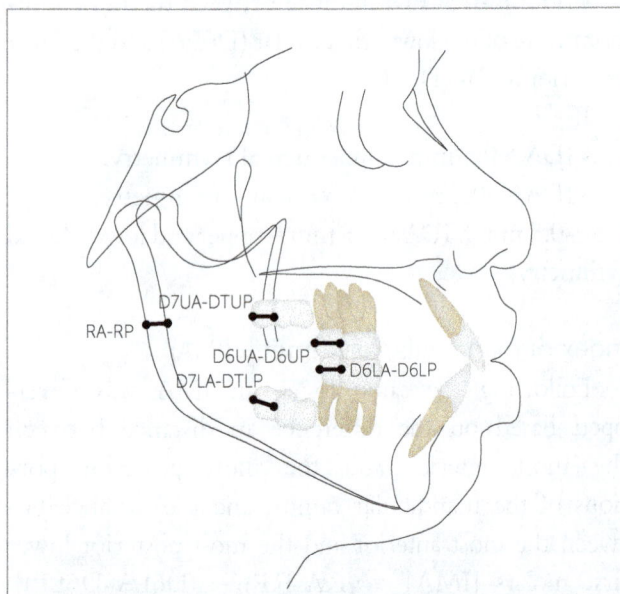

Figure 2 - Skeletal and dental linear cephalometric measurements. RA-RP (Horizontal distance between the anterior (RA) and posterior (RP) images of the posterior mandibular borders), D7UA-D7UP (Horizontal distance between the D7UA and D7UP points), D6UA-D6UP (Horizontal distance between the D6UA and D6UP points), D7LA-D7LP (Horizontal distance between the D7LA and D7LP points), D6LA-D6LP (Horizontal distance between the D6LA and D6LP points).

and skeletal mandibular symmetry. As above, a tolerance criterion of ± 0.5 mm was used to indicate variation from normality. Values greater than 0.5 mm represented skeletal asymmetry, as the anterior-posterior extent of the ramus was greater than that of the lower molars. On the other hand, values of less than -0.5 mm represented dental asymmetry, as the anterior-posterior extent of the lower molars was greater than that of the mandibular ramus.

For example, the IMA using the first molars was described as follows:

» IMA1= (RA-RP) – (D6LA-D6LP), where

» (RA-RP) = distance between the most anterior image of the mandibular ramus (RA) and the most posterior one (RP); and

» (D6LA-D6LP) = distance between the most anterior image of the lower first molar (D6LA) and the most posterior one (D6LP).

If:

» IMA > 0.5 = mandibular skeletal asymmetry;

» IMA < -0.5 = mandibular dental asymmetry;

» -0.5 mm ≥ IMA ≤ 0.5 mm = skeletal and dental mandibular symmetry.

Statistical analysis

To assess consistency of measurements, six radiographs from each group were digitized twice by the same researcher with an interval of two weeks in between. The intra-class correlation coefficient (ICC) was used to assess reliability of the variable measurement process. Measurements were considered adequate when the ICC value was greater than 0.95.

To test the hypothesis that mean angular measurements were equivalent for the three groups, an analysis of variance (ANOVA) was used. When Levene's prior test rejected the hypothesis of homogeneity of variances, Brown-Forsythe test was used to verify equality of means. Scheffé's multiple comparison test was used to detect significant differences between groups.

A chi-square test was used to test the hypothesis that the proportion of subjects with asymmetries did not differ between groups, and to determine whether there was an association between category of asymmetry and group. A 95% confidence level ($p < 0.05$) was considered statistically significant. Statistical analyses were performed using SPSS software, version 16.0 for Windows (release 16.01 – Nov. 2007; SPSS Inc., 1989-2007).

RESULTS

Reliability of the method was satisfactory; ICC values for replicate measurements were greater than 0.99 for angular measurements and greater than 0.96 for linear measurements. The calculated ICC value was greater than 0.98 for all variables.

The analysis of differences between groups (Table 1) confirmed greater mandibular retrusion (smallest SNB) and greater lower incisor inclination (greater L1.GoMe) for Group 2 in comparison to the other groups (1 and 3). Group 1 had smaller maxillomandibular differences (smallest ANB) and lower facial convexity (smallest NAPog) than the other groups (2 and 3). Despite significant ANOVA result for the U1.L1 measurement, Scheffé's multiple comparison test was unable to detect significant differences between groups.

As shown in Table 1, the RA-RP distance was similar for all groups. Therefore, if image distortions or variations in head position occurred, they were similar for all groups. In contrast, the dental measurements differed significantly among groups. Differences in distance between first upper molars (D6UA-D6UP) and second

upper molars (D7UA-D7UP) were smaller in Group 1 than Group 3; yet the values for these groups did not differ from those of Group 2. Distances between first lower molars (D6LA-D6LP) and second lower molars (D7LA-D7LP) were smaller in Group 1 than Groups 2 or 3. All dental measurements were greater in Group 3 than in Groups 1 or 2.

The proportion of subjects with skeletal and dental mandibular symmetry, skeletal mandibular asymmetry and/or dental mandibular asymmetry was determined in the three groups by means of the IMA using first (IMA1) or second (IMA2) molars as reference. Despite the greater proportion of subjects with skeletal asymmetry in Group 1, the greater proportion of subjects with skeletal and dental symmetry in Group 2 and the greater proportion of subjects with dental asymmetry in Group 3, the chi-square test revealed no significant association between asymmetry and group in IMA1 (Table 2). Additionally, there was no statistically significant difference among the means of IMA1 for each asymmetry category. However, a greater incidence of dental mandibular asymmetry was observed in

Table 1 - Mean and standard deviation of measurements and analysis of variance (ANOVA) to test the hypothesis that the means of the three groups are the same

Cephalometric measurement	Group 1 Class I Mean ±SD	Group 2 Class II Mean ±SD	Group 3 Class II Subdivision Mean ±SD	p
Characterization of the groups				
SNA	82.19± 3.54	81.80 ± 2.73	83.43± 4.56	0.208
SNB	79.81[a] ± 3.23	76.04[b] ± 2.82	78.97[a] ± 4.33	0.000
ANB	2.37[a] ± 2.03	5.77[c] ± 2.07	4.46[b] ± 2.05	0.000
SN.PP	7.63 ± 3.14	8.22 ± 3.58	7.62 ± 3.85	0.756
SN.OP	19.95 ± 2.74	19.47 ± 3.59	19.63 ± 4.68	0.884
SN.GoMe	34.99 ± 5.21	34.55 ± 4.17	32.16 ± 5.72	0.073
U1.SN	106.20± 7.88	106.81 ± 6.74	104.93 ± 7.14	0.597
L1.GoMe	91.49[a] ± 8.60	97.50[b] ± 6.12	95.49[ab] ± 6.35	0.005
U1.L1	127.33 ± 12.90	121.15 ± 8.52	127.41 ± 9.84	0.036
NAPog	3.62[a] ± 5.12	9.30[b] ± 5.62	7.11[b] ± 4.91	0.000
Skeletal and dental linear				
RA-RP[1]	1.38 ± 0.88	1.38 ± 1.60	1.37 ± 1.22	1.000
D6UA-D6UP	1.26[a] ± 0.79	1.60[ab] ± 1.19	2.02[b] ± 1.23	0.028
D7UA-D7UP	1.27[a] ± 0.82	1.57[ab] ± 1.15	1.96[b] ± 1.16	0.045
D6LA-D6LP[1]	1.20[a] ± 0.80	1.87[b] ± 1.11	2.51[b] ± 1.78	0.001
D7LA-D7LP[1]	1.15[a] ± 0.75	1.81[b] ± 1.10	2.48[b] ± 1.81	0.001

[1] Brown-Forsythe statistics (Levene's test rejected the hypothesis of homogeneity of variance).

Group 3 than in Groups 1 or 2, and a greater incidence of skeletal asymmetry was observed in Group 2 than in Groups 1 or 3 (Table 3). When the second molar was used to calculate the IMA2, there was no significant association between asymmetry and group membership (Table 2). Finally, the magnitude of dental mandibular asymmetry in Group 1 was smaller than that in Groups 2 or 3 (Table 3).

The proportion of subjects with dental symmetry, upper dental asymmetry and/or lower dental asymmetry was determined in the three groups by IDA1 and IDA2. A chi-square test revealed significant association between asymmetry and group membership. The proportion of individuals with dental symmetry was significantly greater in Groups 1 and 2 than in Group 3. In Group 3, there was a high frequency of lower dental asymmetry (Table 2). The magnitude of lower dental asymmetry was also greater in Group 3 than in Groups 1 or 2 (Table 3).

DISCUSSION

In this study, lateral radiographs were used to assess the nature of asymmetries in individuals with Class II subdivision (Group 3) compared to control groups of individuals with bilateral symmetric Class I (Group 1) or bilateral symmetric Class II (Group 2) relationship. Although other diagnostic methods are more frequently used than lateral radiography, these methods are accompanied by specific disadvantages.[6-9,11-17]

Lateral cephalometric radiographs allow anteroposterior structures to be visualized in a simple manner without additional costs to the orthodontist, as they are traditionally required for diagnostic and treatment planning. However, as other radiographic methods, errors in head positioning may occur.[20] The head may rotate along transverse, anteroposterior, or vertical axes. Rotations along the transverse axis do not cause image distortions because the head remains parallel to the X-ray source. Rotation produces relative changes in the location of images on the film, but none in

Table 2 - Number and proportion of individuals according to group and category of the index of asymmetry and results of chi-square test for the association between asymmetry and group

Index / Category of asymmetry	Group 1		Group 2		Group 3	
	n	%	n	%	n	%
IMA1 (χ^2= 8.66; df=4; p=0.070)						
Dental asymmetry	10	33.3	14	46.7	20	66.7
Symmetry	7	23.3	9	30	4	13.3
Skeletal asymmetry	13	43.3	7	23.3	6	20
Total	30	100	30	100	30	100
IMA2 (χ^2= 9.15; df=4; p=0.057)						
Dental asymmetry	11	36.7	13	43.3	20	66.7
Symmetry	6	20.0	10	33.3	4	13.3
Skeletal asymmetry	13	43.3	7	23.3	6	20.0
Total	30	100.0	30	100.0	30	100.0
IDA1 (χ^2 = 16.33; df=4; p=0.003)						
Dental asymmetry	3	10.0	8	26.7	13	43.3
Symmetry	23	76.7	18	60.0	8	26.7
Skeletal asymmetry	4	13.3	4	13.3	9	30.0
Total	30	100.0	30	100.0	30	100.0
IDA2 (χ^2= 14.60; df=4; p=0.006)						
Dental asymmetry	3	10.0	7	23.3	12	40.0
Symmetry	23	76.7	19	63.3	9	30.0
Skeletal asymmetry	4	13.3	4	13.3	9	30.0
Total	30	100.0	30	100.0	30	100.0

IMA = index of mandibular asymmetry; IMA1 = (RA-RP) – (D6LA - D6LP); IMA 2 = (RA-RP) – (D7LA – D7LP).
IDA = index of dental asymmetry; IDA1 = (D6UA-D6UP)–(D6LA-D6LP); IDA 2 = (D7UA-D7UP)–(D7LA-D7LP).

Table 3 - Mean and standard deviation of the index of asymmetry and results of the analysis of variance (ANOVA) to test the hypothesis of equality of the means of the three groups, according to the category of asymmetry.

Index / Category of asymmetry	Group 1 Mean ± SD	Group 2 Mean ± SD	Group 3 Mean ± SD	p
IMA1 (RA-RP) − (D6LA − D6LP)				
Dental asymmetry	-1.35 ± 0.54	-1.89 ± 0.85	-2.23 ± 1.12	0.064
Symmetry	-0.21 ± 0.42	-0.04 ± 0.28	0.25 ± 0.29	0.120
Skeletal asymmetry	1.57 ± 0.68	1.74 ± 0.57	1.57 ± 0.73	0.840
IMA2 (RA-RP) − (D7LA − D7LP)				
Dental asymmetry	-1.18[a] ± 0.47	-1.97[b] ± 0.8	-2.16[b] ± 1.22	**0.031**
Symmetry	-0.12 ± 0.44	-0.02 ± 0.31	0.18 ± 0.21	0.429
Skeletal asymmetry	1.58 ± 0.67	1.83 ± 0.78	1.55 ± 0.73	0.721
IDA1 (D6UA − D6UP) − (D6LA − D6LP))				
Dental asymmetry	-0.80[a] ± 0.20	-1.28[a] ± 0.24	-2.52[b] ± 0.40	0.002
Symmetry	-0.01 ± 0.57	-0.08 ± 0.27	0.18 ± 0.16	0.050
Skeletal asymmetry	1.13 ± 1.03	0.90 ± 0.16	1.86 ± 0.84	0.058
IDA2 (D7UA-D7UP)−(D7LA-D7LP)				
Dental asymmetry	-0.73[a] ± 0.23	-1.31[a] ± 0.39	-2.70[b] ± 1.00	**0.001**
Symmetry	0.07[ab] ± 0.26	-0.05[a] ± 0.25	0.21[b] ± 0.19	**0.031**
Skeletal asymmetry	1.05 ± 0.47	0.75 ± 0.17	1.66 ± 0.82	0.082

the relationships of structures that could cause errors in the process of radiographic measurement. Rotation along the anteroposterior axis affects vertical measurements. Although bilateral structures move equally, vertical measurements increase or decrease based on the direction of rotation. Rotation along the vertical axis could influence horizontal measurements, as analyzed in this study.[20] When the head rotates along the vertical axis, the length of the mandibular body gradually decreases as the rotation angle increases along the direction of the film. Alteration in length is typically approximately 1%; however, this percentage may increase to -5.78% when the angle of head rotation varies between -5 and -15 degrees.[20] The effects of head rotation on measurements of mandible and molars are equal in magnitude. Therefore, the absolute but not relative distance between these structures is affected, as demonstrated by the indexes of asymmetry of this current study.

According to Kjellberg et al,[19] radiographic extent, head position and distortions can be ignored when an index is used to calculate linear measurements. Habets et al[20] also believe that morphological differences of size, calculation and interpretation of findings can be excluded by certain indexes such as those used in the current study.

Our sample showed a few cephalometric differences related to the characteristics of malocclusion.

For example, individuals in Group 1 presented smaller ANB and less facial convexity. These differences reflect the characteristics of the groups, confirming that individuals in Group 2 presented greater mandibular retrusion than those in Groups 1 and 3. Although Group 3 has a Class II relationship on one side, the Class I relationship on the other side produces smaller retrusion than in individuals with bilateral Class II (Group 2). Azevedo et al[4] reported that skeletal involvement in individuals with Class II subdivision is typically small. Greater buccal positioning of lower incisors in individuals with Class II arises due to dentoalveolar compensation for their greater mandibular retrusion, which results in a significantly more closed interincisal angle.

Distances between first and second upper or lower molars (Table 2) were always smaller in Group 1 than in Groups 2 and 3, thus revealing that this type of relationship is associated with greater dental symmetry. IDA1 and IDA2 identified greater dental symmetry in Groups 1 and 2, indicating great concordance between our direct measurements and the results of these indexes.

Similarly, IMA1 and IMA2 revealed greater skeletal mandibular asymmetry in Group 1 (Table 2). This result is supported by the findings by Sezgin et al[21] who found greater asymmetry in individuals with Class I than those with normal occlusion. They also found[22] asymmetry in Class I patients, with the mandible less anterior and highly positioned in hyperdivergent patients than in hypodivergent.

IMA revealed greater skeletal and dental mandibular symmetry in Group 2 than in Groups 1 and 3. Although Group 2 tended to show greater symmetry than individuals in the other groups, their skeletal asymmetry (when present) was greater in magnitude than that of Groups 1 and 3.

IMA revealed greater dental mandibular asymmetry in Group 3 than those in Groups 1 and 2. IDA also showed individuals in Group 3 to have greater lower dental asymmetry than Groups 1 and 2. These results corroborate those presented by authors[4,7-11] using other diagnostic methods, such as posteroanterior radiography, submentovertex radiography, 45° radiography, study models and photographs. Alavi et al[6] used lateral radiograph to investigate asymmetries in individuals with Class II subdivision. Nevertheless, the authors were not able to determine whether these changes arose due to dentoalveolar or skeletal etiology.

CONCLUSION

» Two indexes of asymmetry and direct measurements were presented as part of a new evaluation method used to identify dental and skeletal asymmetries by means of lateral cephalometric radiography.

» Distances between first and second upper or lower molars were always less in the Class I group and greater in the Class II subdivision group, in accordance with new IDA indexes which identified greater dental asymmetry in individuals with Class II subdivision than those with Class I and Class II.

» New IMA indexes revealed less skeletal and dental mandibular asymmetry in individuals with Class II, and greater skeletal mandibular asymmetry in individuals with Class I.

» IMA and IDA suggested that Class II subdivision individuals had greater mandibular dental asymmetry than Class I or Class II.

REFERENCES

1. Janson GRP, Pereira ACJ, Dainesi EA, Freitas MR. The dental asymmetry and implication in the orthodontic treatment: a clinical case. Ortodontia. 1995;28:68-73.

2. Thompson JR. Asymmetry of the face. J Am Dent Assoc. 1943;30:1859-71.

3. Alkofide EA. Class II division 1 malocclusion: the subdivision problem. J Clin Pediatr Dent. 2001;26(1):37-40.

4. Azevedo ARP, Janson G, Henriques JFC, Freitas MR. Evaluation of asymmetries between subjects with Class II subdivision and apparent facial asymmetry and those with normal occlusion. Am J Orthod Dentofacial Orthop. 2006;129(3):376-83.

5. Brin I, Bem-Bassat Y, Blustein Y, Ehriich J, Hochman N, Marmary Y, et al. Skeletal and functional effects of treatment for unilateral posterior crossbite. Am J Orthod Dentofacial Orthop. 1996;109(2):173-9.

6. Alavi DG, BeGole EA, Schneider BJ. Facial and dental arch asymmetries in Class II subdivision malocclusion. Am J Orthod Dentofacial Orthop. 1988;93(1):38-46.

7. Rose JM, Sadowsky C, BeGole EA, Moles R. Mandibular skeletal and dental asymmetry in Class II subdivision malocclusions. Am J Orthod Dentofacial Orthop. 1994;105(5):489-95.

8. Araujo TM, Wilhelm RS, Almeida MA. Skeletal and dental arch asymmetries in Class II division 1 subdivision malocclusions. J Clin Pediatr Dent. 1994;18(3):181-5.

9. Janson GRP, Metaxas A, Woodside DG, Freitas MR, Pinzan A. Three-dimensional evaluation of skeletal and dental asymmetries in Class II subdivision malocclusions. Am J Orthod Dentofacial Orthop. 2001;119(4):406-18.

10. Janson G, Lima KJRS, Woodside DG, Metaxas A, Freitas MR, Henriques JFC. Class II subdivision malocclusion types and evaluation of their asymmetries. Am J Orthod Dentofacial Orthop. 2007;131(1):57-66.

11. Sabah ME. Submentovertex cephalometric analysis of Class II subdivision malocclusions. J Oral Sci. 2002;44(3-4):125-7.

12. Palomo JM, Hunt DW Jr, Hans MG, Broadbent BH Jr. A longitudinal 3-dimensional size and shape comparison of untreated Class I and Class II subjects. Am J Orthod Dentofacial Orthop. 2005;127(5):584-91.

13. Lima KJRS, Janson G, Henriques JFC, Freitas MR, Pinzan A. Avaliação da concordância entre a classificação dos tipos de Classe II subdivisão em fotografias e em radiografias póstero-anteriores. Rev Dental Press Ortod Ortop Facial. 2005;10(3):46-55.

14. Edler R, Wertheim D, Greenhill D. Comparison of radiographic and photographic measurement of mandibular asymmetry. Am J Orthod Dentofacial Orthop. 2003;123(2):167-74.

15. Azevedo ARP. Correlação entre assimetria clínica e assimetria radiográfica na Classe II, Subdivisão [dissertação]. Bauru (SP): Universidade de São Paulo; 2003.

16. Lew KKK, Tay DKL. Submentovertex cephalometric norms in male Chinese subjects. Am J Orthod Dentofacial Orthop 1993;103(3):247-52.

17. Arnold TG, Anderson GC, Liijemark WF. Cephalometric norms for craniofacial asymmetry using submental-vertical radiographs. Am J Orthod Dentofacial Orthop. 1994;106(3):250-6.

18. Yoon Y-J, Kim K-S, Hwang M-S, Kim H-J, Choi E-H, Kim K-W. Effect of head rotation on lateral cephalometric radiographs. Angle Orthod 2001;71(5):396-403.

19. Kjellberg H, Ekestubbe A, Kiliaridis S, Thilander B. Condylar height on panoramic radiographs: a methodologic study with a clinical application. Acta Odontol Scand. 1994;52(1):43-50.

20. Habets LLMH, Bezuur JN, Naeiji M, Hansson TL. The orthopantomogram and aid in diagnosis of temporomandibular joint problems. II. The vertical symmetry. J Oral Rehabil. 1988;15(5):465-71.

21. Sezgin OS, Celenk P, Arici S. Mandibular asymmetry in different occlusion patterns: a radiological evaluation. Angle Orthod. 2007;77(5):803-7.

22. Ferrario VF, Sforza C, De Franco DJ. Mandibular shape and skeletal divergency. Eur J Orthod. 1999;21:145-53.

6

Therapeutic approach to Class II, Division 1 malocclusion with maxillary functional orthopedics

Aristeu Corrêa de Bittencourt Neto[1], Armando Yukio Saga[2], Ariel Adriano Reyes Pacheco[3], Orlando Tanaka[4]

Introduction: Interceptive treatment of Class II, Division 1 malocclusion is a challenge orthodontists commonly face due to the different growth patterns they come across and the different treatment strategies they have available. **Objective:** To report five cases of interceptive orthodontics performed with the aid of Klammt's elastic open activator (KEOA) to treat Class II, Division 1 malocclusion. **Methods:** Treatment comprehends one or two phases; and the use of functional orthopedic appliances, whenever properly recommended, is able to minimize dentoskeletal discrepancies with consequent improvement in facial esthetics during the first stage of mixed dentition. The triad of diagnosis, correct appliance manufacture and patient's compliance is imperative to allow KEOA to contribute to Class II malocclusion treatment. **Results:** Cases reported herein showed significant improvement in skeletal, dental and profile aspects, as evinced by cephalometric analysis and clinical photographs taken before, during and after interceptive orthodontics.

Keywords: Interceptive orthodontics. Class II. Klammt. Activator.

[1] MSc in Dentistry, Orthodontics, Uningá, Maringá, Paraná, Brazil.
[2] Professor at the Specialization course in Orthodontics, Pontifícia Universidade Católica do Paraná (PUCPR) and ABO-PR, Curitiba, Paraná, Brazil.
[3] PhD resident in Dentistry, Orthodontics, Pontifícia Universidade Católica do Paraná (PUCPR), Curitiba, Paraná, Brazil.
[4] Full professor of Dentistry, Orthodontics, Pontifícia Universidade Católica do Paraná (PUCPR), School of Health and Biosicences, Curitiba, Paraná, Brazil..

Orlando Tanaka
Rua Imaculada Conceição, 1155, Bairro Prado Velho
CEP: 80.215-901 – Curitiba, PR - Brazil
E-mail: tanakaom@gmail.com

» The authors report no commercial, proprietary or financial interest in the products or companies described in this article.

INTRODUCTION

Class II malocclusion is often associated with one of the following: mandibular retrognathism, anterior displacement of the maxilla, increased vertical dimension of posterior maxilla, mandibular fossa in posterior position, maxillary constriction and a combination of factors. In general, maxilla and mandibular incisors are well-positioned, differently from maxillary incisors which tend to be protrusive.[1-4] In Class II skeletal malocclusion, mandibular retrognathism seems to be the major contributing factor.[3]

Kingsley (1879) was the first to use forward positioning of the mandible in orthodontic treatment. The removable appliance developed by the author comprises a continuous labial wire, a bite plane extending posteriorly and molar clasps, and is considered the prototype of functional orthopedic appliances. As he described it, the objective was not to protrude mandibular teeth, but to change or jump the bite in case of an excessively retrusive mandible.[5]

Functional orthopedic appliances have been widely used in Europe since the 1930s,[6,7] particularly focusing on changing the muscle conditions that affect mandibular position and function. These appliances, whether fixed or removable, are used to correct Class II malocclusion while improving shape and function of the maxilla and mandible, stimulating natural growth by transduction of forces from muscles to basal bones and dentoalveolar process, affecting the neuromuscular complex, and treating mandibular deficiency.[6,8-11] Since forward mandibular growth is often limited by a narrow maxillary arch, functional orthopedics considers correcting sagittal discrepancy by maxillary expansion which allows the mandible to be placed forward.[12,13]

In mixed dentition, children or preadolescents might develop esthetically unfavorable malocclusion and, for this reason, be exposed intentionally and repeatedly to acts of physical or psychological violence by one person or a group of people (bullying). This might cause victims to feel pain, anxiety and low self-esteem, which significantly affects their psychosocial development.[14] The use of functional orthopedic appliances, whenever properly recommended, is able to minimize dentoskeletal discrepancies with consequent improvement in patient's facial esthetics.

Class II, Division 1 malocclusion treatment comprehends one or two phases. In 2-phased treatment, the first phase is carried out in mixed dentition with potential application of maxillary functional orthopedics (MFO), followed by a corrective phase in the early permanent dentition.[15]

This special article aims at reporting five cases of interceptive orthodontics performed with the aid of Klammt's elastic open activator (KEOA) during the first phase of treatment. Clinical outcomes minimized dental and skeletal discrepancies and proved a feasible alternative that contributes to orthodontically treat Class II skeletal malocclusion and Angle Class II, Division 1 malocclusion.

RECOMMENDATION AND ADVANTAGES

MFO success relies on compliant patients not referred for treatment with tooth extraction, who are short-faced (brachycephalic), with increased posterior facial height, mild to moderate overjet, excess overbite, active facial growth and counterclockwise rotation of the mandible.[6,8,10,16] The advantages provided by the activator include: (1) potential for treatment in primary dentition, early or late mixed dentition; (2) appointments spread out to two months or more; (3) tissues are not easily injured; (4) the appliance is used at night which renders it esthetically acceptable and favors hygiene control; and (5) it contributes to eliminate mouth breathing and tongue thrusting habits.[5]

SIDE EFFECTS AND DISADVANTAGES

Side effects commonly found at treatment completion include posterior open bite,[17] increased anterior facial height, protrusion of mandibular incisors and proclined maxillary incisors.[1,18-21] The disadvantages include: (1) treatment success relies on patient's compliance; (2) activators are of little value in cases of marked crowding; (3) the appliance does not provoke response from older patients; (4) forces exerted on teeth cannot be controlled precisely as in fixed appliances;[5] and (5) there is a risk of patients accidently swallowing the appliance.[22]

KLAMMT APPLIANCE

The appliance developed by Klammt (1969) derived from Andresen and Häupl's appliance, and was termed "open activator" of three different types: the first had an expansion screw with palatal support, used when there was a need for maxillary expansion greater than 3 mm; the second had a one-piece lower appliance combined with a transpalatal arch, used when there was no need for significant expansion; and the third, termed elastic open activator, provided plenty of space for the tongue and could also be used during the day without bringing discomfort to patient's cheeks, lips and tongue. As such, the appliance remains in function without causing any tension and while following all movements performed by the mandible.[23]

CONSTRUCTION BITE

Appliance manufacture requires a construction bite or working casts mounted in semi-adjustable articulators. A U-shaped construction bite wax is prepared to be inserted between dental arches and acquire the shape of the arch. It should be of adequate width and between 2-3 mm thick. The wax is slightly softened and placed onto the mandibular arch; dentally-guided forward (sagittal) mandibular movement is then performed so as to achieve maximal intercuspation (case 3). During construction bite, forward movement of the mandible does not exceed 10 mm at each stage. Advancement greater than 10 mm requires a second stage, during which a new appliance is manufactured.[24] Gradual advancement of the mandible demands adaptation to the appliance within a shorter period of time, which favors patient's comfort. Maximum advancement performed at one single stage provides patients with greater discomfort after appliance placement; however, with no further biological effects. Nevertheless, when variables of overjet, overbite and molar and canine relationship are assessed, both types of advancement result in similar improvement.[17]

APPLIANCE USE PROTOCOL

At the time of appliance placement, patient and parents are informed about the time of appliance use and appliance hygiene, as well as swallowing and speech issues. The appliance should be worn for as long as possible, except during meals and sports practice involving physical contact. At the following appointments, it is possible to assess whether the appliance is being correctly used or not by monitoring patient's speech, swallowing movements and the marks left on the mucosa by buccal archwires, which is an obvious sign of use. Patient's compliance is key to treatment success.

Activation control might be performed every 15 days or on a monthly basis. Adjustments might be rendered necessary so as to provide patient with comfort. Once KEOA

treatment objectives are achieved, patients are advised to wear the appliance as a retainer (at night) during a period equivalent to half the active period.

KEOA placement comprehended an initial adaptation period that ranged from two to four weeks. Soon after that, patients were advised to wear the appliance full-time, except during meals and sports practice. Appointments were scheduled every 15 days, with monthly activations of coffin springs (approximately 0.25 mm activation with the aid of a bird beak plier) during treatment.

TREATMENT OBJECTIVES

Correcting skeletal and dental discrepancies resulting from Class II, Division 1 malocclusion during growth acceleration, and reducing the need for biomechanics during the corrective phase of orthodontic treatment. All patients reported herein were growing patients; however, at different phases.

DIAGNOSIS, TREATMENT PROGRESS AND INTERCEPTIVE ORTHODONTICS OUTCOMES
Case report 1

Female 10.9-year-old patient in the second transitional period of mixed dentition. She presented with increased lower facial height and a convex profile, Class II skeletal malocclusion (ANB = 8°) and Class II, Division 1 malocclusion, 6.5-mm overjet and moderate overbite. Cephalometric measurements revealed the patient had a well-positioned maxilla (SNA = 81°), mandibular retrognathism relative to the cranial base (SNB = 73°) and predominantly vertical facial growth pattern (SN.GoGn = 42°). Maxillary incisors were slightly proclined (1-NA = 21°) and retrusive (1-NA = 3°), whereas mandibular incisors were labially proclined (1-NB = 34°) and protrusive (1-NB = 8°). In addition, she presented with lip incompetence and predominantly mouth breathing.

Skeletal changes resulting from KEOA treatment included mild protrusion of the mandible expressed in a SNB value of 74°, with consequent reduction in the relationship between the maxilla and mandible (ANB = 7°) during treatment. As for facial growth pattern (SN-GoGn = 42° and FMA = 32°), there was a slight increase in the vertical plane of both vectors (SN-GoGn = 44° and FMA = 34°). Maxillary incisors ended up proclined and retrusive, whereas mandibular incisors were slightly proclined and retrusive. Patient's profile was less convex (Z-angle = 57°).

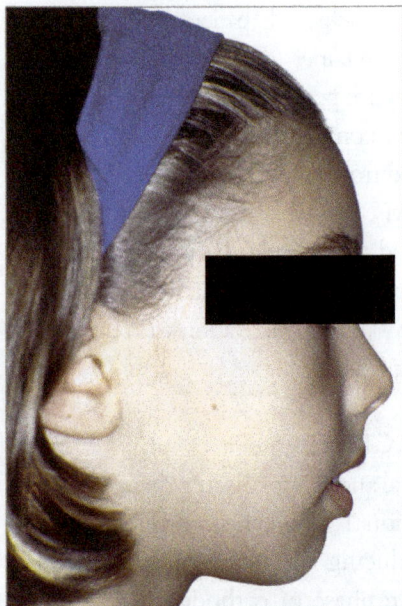
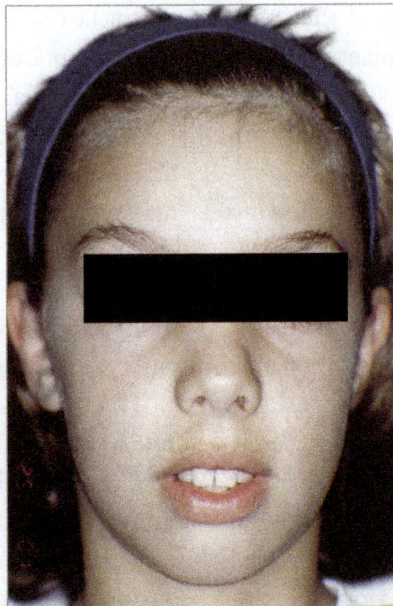

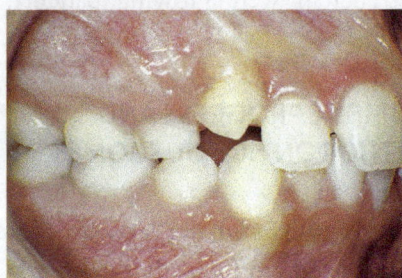
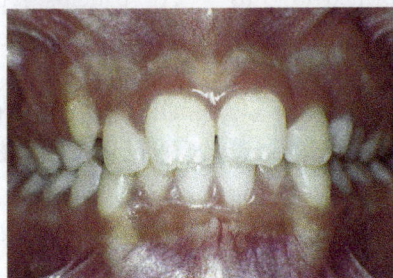
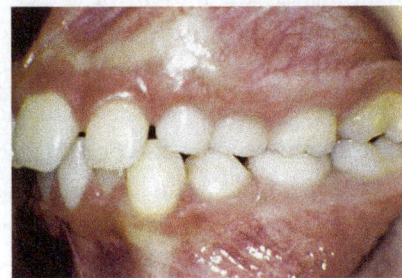

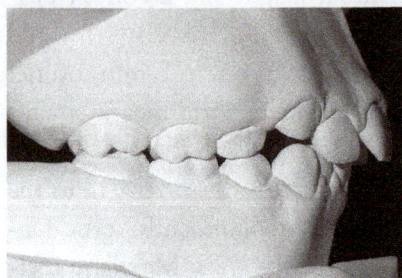
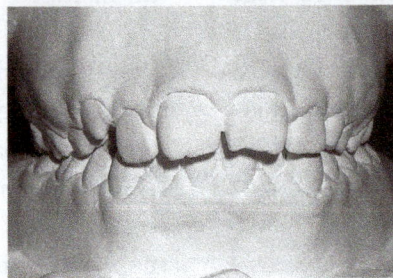
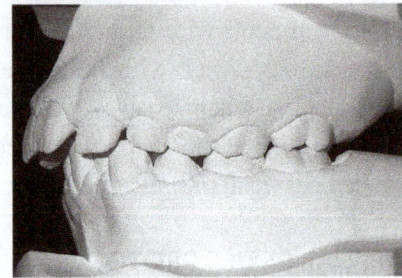

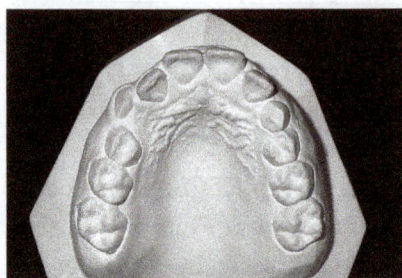
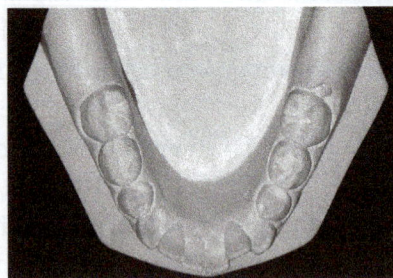
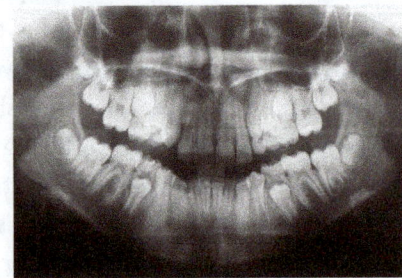

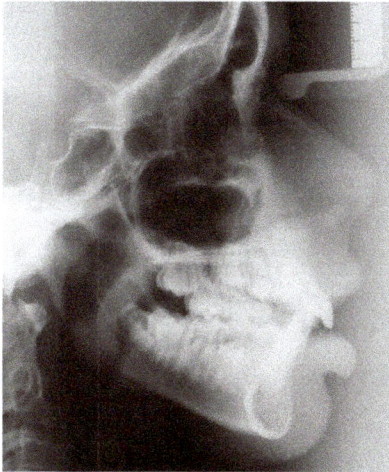

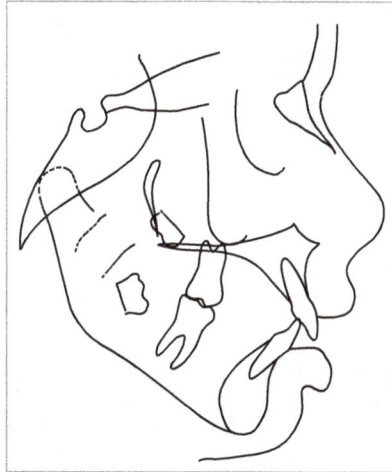

	Nor.	Author	10.9 y
SNA	82	Steiner	81
SNB	80	Steiner	73
ANB	2	Steiner	8
Convex.	0	Downs	18
Y-axis	59	Downs	62
Facial	87	Downs	83
SN-GoGn	32	Steiner	42
FMA	25	Tweed	32
IMPA	90	Tweed	96
1.NA	22	Steiner	21
1-NA	4	Steiner	3
$\overline{1}$.NB	25	Steiner	34
$\overline{1}$-NB	4	Steiner	8
Pog-NB		Holdaway	-1
$1-\overline{1}$	130	Downs	118
$\overline{1}$-APo	1	Ricketts	3
UL-S	0	Steiner	2
LL-S	0	Steiner	5
Z-angle	75	Merrifield	52

Case 1. Initial examination: 10.9-year-old patient, Class II skeletal malocclusion and Class II, Division 1 malocclusion; 5-mm overjet and moderate overbite.

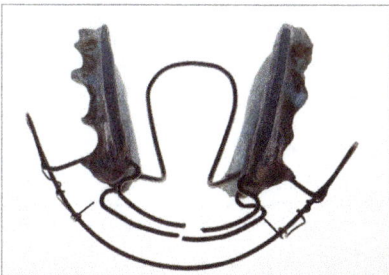

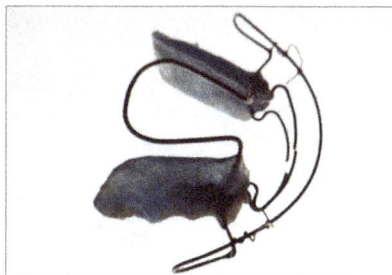

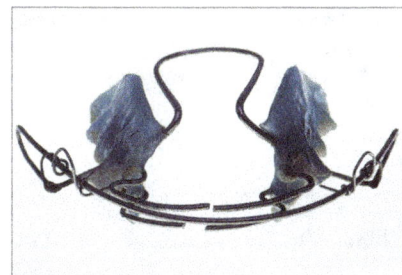

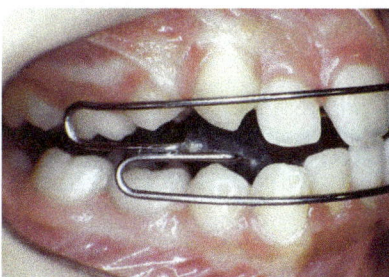

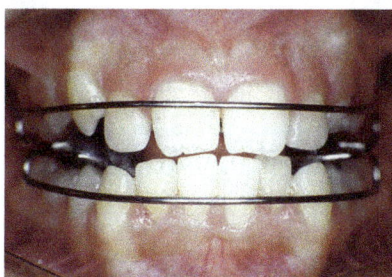

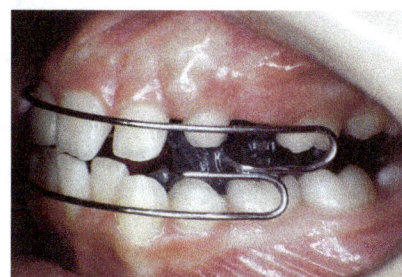

Case 1. Treatment progress: Klammt's elastic open activator (KEOA).

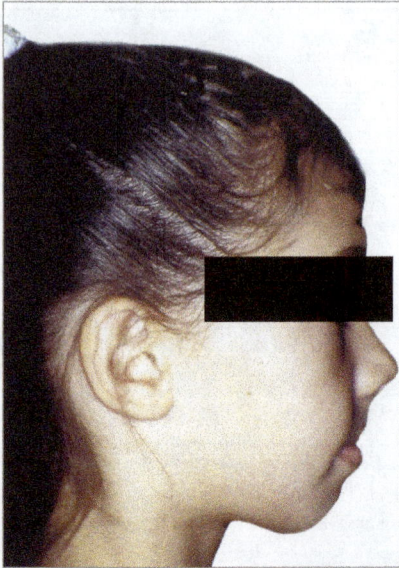
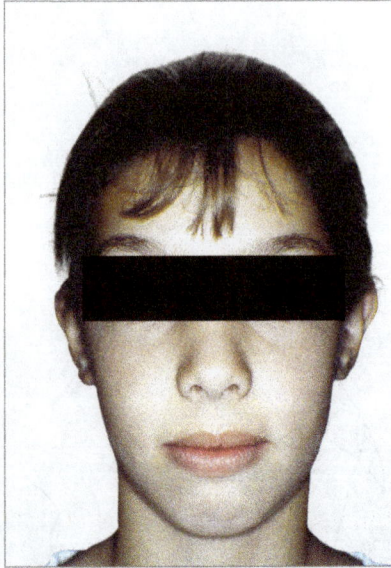

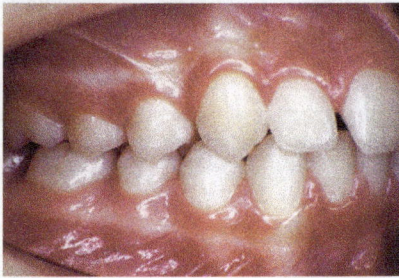
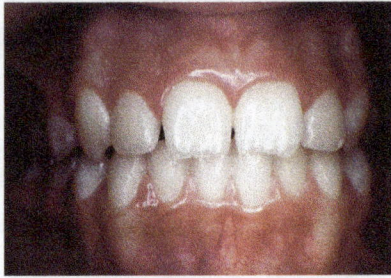
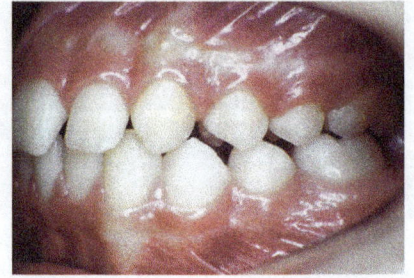

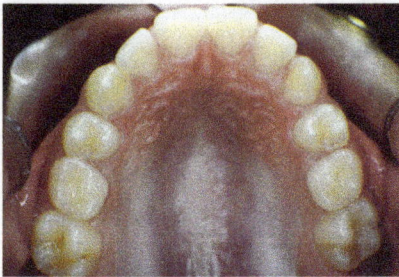
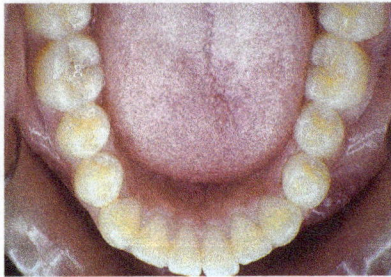

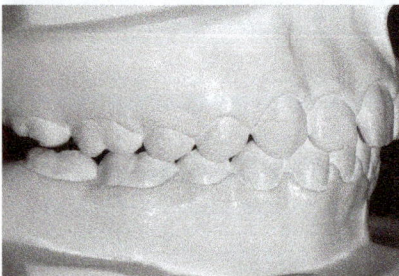
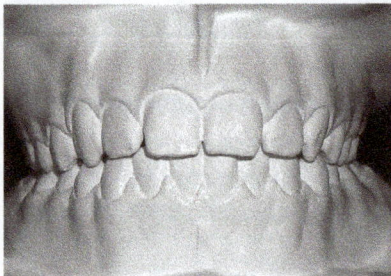
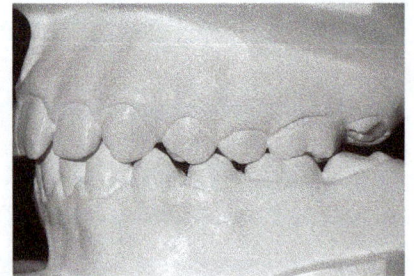

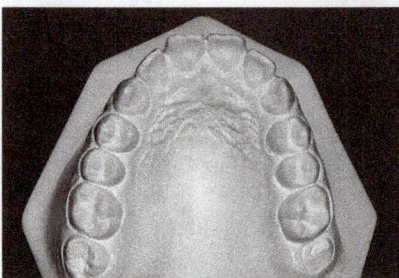
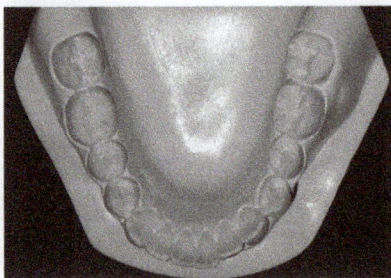
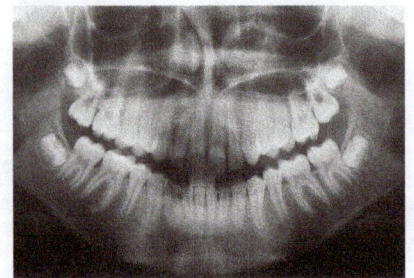

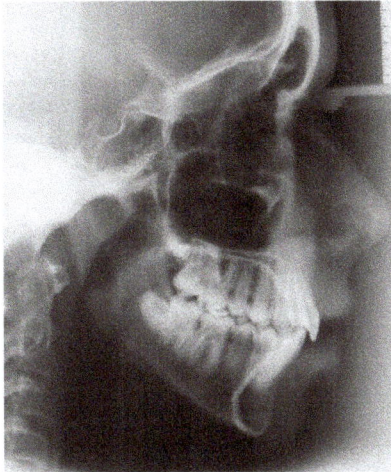

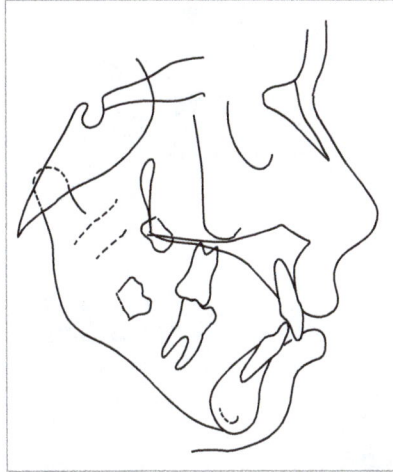

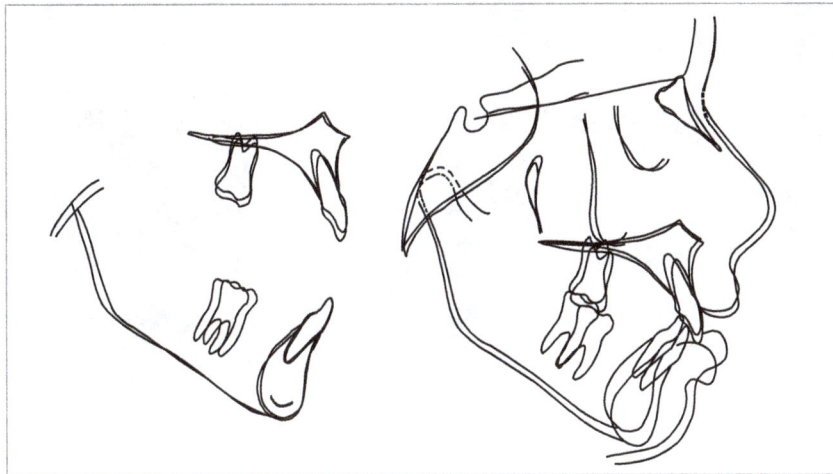

	Nor.	Author	12.2 y
SNA	82	Steiner	81
SNB	80	Steiner	74
ANB	2	Steiner	7
Convex.	0	Downs	17
Y-axis	59	Downs	64
Facial	87	Downs	83
SN-GoGn	32	Steiner	44
FMA	25	Tweed	34
IMPA	90	Tweed	95
1.NA	22	Steiner	15
1-NA	4	Steiner	2
$\overline{1}$.NB	25	Steiner	33
$\overline{1}$-NB	4	Steiner	7
Pog-NB		Holdaway	-2
$1-\overline{1}$	130	Downs	129
$\overline{1}$-A-Po	1	Ricketts	3
UL-S	0	Steiner	1
LL- S	0	Steiner	4
Z-angle	75	Merrifield	57

Case 1. 12.2-year-old patient, Class I relationship, adequate overbite and overjet.

Case report 2

Female 9.7-year-old patient in transitional mixed dentition. She presented with short lower facial height, convex profile, mandibular retrognathism, balanced vertical and horizontal growth patterns (SN.GoGn = 30°; FMA = 23°; Y-axis= 59°), Class II skeletal malocclusion (ANB = 7°) and Class II, Division 1 malocclusion with 9.0-mm overjet and moderate overbite. Maxillary and mandibular incisors were slightly proclined. There was mandibular midline deviation to the right and maxillary constriction in the region of primary molars; however, without posterior crossbite. Palatal inclination of maxillary right lateral incisor. In addition, she presented with lip incompetence and predominantly mouth breathing.

As for skeletal changes, the maxilla remained in unchanged position (SNA = 85°), since SNA angle remained stable. However, there was an increase in SNB angle (SNB = 80°), which revealed that the mandible was positioned forward, with consequent reduction in the relationship between the maxilla and mandible (ANB = 5°) during treatment. As for facial growth pattern (SN-GoGn = 26° and FMA = 20°), there was a slight decrease in the vertical plane.

Maxillary incisors were proclined and retrusive (1-NA = 15 and 1-NA = 7 mm), whereas mandibular incisors were slightly buccaly proclined (1-NB = 26). There was significant improvement in patient's facial profile, as revealed by Z-angle values (Z = 74°).

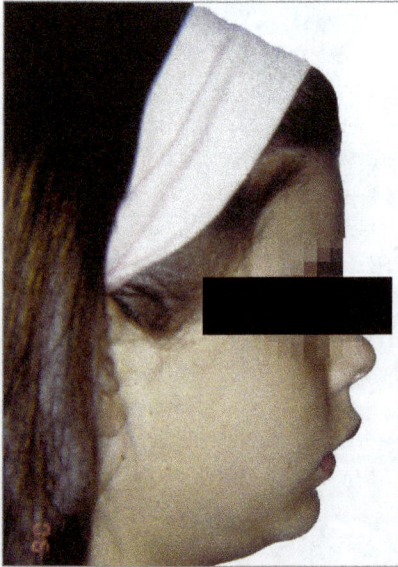
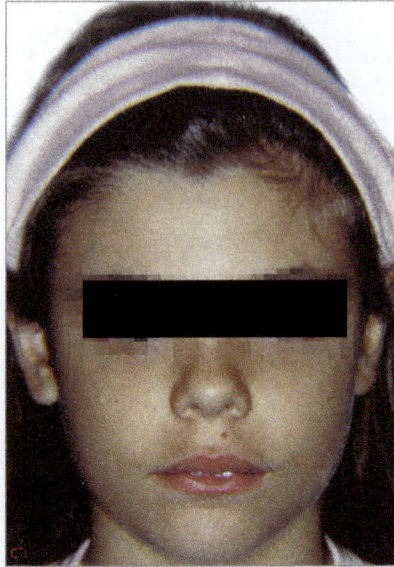

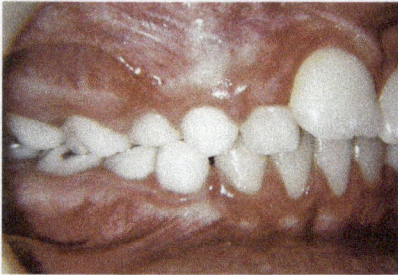
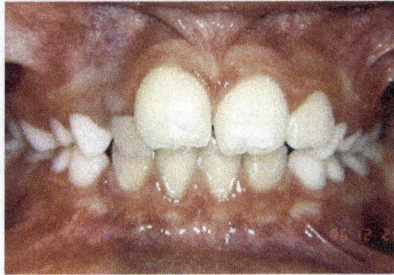
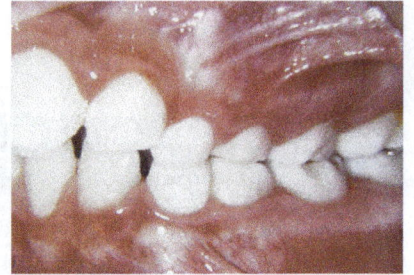

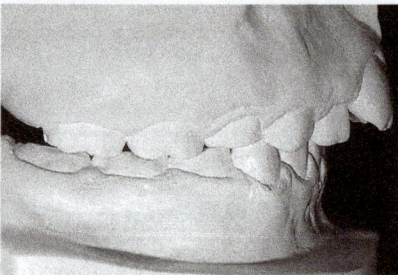
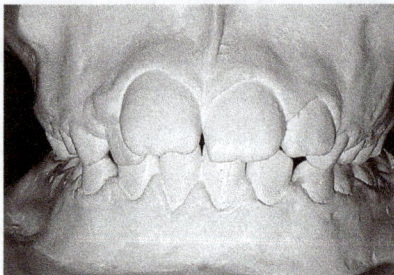
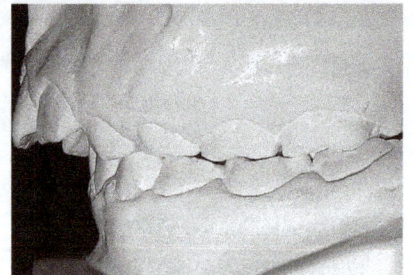

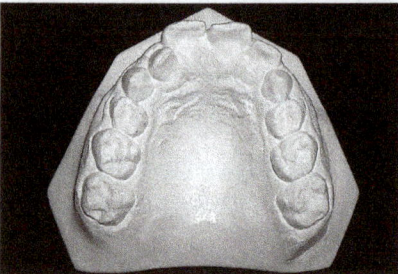
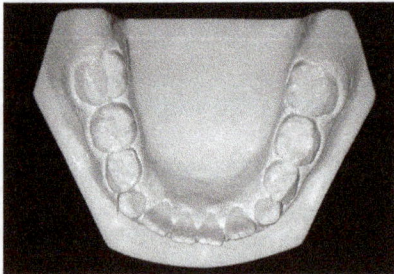
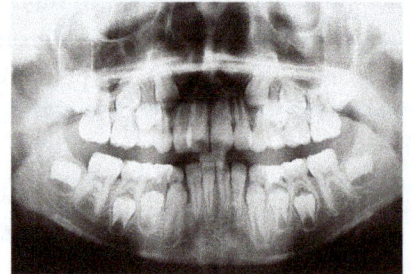

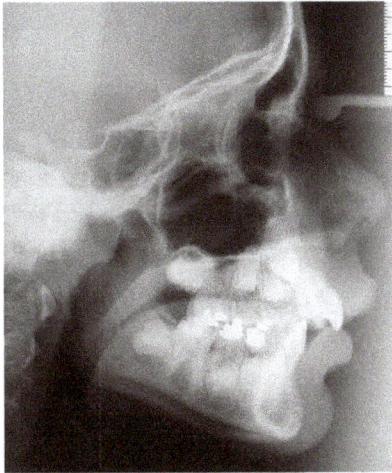

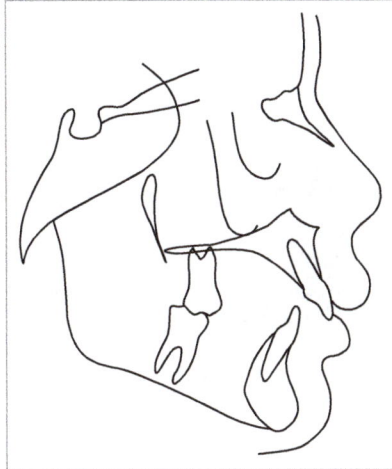

	Nor.	Author	9.7 y
SNA	82	Steiner	85
SNB	80	Steiner	78
ANB	2	Steiner	7
Convex.	0	Downs	12
Y-axis	59	Downs	59
Facial	87	Downs	87
SN-GoGn	32	Steiner	30
FMA	25	Tweed	23
IMPA	90	Tweed	94
1.NA	22	Steiner	22
1-NA	4	Steiner	4
$\overline{1}$.NB	25	Steiner	22
$\overline{1}$-NB	4	Steiner	3
Pog-NB		Holdaway	3
$1 - \overline{1}$	130	Downs	129
$\overline{1}$-APo	1	Ricketts	-1
UL-S	0	Steiner	5
LL-S	0	Steiner	2
Z-angle	75	Merrifield	69

Case 2. Initial examination: 9.7-year-old patient, Class II skeletal malocclusion and Class II, Division 1 malocclusion, 8-mm overjet and moderate overbite.

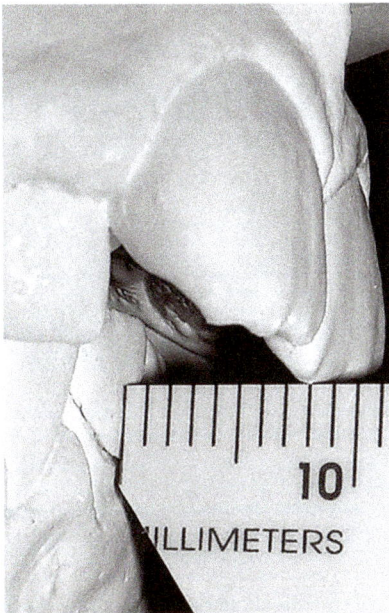

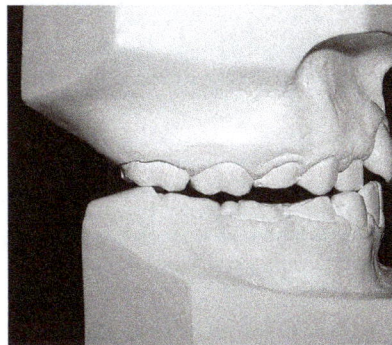

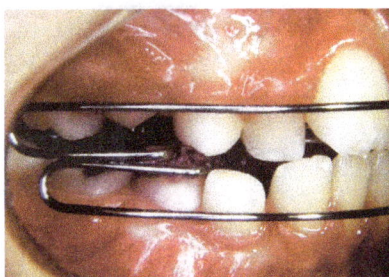

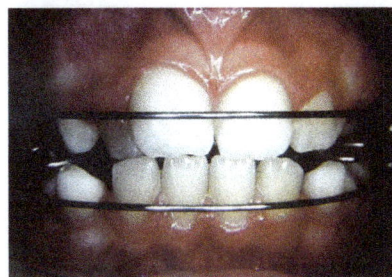

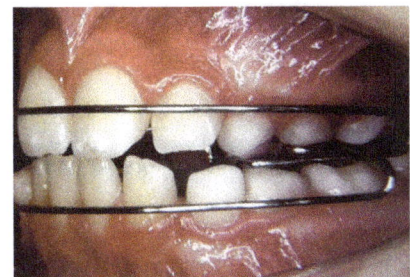

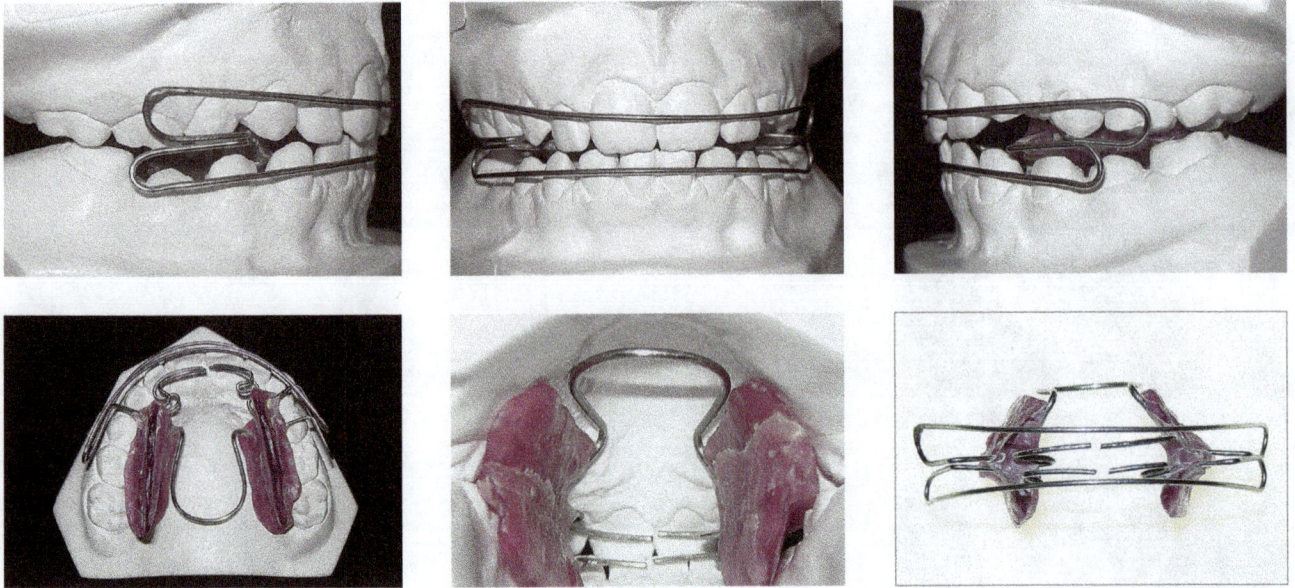

Case 2. Treatment progress: constructive bite, Klammt's elastic open activator (KEOA).

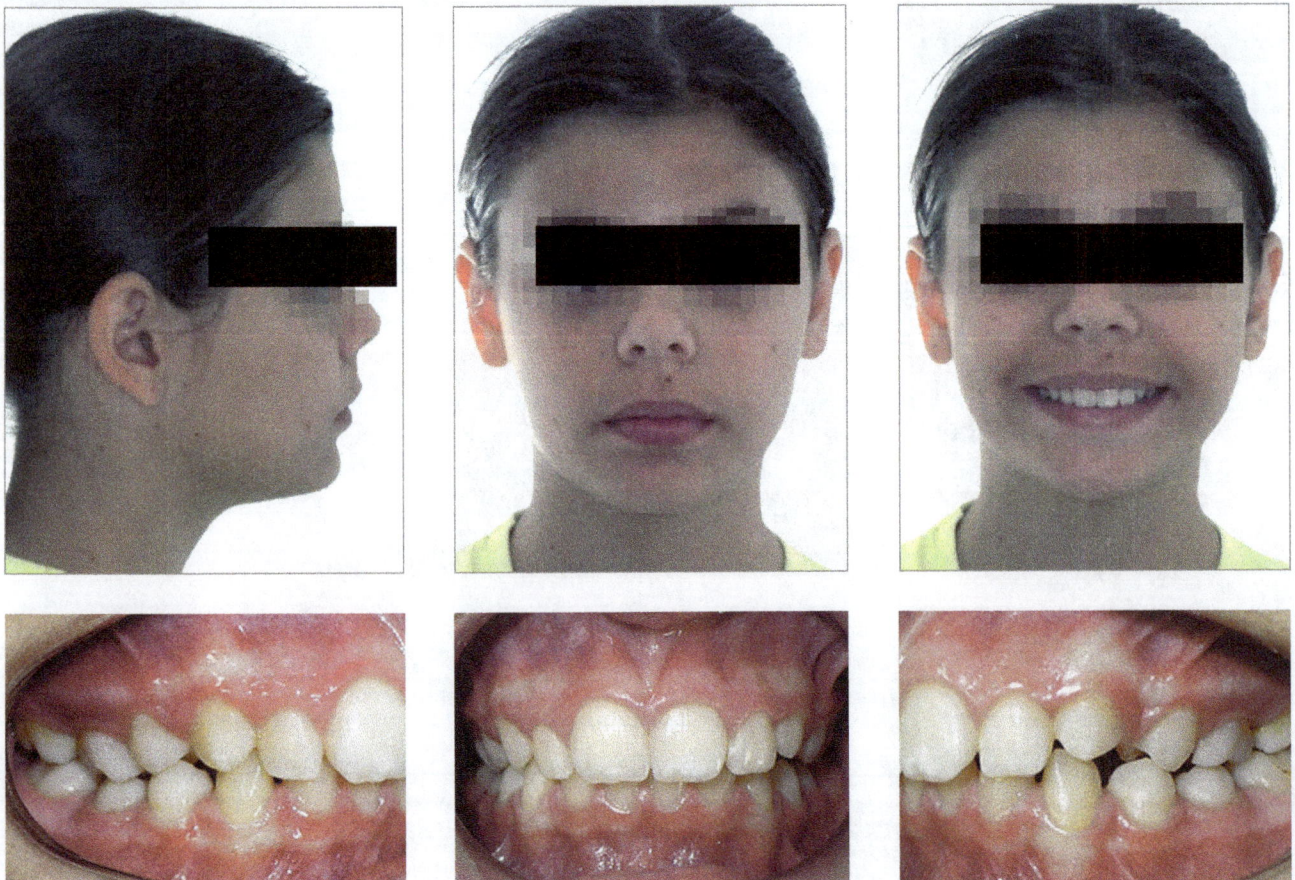

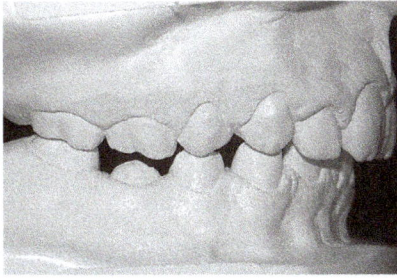

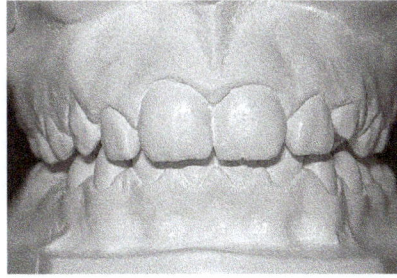

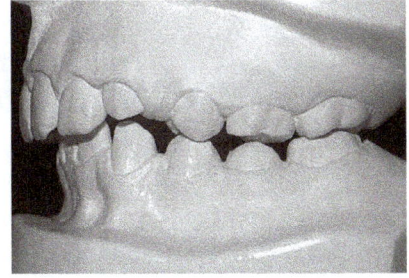

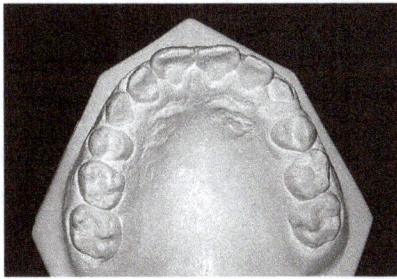

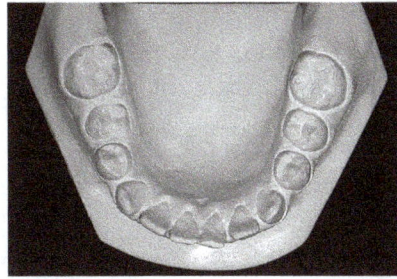

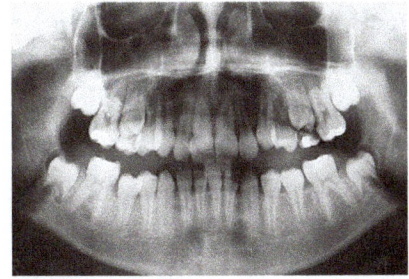

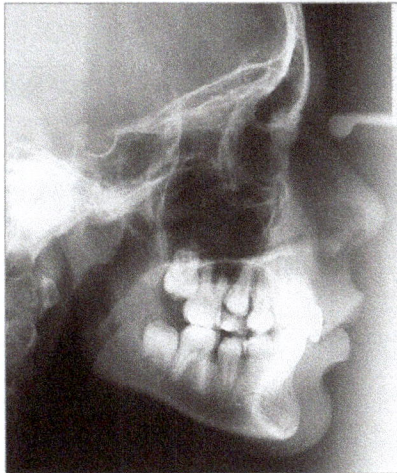

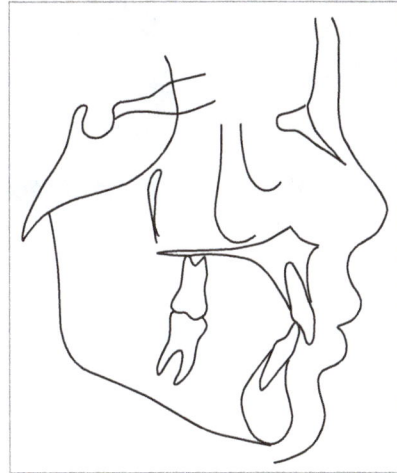

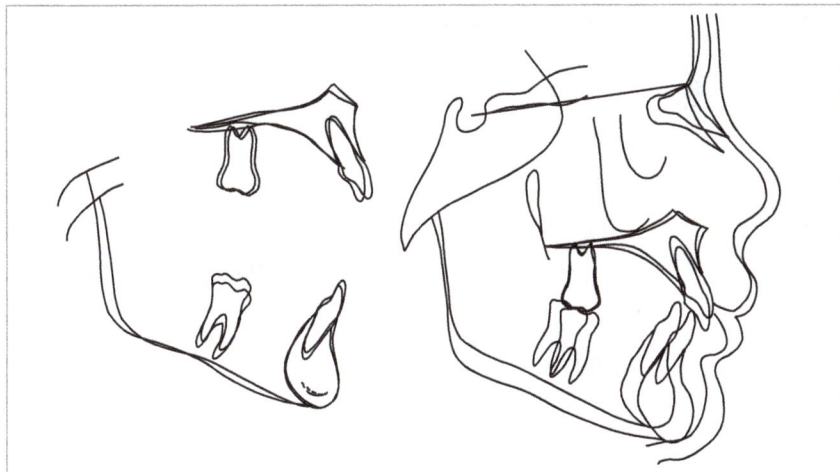

	Nor.	Author	12.6 y
SNA	82	Steiner	85
SNB	80	Steiner	80
ANB	2	Steiner	5
Convex.	0	Downs	8
Y-axis	59	Downs	57
Facial	87	Downs	89
SN-GoGn	32	Steiner	26
FMA	25	Tweed	20
IMPA	90	Tweed	98
1.NA	22	Steiner	15
1-NA	4	Steiner	7
1̄.NB	25	Steiner	26
1̄-NB	4	Steiner	3
Pog-NB		Holdaway	2
1 – 1̄	130	Downs	135
1̄-APo	1	Ricketts	0
UL-S	0	Steiner	3
LL-S	0	Steiner	1
Z-angle	75	Merrifield	74

Case 2. Finished case: 12.6-year-old patient, Class I relationship, moderate overbite and overjet.

Case report 3

Male 8.7-year-old patient in the first transitional period of mixed dentition. He presented with increased lower facial height and convex profile (Z = 52°), mandibular retrognathism (SNB = 74°) and predominantly vertical growth pattern (Y-axis = 64°, SN-GoGn = 43°). Class II skeletal malocclusion (ANB = 6°), Class II, Division 1 malocclusion, 12-mm overjet and normal overbite. Maxillary (1-NA = 27°) and mandibular incisors (1-NB = 27°) were slightly protrusive. In addition, he presented with predominantly mouth breathing and maxillary constriction; however, without posterior crossbite. Torsiversion of maxillary and mandibular central incisors.

Skeletal changes resulting from KEOA treatment were practically nonexistent, as SNA slightly decreased, which revealed restriction of maxillary anterior displacement with a slight decrease in SNB. This case experienced more marked dental changes in the maxilla, with proclined, retrusive maxillary incisors and mandibular incisors remaining stable.

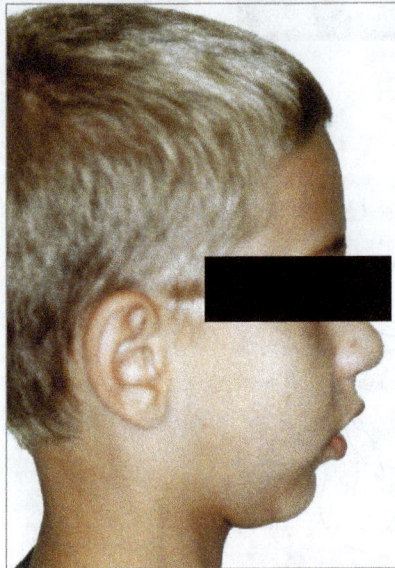

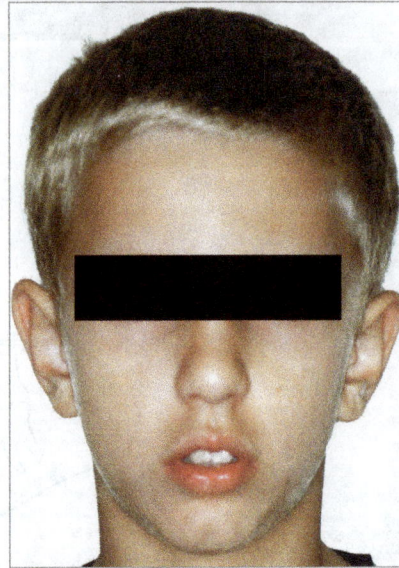

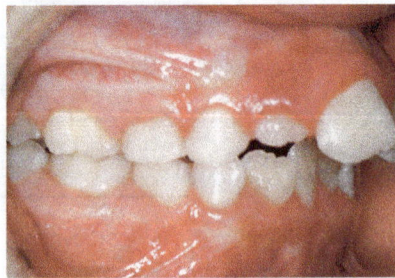

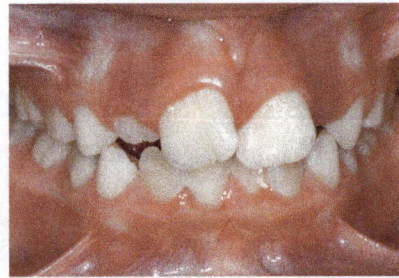

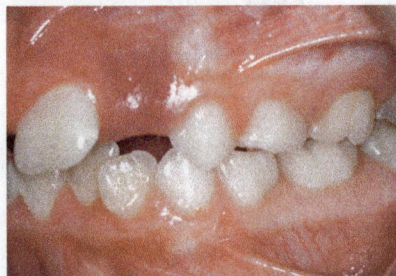

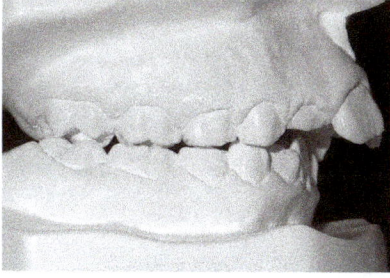

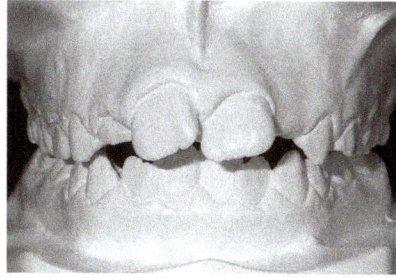

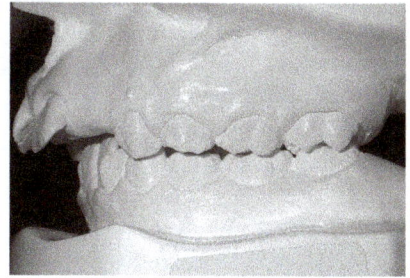

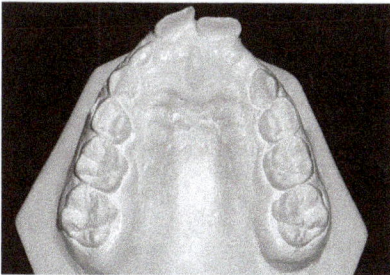

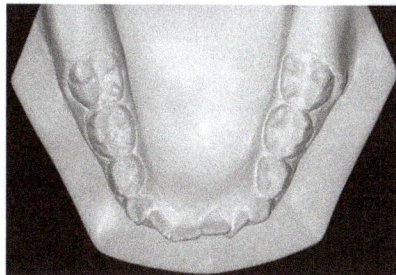

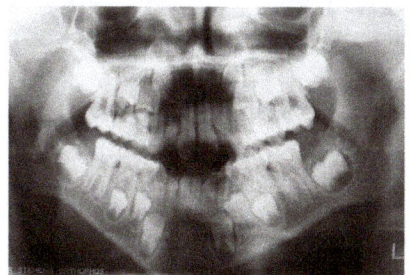

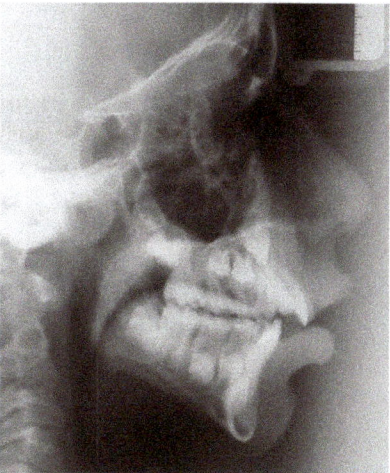

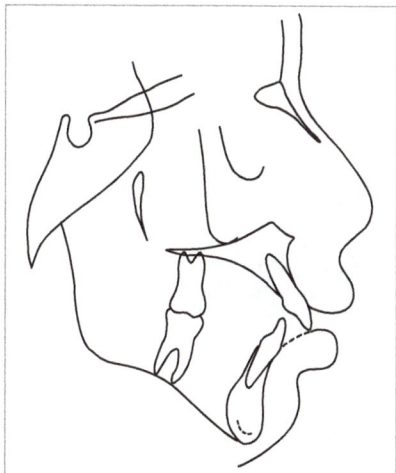

	Nor.	Author	8.7 y
SNA	82	Steiner	80
SNB	80	Steiner	74
ANB	2	Steiner	6
Convex.	0	Downs	7
Y-axis	59	Downs	64
Facial	87	Downs	83
SN-GoGn	32	Steiner	43
FMA	25	Tweed	34
IMPA	90	Tweed	89
1.NA	22	Steiner	27
1-NA	4	Steiner	7
$\overline{1}$.NB	25	Steiner	27
$\overline{1}$-NB	4	Steiner	6
Pog-NB		Holdaway	2
$\underline{1}$ – $\overline{1}$	130	Downs	119
$\overline{1}$-APo	1	Ricketts	4
UL-S	0	Steiner	5
LL-S	0	Steiner	6
Z-angle	75	Merrifield	52

Case 3. Initial examination: 8.7-year-old patient, 12-mm overjet and mild overbite.

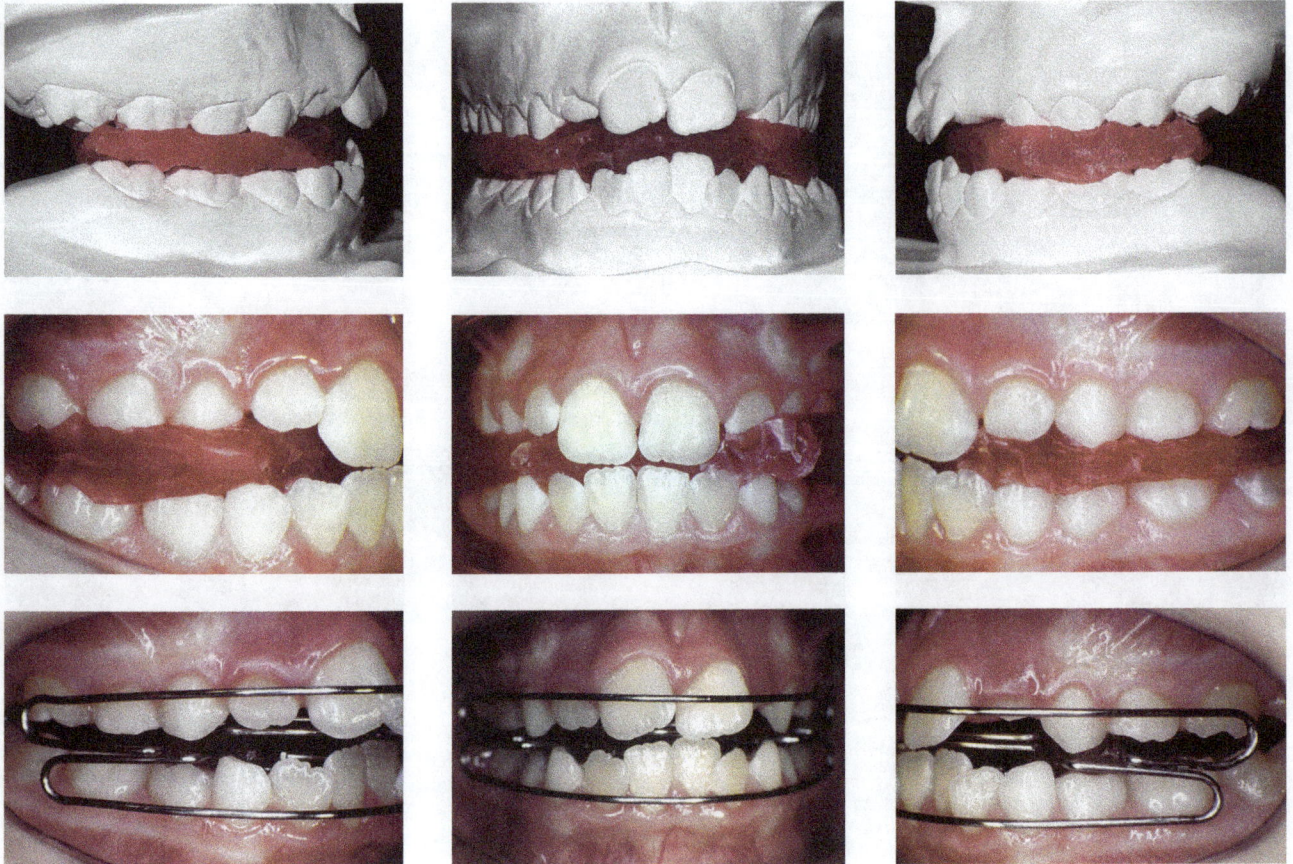

Case 3. Constructive bite and intraoral cast with erupted maxillary lateral incisors, for illustration purposes, only.

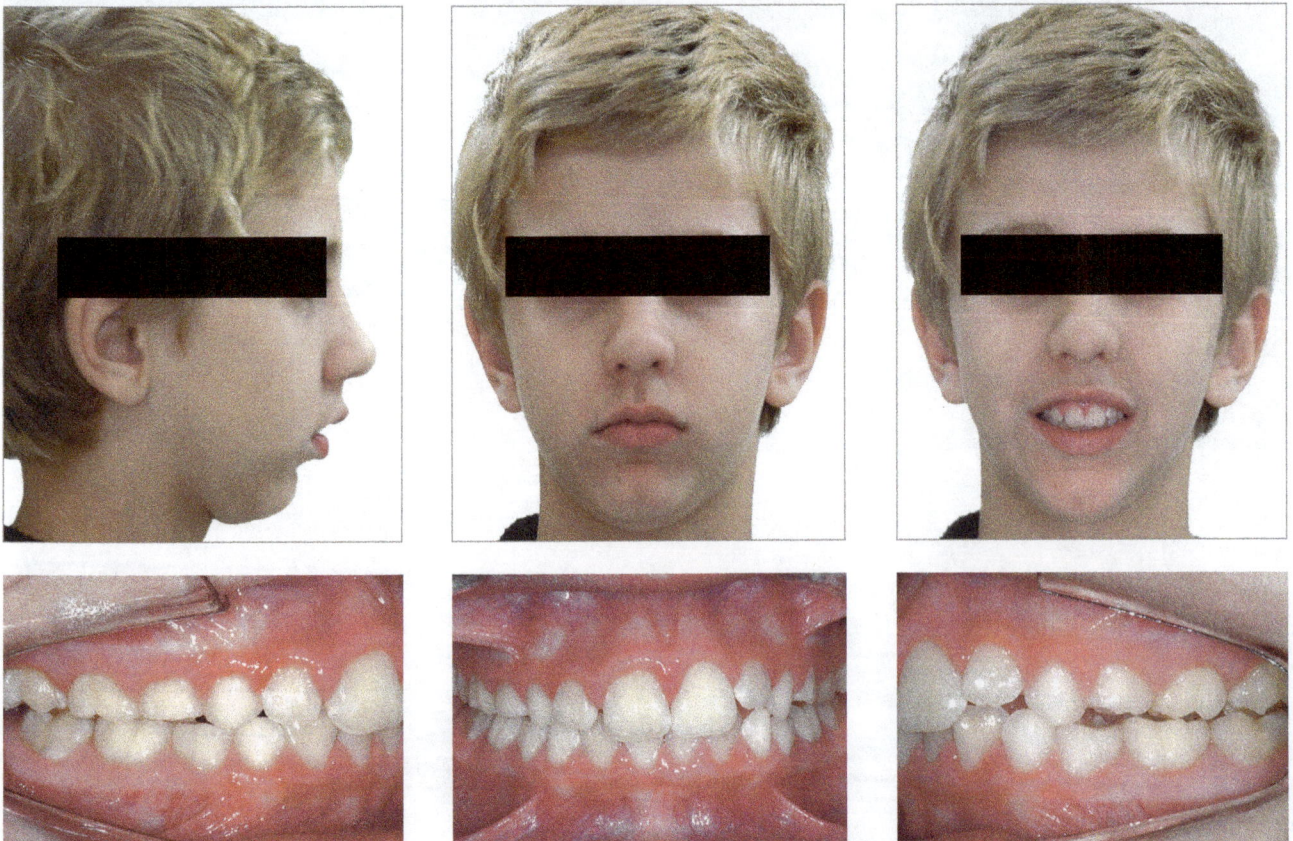

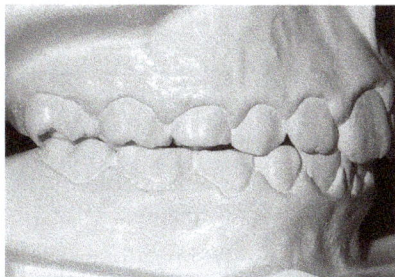

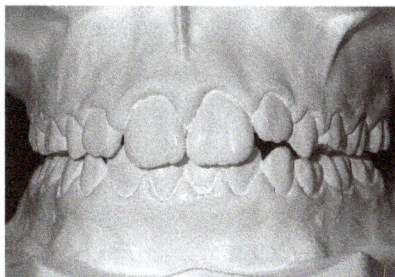

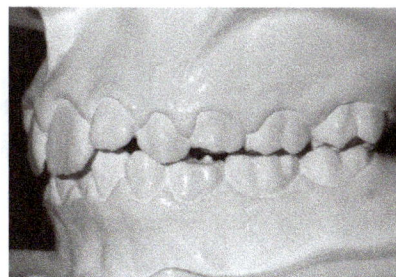

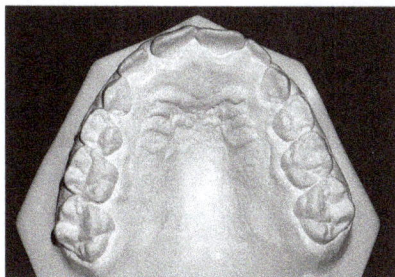

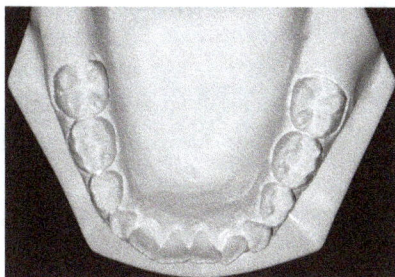

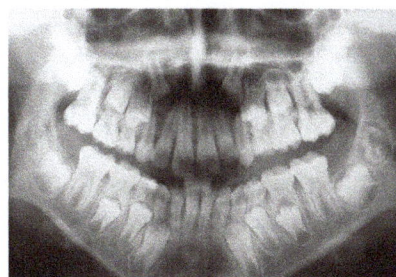

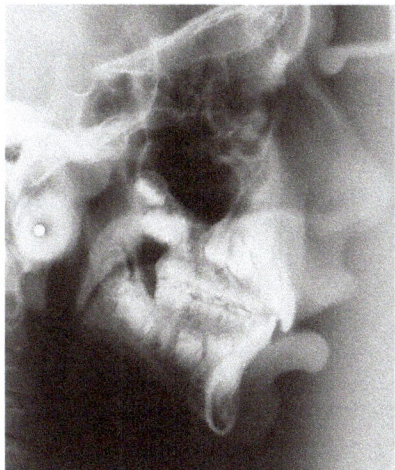

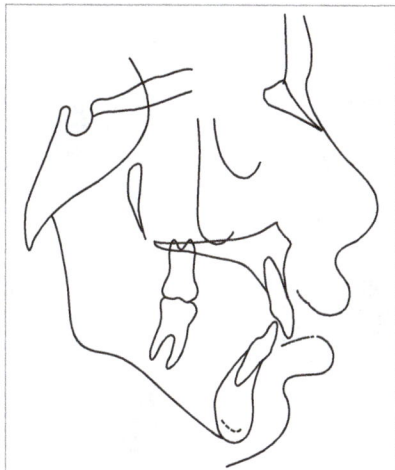

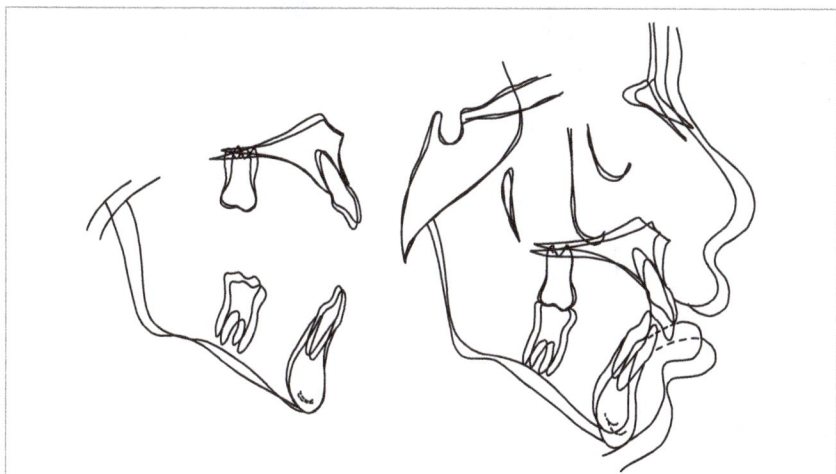

	Nor.	Author	9.11 y
SNA	82	Steiner	79
SNB	80	Steiner	73
ANB	2	Steiner	6
Convex	0	Downs	12
Y-axis	59	Downs	65
Facial	87	Downs	82
SN-GoGn	32	Steiner	42
FMA	25	Tweed	34
IMPA	90	Tweed	90
1.NA	22	Steiner	13
1-NA	4	Steiner	4
$\overline{1}$.NB	25	Steiner	27
$\overline{1}$-NB	4	Steiner	8
Pog-NB		Holdaway	7
$\underline{1}-\overline{1}$	130	Downs	133
$\overline{1}$-APo	1	Ricketts	4
UL-S	0	Steiner	4
LL-S	0	Steiner	6
Z-angle	75	Merrifield	49

Case 3. Finished case: Class I molar relationship, adequate overjet and moderate overbite.

Case report 4

Female 9.9-year-old patient in transitional mixed dentition. She presented with short lower facial height and tendency towards predominantly sagittal growth pattern (Y-axis = 57°, SN-Gn = 31°), lip incompetence and predominantly mouth breathing. Convex profile (Z = 67°). Class II skeletal malocclusion (ANB = 10°) and Class II, Division 1 malocclusion, 9-mm overjet and overbite with a tendency towards anterior open bite. Maxillary prognathism (SNB = 90°), relatively well-positioned maxillary incisors (1-NA = 24°) and mandibular incisors significantly protrusive (1-NB = 32°). Maxillary constriction in the region of primary molars; however, without posterior crossbite, in addition to diastema between maxillary incisors. Skeletal changes and SNA angle analysis of this case suggest no increase in maxillary protrusion and no partial restriction of anterior maxillary displacement. Meanwhile, SNB angle presented with an increase in mandibular protrusion, with consequent reduction in the relationship between the maxilla and mandible during the orthopedic phase of treatment. In terms of patient's horizontal growth pattern, all variables had values within normality.

Dental changes derived from treatment included marked lingual inclination and retrusion of maxillary incisors, and buccal inclination and protrusion of mandibular incisors. In addition, there was significant improvement in lower facial midlines.

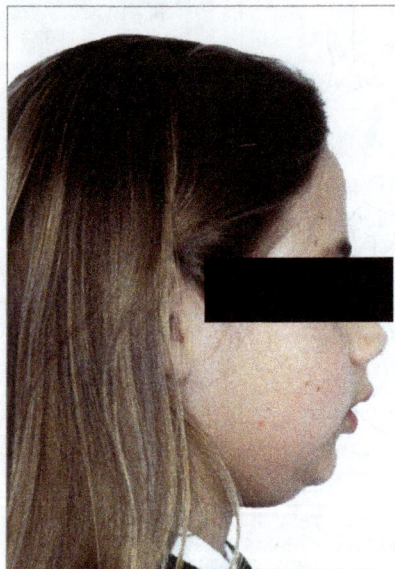

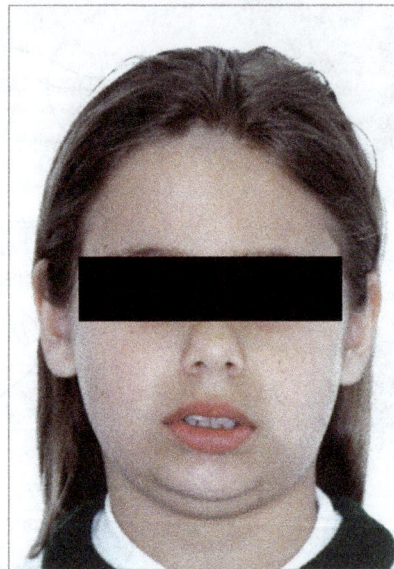

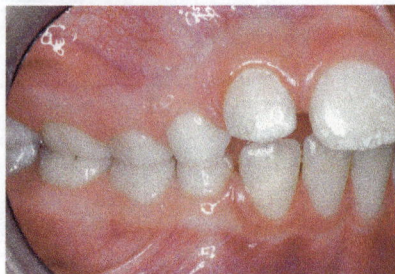

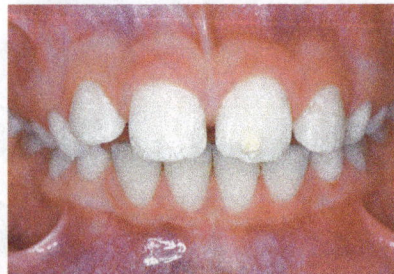

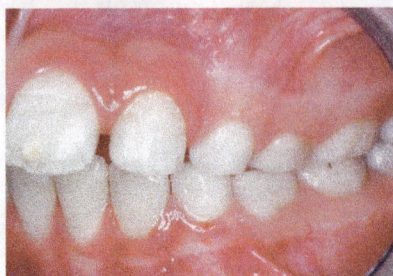

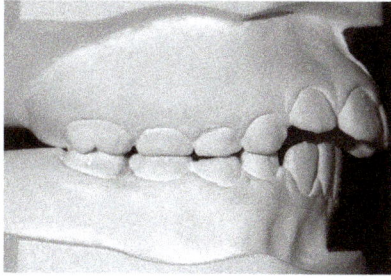

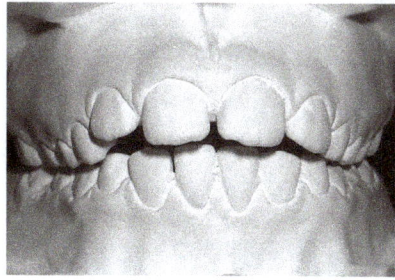

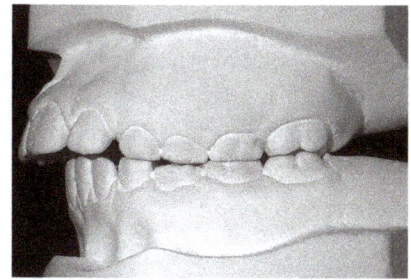

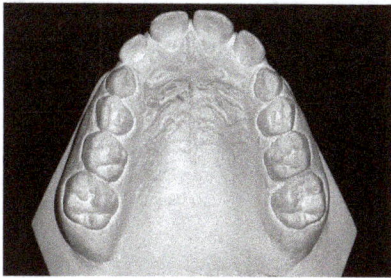

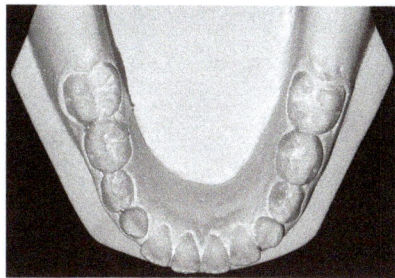

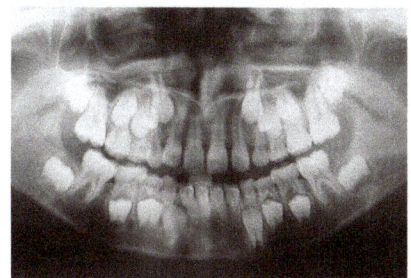

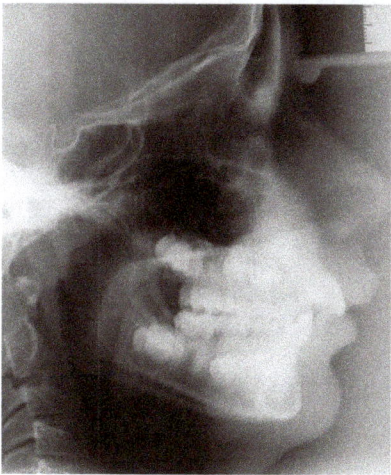

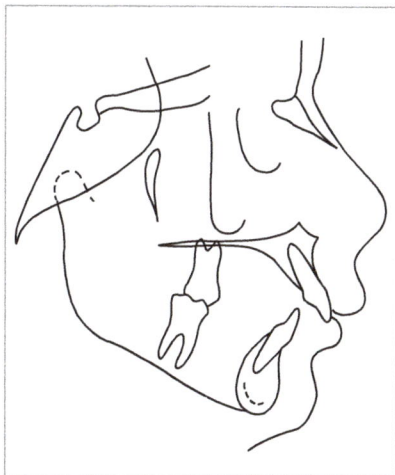

	Nor.	Author	8.9 y
SNA	82	Steiner	90
SNB	80	Steiner	80
ANB	2	Steiner	10
Convex.	0	Downs	20
Y-axis	59	Downs	57
Facial	87	Downs	87
SN-GoGn	32	Steiner	31
FMA	25	Tweed	23
Co-Gn		McNamara	101
Co-A		McNamara	86
IMPA	90	Tweed	100
1.NA	22	Steiner	24
1-NA	4	Steiner	5
$\overline{1}$.NB	25	Steiner	32
$\overline{1}$-NB	4	Steiner	6
Pog-NB		Holdaway	1
$1-\overline{1}$	130	Downs	117
$\overline{1}$-APo	1	Ricketts	0
UL-S	0	Steiner	3
LL-S	0	Steiner	1
Z-angle	75	Merrifield	67

Case 4. Initial examination: 8.9-year-old patient, Class II dental and skeletal malocclusion, 9-mm overjet and tendency towards anterior open bite.

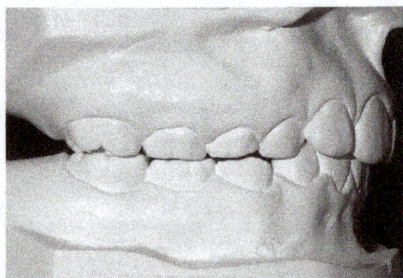

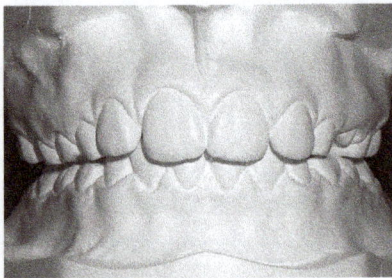

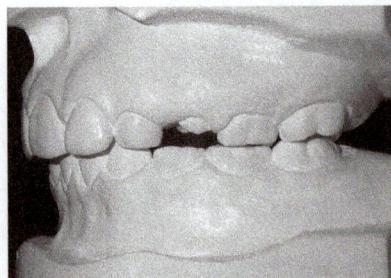

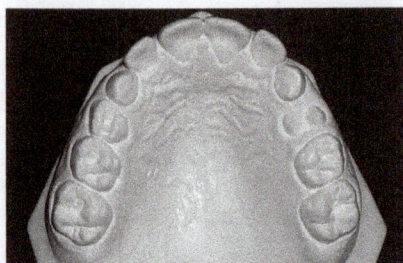

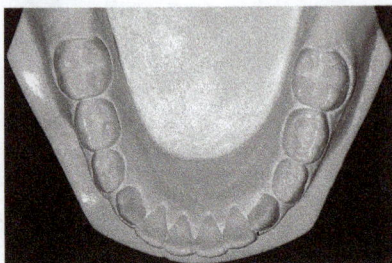

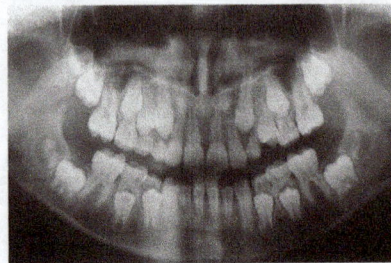

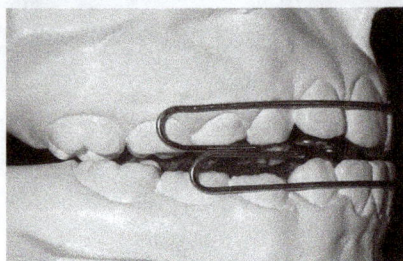

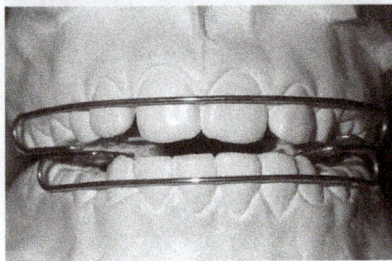

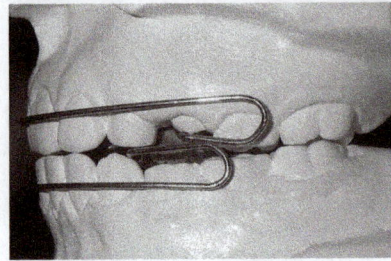

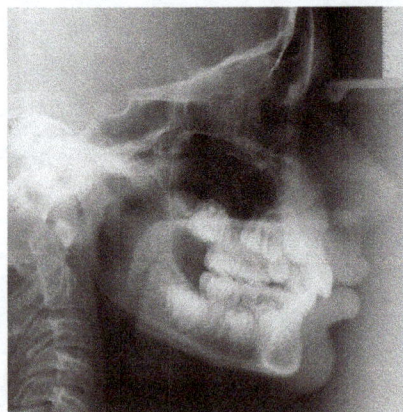

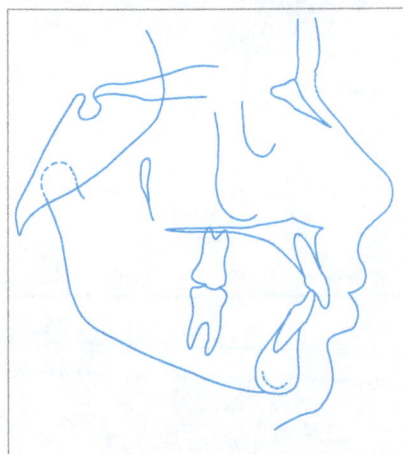

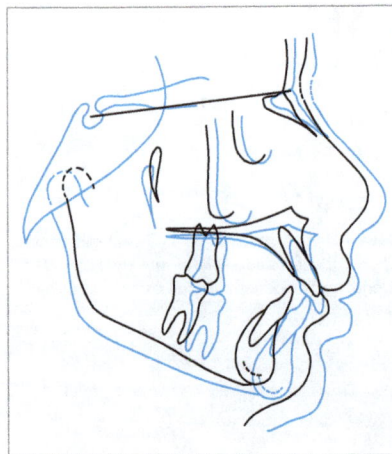

	Nor.	Author	10.7 y
SNA	82	Steiner	90
SNB	80	Steiner	83
ANB	2	Steiner	7
Convex.	0	Downs	14
Y-axis	59	Downs	56
Facial	87	Downs	89
SN-GoGn	32	Steiner	28
FMA	25	Tweed	21
Co-Gn		McNamara	122
Co-A		McNamara	96
IMPA	90	Tweed	102
1.NA	22	Steiner	14
1-NA	4	Steiner	3
$\overline{1}$.NB	25	Steiner	32
$\overline{1}$-NB	4	Steiner	6
Pog-NB		Holdaway	0
$1-\overline{1}$	130	Downs	126
$\overline{1}$-APo	1	Ricketts	3
UL-S	0	Steiner	1
LL-S	0	Steiner	2
Z-angle	75	Merrifield	67

Case 4. Treatment progress: 10.7-year-old patient, Klammt's elastic open activator placed on the study cast.

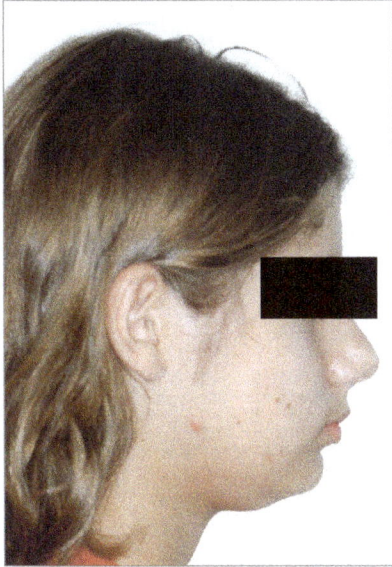
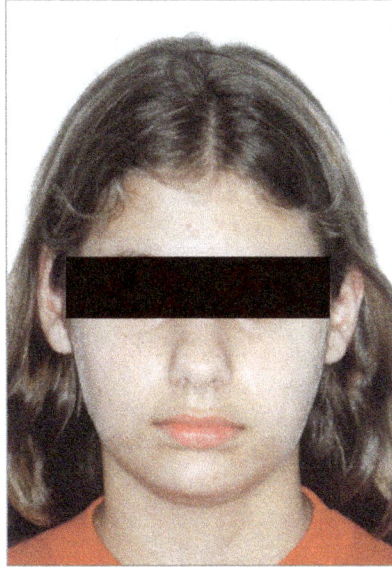

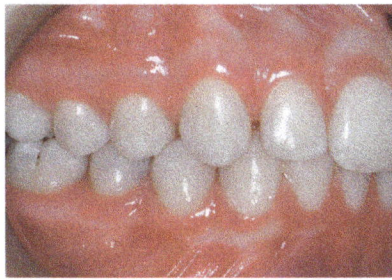
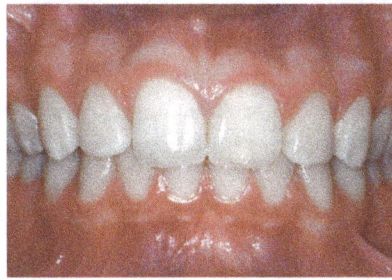
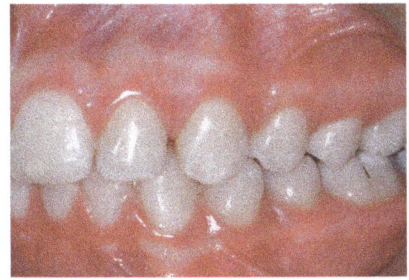

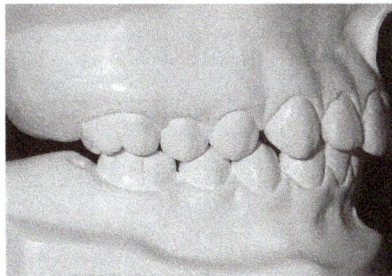
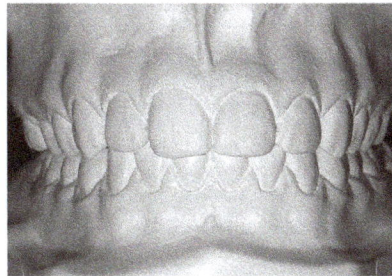
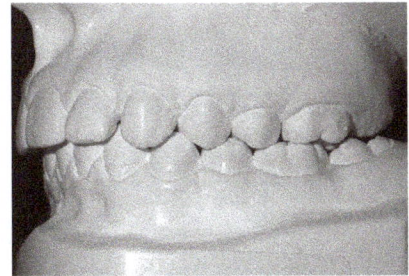

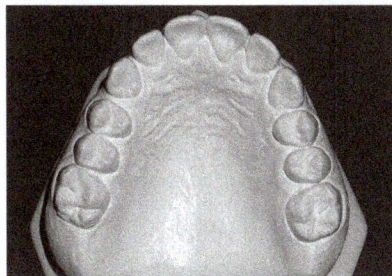
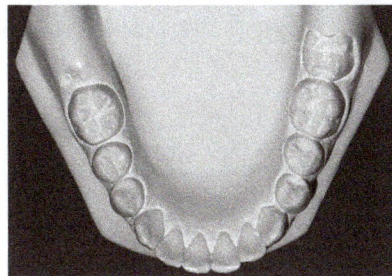
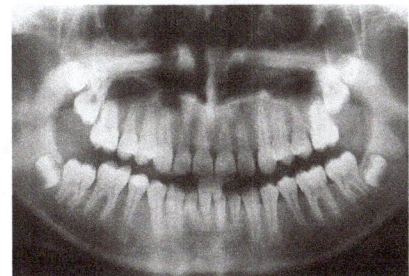

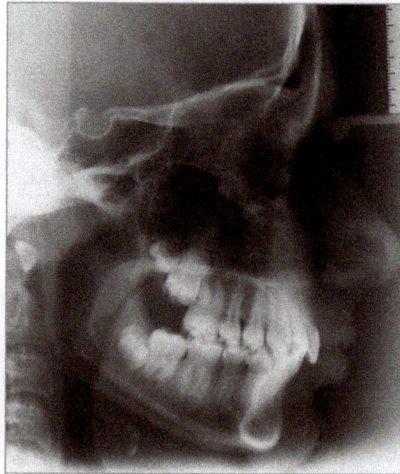

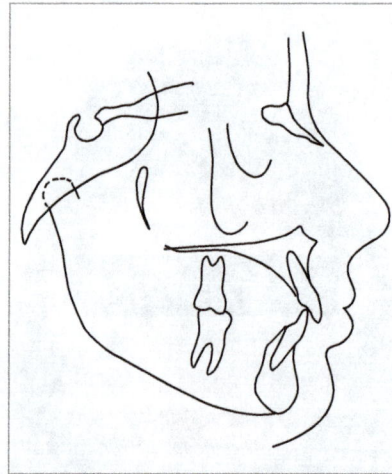

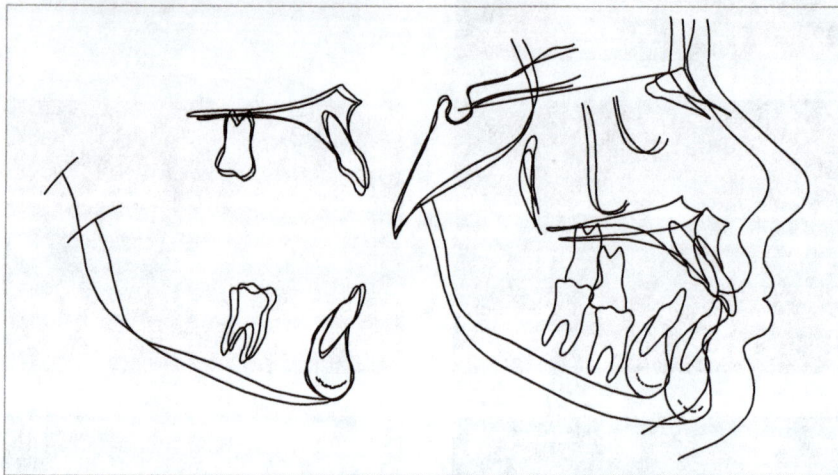

	Nor.	Author	13.1 y
SNA	82	Steiner	90
SNB	80	Steiner	84
ANB	2	Steiner	6
Convex.	0	Downs	12
Y-axis	59	Downs	54
Facial	87	Downs	92
SN-GoGn	32	Steiner	26
FMA	25	Tweed	21
Co-Gn		McNamara	122
Co-A		McNamara	99
IMPA	90	Tweed	100
1.NA	22	Steiner	16
1-NA	4	Steiner	3
Ī.NB	25	Steiner	31
Ī-NB	4	Steiner	7
Pog-NB		Holdaway	2
1 – Ī	130	Downs	127
Ī-APo	1	Ricketts	3
UL-S	0	Steiner	-1
LL-S	0	Steiner	1
Z-angle	75	Merrifield	72

Case 4. Finished case: 13.1-year-old patient, Class II skeletal relationship, Class I relationship, adequate overbite and overjet.

Case report 5

Male 8.9-year-old patient in the first transitional period of mixed dentition. He presented with increased lower facial height, convex profile and mandibular retrognathism (SNB = 72°). Class II skeletal malocclusion (ANBv = 6°), Class II, Division 1 malocclusion, 9-mm overjet and anterior open bite. Protrusive maxillary incisors (1NA = 34°) and proclined mandibular incisors (1NB = 18°). In addition, the patient had a tendency towards vertical growth greater than anteroposterior growth (Y-axis = 63°, SN-GoGn = 43°) and maxillary constriction in the region of primary molars; however, without posterior crossbite. Diastema between maxillary incisors, lack of space for eruption of maxillary lateral incisors and mandibular right canine. Mandibular midline slightly deviated to the right and impaction of teeth #16 and 46 in the distal curvature of primary second molars.

Nine months after treatment onset, Klammt's elastic open activator (KEOA) improved the relationship between the maxilla and mandible, as well as overjet and overbite. In addition, Class I molar relationship was achieved, with space gain that allowed mandibular right second premolar to erupt and considerable change in facial profile.

Post-treatment lateral cephalogram revealed dentoalveolar and skeletal changes, in addition to a decrease in the ANB angle to 5° due to restriction of anterior maxillary growth and mandibular response. It also revealed lingual inclination of maxillary incisors (1-NA = 22°), protrusion of mandibular incisors within normality standards, and improvement in facial profile (Z = 64°).

The appliance remained in use for another six months, with occasional use during the day going to constant use at night. During the retention phase, permanent teeth erupted and treatment outcomes remained unchanged.

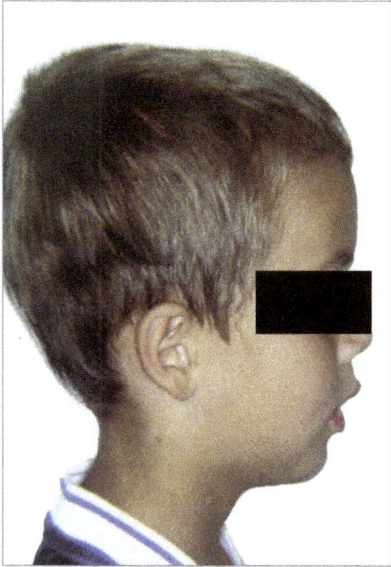
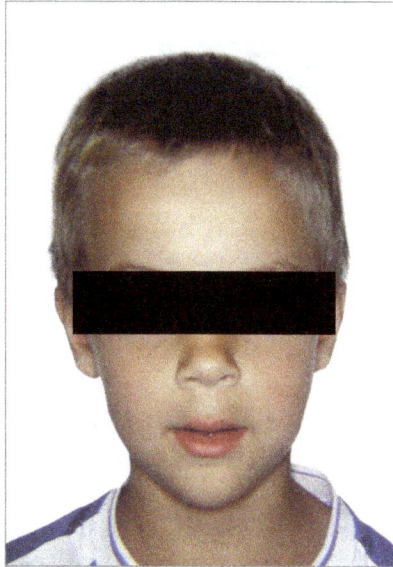

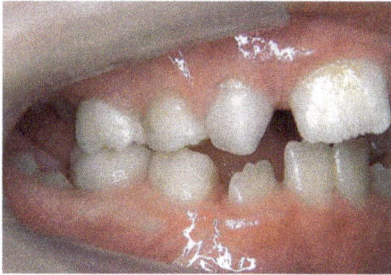
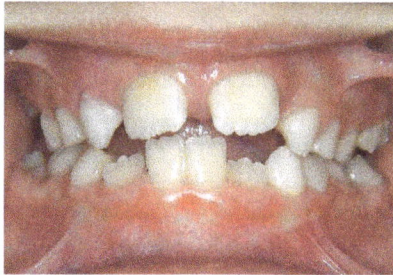
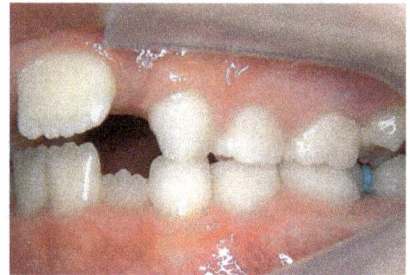

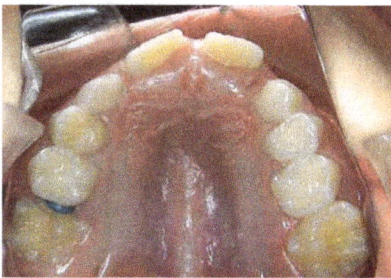
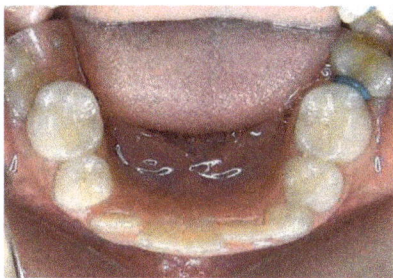

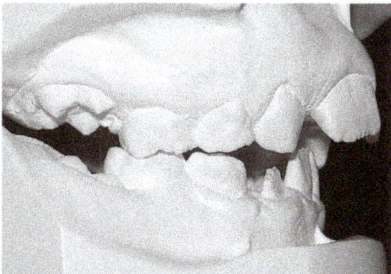
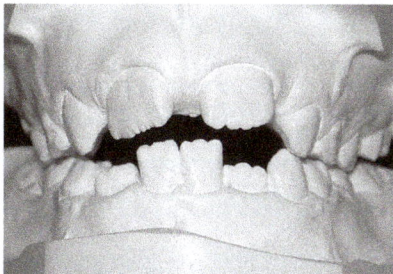
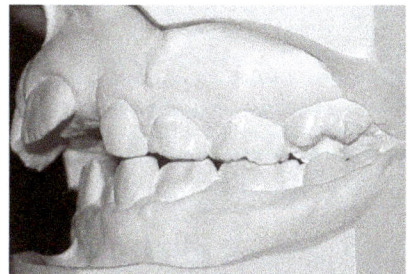

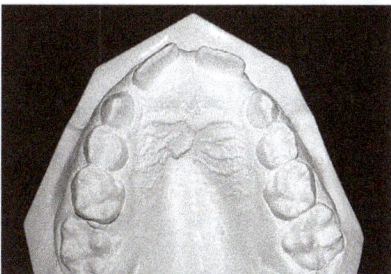
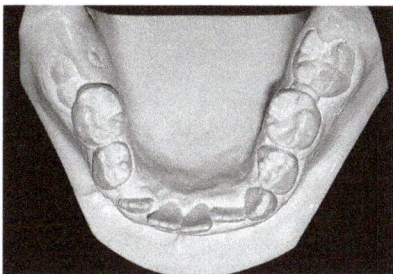
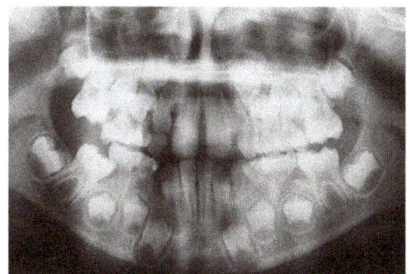

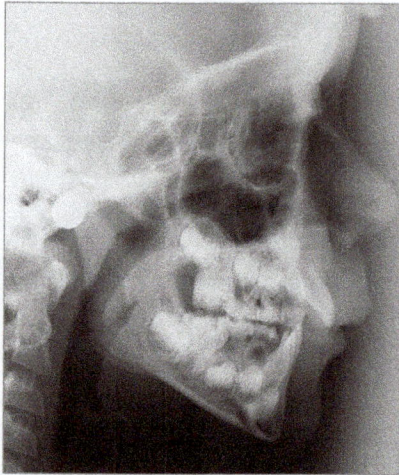

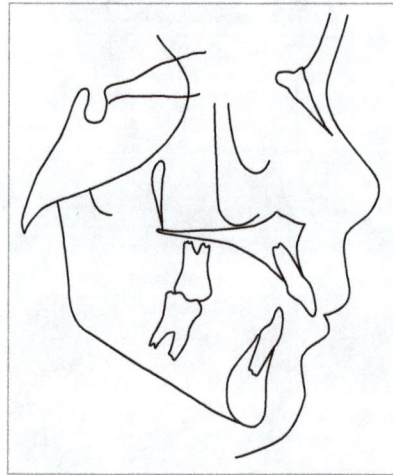

	Nor.	Author	8.9 y
SNA	82	Steiner	78
SNB	80	Steiner	72
ANB	2	Steiner	6
Convex.	0	Downs	11
Y-axis	59	Downs	63
Facial	87	Downs	83
SN-GoGn	32	Steiner	43
FMA	25	Tweed	31
IMPA	90	Tweed	86
1.NA	22	Steiner	34
1-NA	4	Steiner	6
$\overline{1}$.NB	25	Steiner	18
$\overline{1}$-NB	4	Steiner	4
Pog-NB		Holdaway	2
$\underline{1} - \overline{1}$	130	Downs	125
$\overline{1}$-APo	1	Ricketts	2
UL-S	0	Steiner	3
LL-S	0	Steiner	0
Z-angle	75	Merrifield	55

Case 5. Initial examination: 8.9-year-old patient, Class II dental and skeletal malocclusion, 9-mm overjet. anterior open bite.

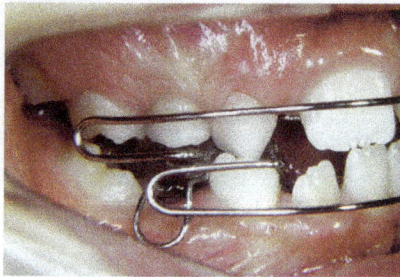

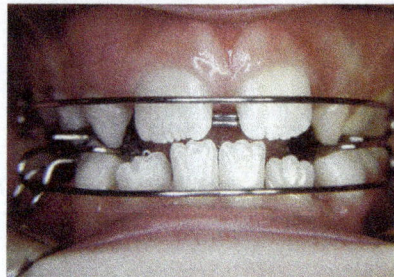

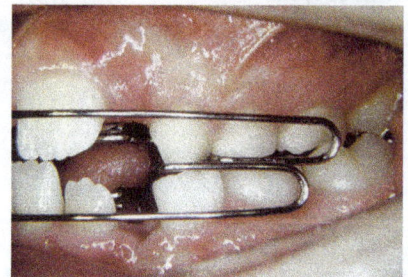

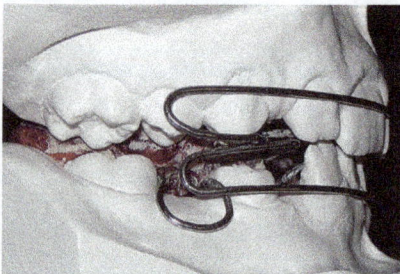

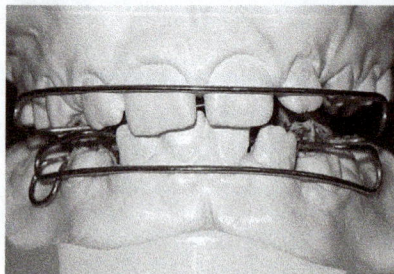

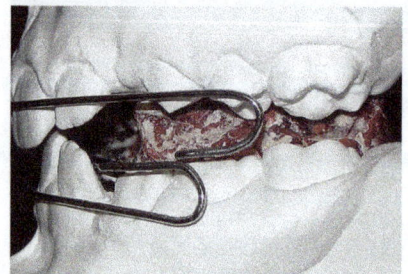

Case 5. Klammt's elastic open activator in function and placed in the dental cast for illustrative purposes, only.

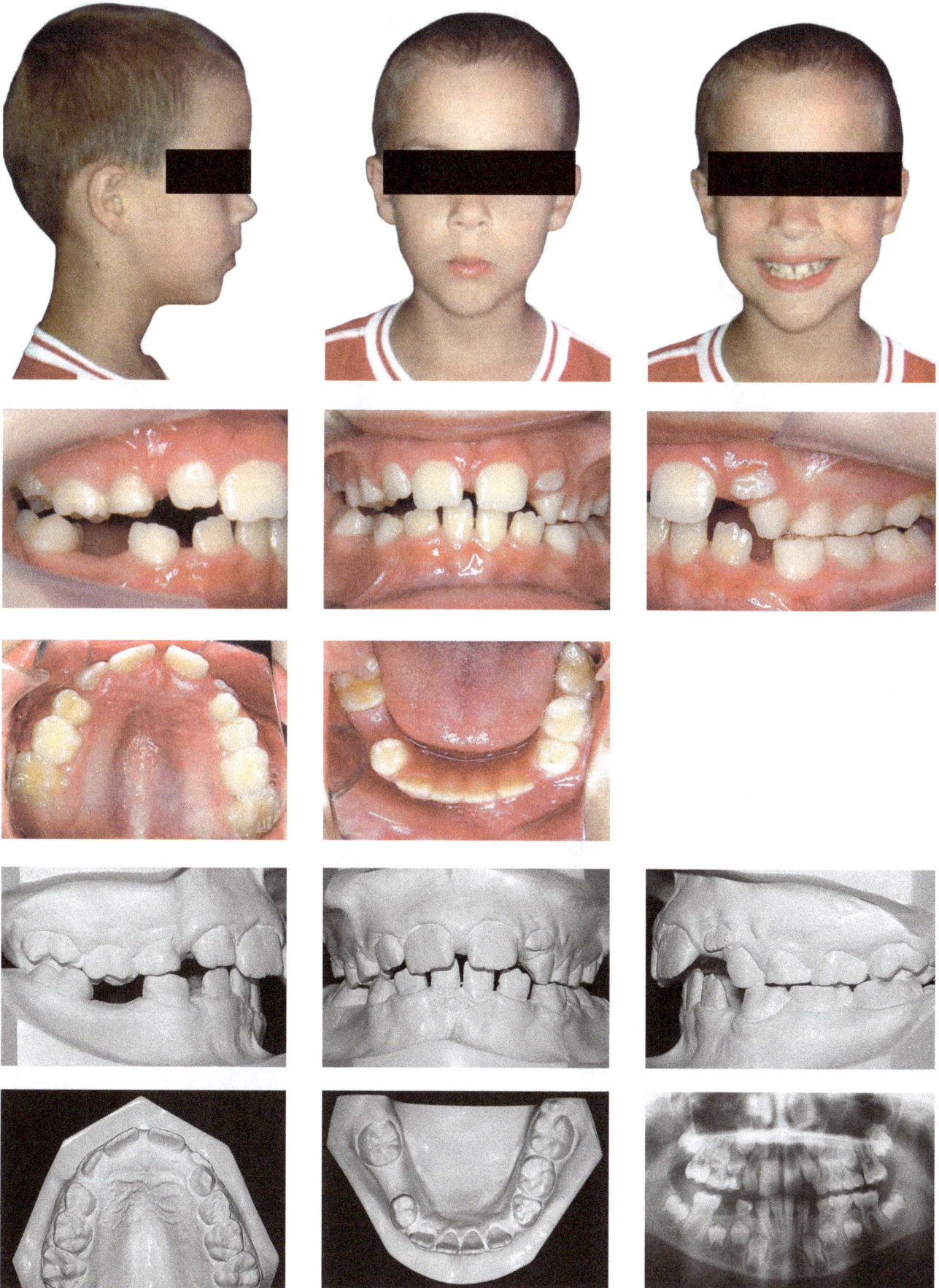

Case 5. Treatment progress: 9.9-year-old patient.

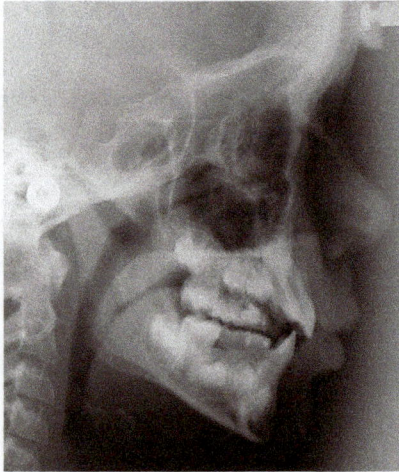

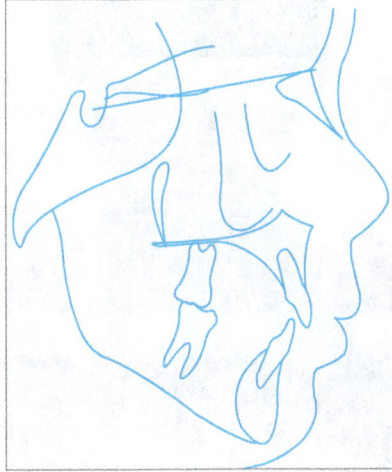

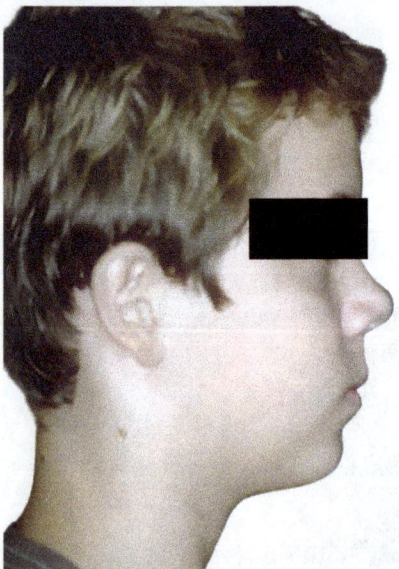

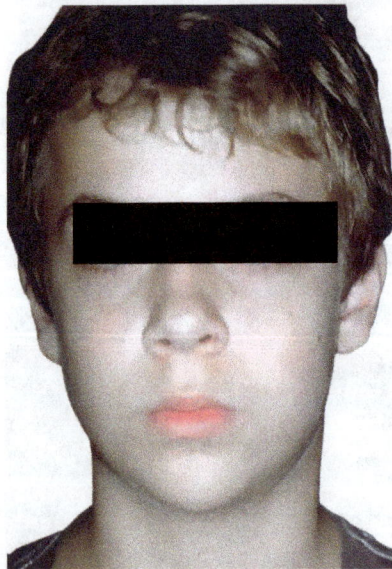

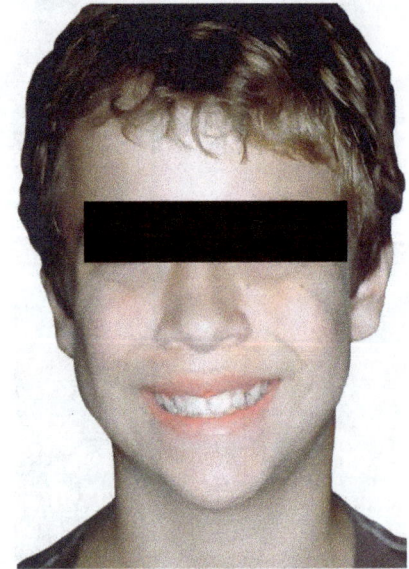

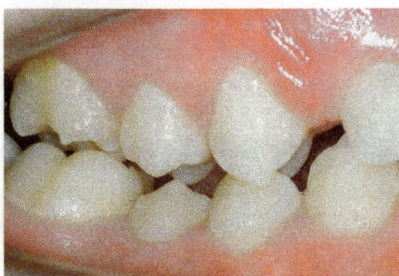

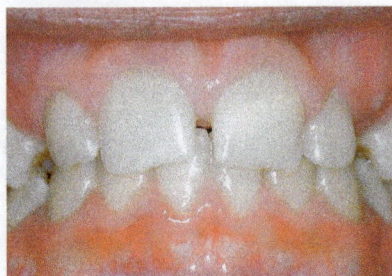

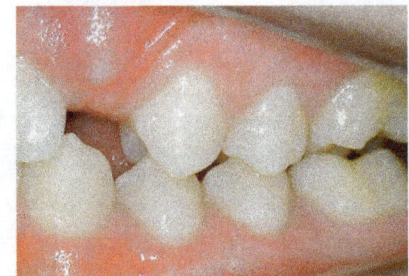

	Nor.	Author	9.9 y
SNA	82	Steiner	79
SNB	80	Steiner	74
ANB	2	Steiner	5
Convex.	0	Downs	8
Y-axis	59	Downs	62
Facial	87	Downs	83
SN-GoGn	32	Steiner	40
FMA	25	Tweed	28
IMPA	90	Tweed	88
1.NA	22	Steiner	23
1-NA	4	Steiner	3
$\overline{1}$.NB	25	Steiner	20
$\overline{1}$-NB	4	Steiner	4
Pog-NB		Holdaway	1
$\underline{1}-\overline{1}$	130	Downs	133
$\overline{1}$-APo	1	Ricketts	0
UL-S	0	Steiner	3
LL-S	0	Steiner	4
Z-angle	75	Merrifield	62

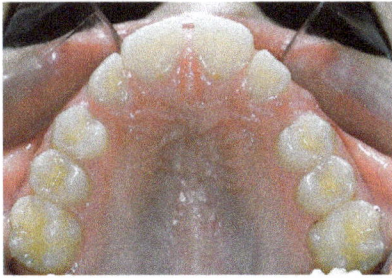

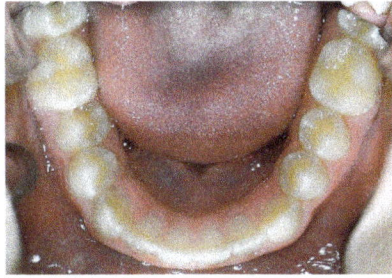

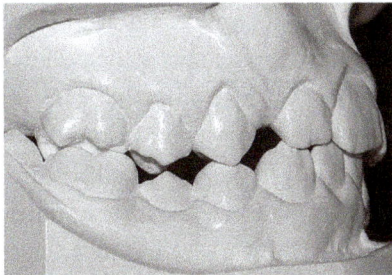

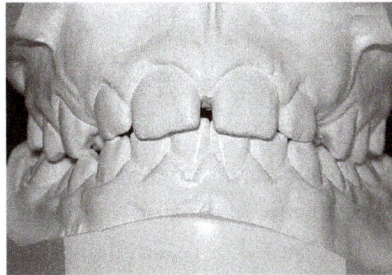

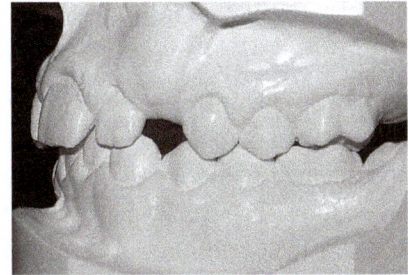

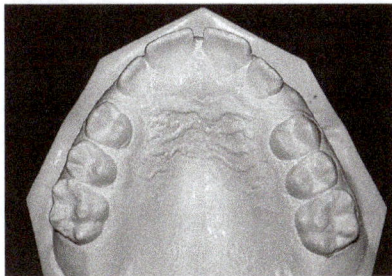

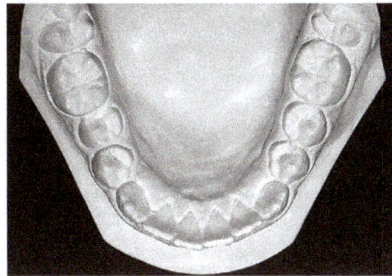

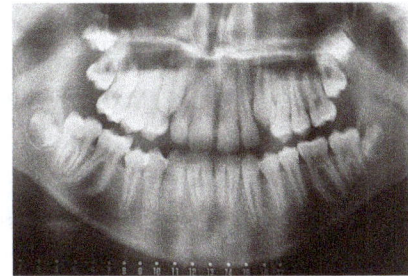

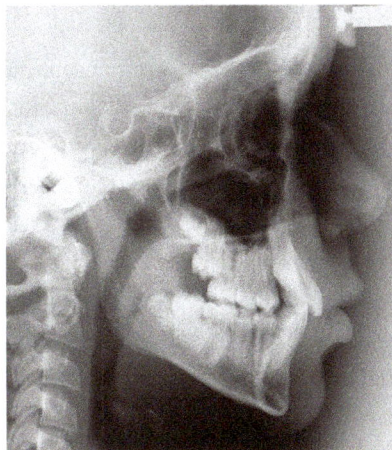

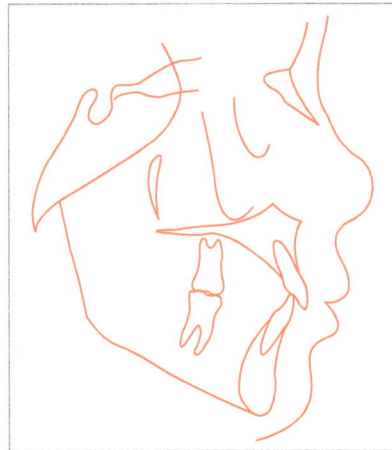

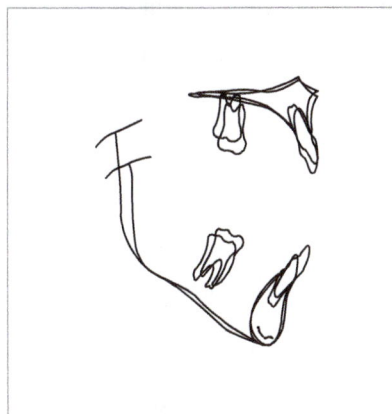

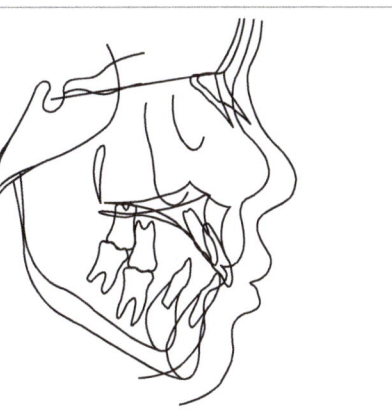

	Nor.	Author	13.1 y
SNA	82	Steiner	81
SNB	80	Steiner	76
ANB	2	Steiner	5
Convex.	0	Downs	8
Y-axis	59	Downs	62
Facial	87	Downs	85
SN-GoGn	32	Steiner	38
FMA	25	Tweed	27
IMPA	90	Tweed	92
1.NA	22	Steiner	22
1-NA	4	Steiner	5
$\overline{1}$.NB	25	Steiner	24
$\overline{1}$-NB	4	Steiner	6
Pog-NB		Holdaway	1
1 – $\overline{1}$	130	Downs	130
$\overline{1}$-APo	1	Ricketts	2
UL-S	0	Steiner	4
LL-S	0	Steiner	4
Z-angle	75	Merrifield	64

Case 5. Finished case: 13.11-year-old patient, Class II skeletal relationship, Class I relationship, adequate overbite and overjet.

DISCUSSION

The potential effects produced by correcting Class II, Division 1 malocclusion might derive from one of the following factors: restricted maxillary or dentoalveolar components, increased growth of the mandible or mesial and vertical alveolar growth, anterior relocation of the mandibular fossa, and protrusion of mandibular incisors, thereby correcting overjet.[2,6,25,26]

The ideal time for malocclusion treatment onset remains controversial. A 2-phased treatment is advocated by some clinicians as advantageous, while others consider it to be a waste of time and money. The 2-phased treatment should be recommended on a case-by-case basis, not as a treatment option to the majority of Class II malocclusion cases. Additionally, it is considered an option only when it provides patients with additional benefits.[15] All patients reported in the present study gained clinically significant esthetic benefits.

Even though only 0.2% of patients aged between 8 and 11 years old have overjet greater than 10 mm, these children are most likely to be looked down and experience social discrimination. They also present a higher risk of trauma of anterior teeth during accidents due to having protrusive maxillary incisors. Thus, treatment at an early age might have a positive psychological impact over patient's self-esteem. To this end, the resources provided by MFO followed by corrective orthodontics are an option.[27]

MFO is a clinical activity that provides benefits to growing patients, provided that they comply with the use of the appliances (10 to 15 hours a day during 1.5 to 2 years), as illustrated by the cases reported herein. Potential and direction of growth are also important.[28] The ideal time for orthopedic appliance use is during the phase of active growth, which allows facial growth pattern to be restores to normality.[6,7,8,10,16]

In general, as illustrated by the cases reported in the present study, changes produced by KEOA over Class II malocclusion are due to a combination of skeletal and dental factors. There was a reduction in SNA angle, in addition to mandibular protrusion (increased SNB angle), retrusion of maxillary incisors, maintenance of mandibular incisors inclination, unchanged facial vertical dimensions, and improvement in facial profile.

In case 1, the Klammt appliance did not cause any changes in maxillary growth; this basal bone remained stable, with only slight anterior displacement of the mandible. As reported in the literature,[29] the increase in

SN-GoGn and FMA was due to the fact that the appliance was mounted in construction bite with increased interocclusal space between teeth. This process is rather common in functional appliance manufacture.

In case 2, the vertical variables most likely decreased due to counterclockwise mandibular rotation associated with two aspects inherent to the Klammt appliance: impaired eruption of maxillary molars caused by the block of acrylic in the occlusal region; and absence of the same block in the anterior region, which allows greater vertical development of anterior teeth.

In case 3, there was a decrease in the SNA angle, which suggested restriction of anterior maxillary displacement caused by retractor muscles of the mandible, and slight decrease in the SNB angle due to vertical mandibular displacement during facial growth, which caused clockwise rotation of the mandible. These values were already expected due to patient's vertical growth pattern, as indicated by Y-axis, FMA and SN-GoGn variables. This case experienced more marked dental changes in the maxilla, with proclined, retrusive maxillary incisors and mandibular incisors remaining stable.

In case 4, there was restriction of anteroposterior maxillary growth, evinced by a decrease in the SNA angle. According to Webster,[30] who requotes Blau,[31] functional appliances affect the maxilla and mandible at the same time, and are mounted in construction bite, which requires masticatory muscles to act in a different direction (posteriorly), thereby leading to restriction of maxillary growth.

In case 5, the relationship between the maxilla and mandible was effectively restored to normality by the activator, as a result of an increase in mandibular protrusion. Changes were practically nonexistent for the facial growth pattern variables assessed.[32] Nevertheless, dental changes derived from treatment resulted in proclined and retrusive maxillary incisors, in addition to slight buccal inclination and protrusion of mandibular incisors.

KEOA is particularly effective in contributing to Angle Class II, Division 1 malocclusion treatment. It is recommended to patients with a tendency towards favorable growth, mandibular retrognathism, marked overjet and relatively adequate arch circumference, both lower and upper arches, during the phase of active growth. This is because it results in dentoalveolar changes and improved relationship between the maxilla and mandible, with satisfactory clinical outcomes and minimal correction of skeletal discrepancies restricted to the second phase of treatment performed with a fixed appliance. All the above has been reported for the five cases presented herein.

FINAL CONSIDERATIONS

Klammt's elastic open activator (KEOA), used to treat Class II, Division 1 malocclusion, achieved the objectives of intercepting or minimizing the existing problem, in addition to reducing the risk of trauma involving maxillary

incisors labially proclined and providing patients with psychological benefits and self-esteem. Treatment finishing was performed with fixed orthodontic appliances, which allowed proper function and balance to be achieved, both of which should be part and parcel of treatment planning.

Acknowledgements

The authors thank Prof. Dr. Telma Martins (full professor of Orthodontics, Universidade Federal da Bahia) for reviewing and giving further suggestions to improve this article.

REFERENCES

1. McNamara J, Peterson J, Alexander R. Three-dimensional diagnosis and management of class II malocclusion in the mixed dentition. Semin Orthod. 1996;2(2):114-37.
2. Vargervik K, Harvold E. Response to activator treatment in Class II malocclusions. Am J Orthod. 1985;88(3):242-51.
3. McNamara JA Jr. Components of Class II malocclusion in children 8-10 years of age. Angle Orthod. 1981;51(3):177-202.
4. Marsico E, Gatto E, Burrascano M, Matarese G, Cordasco G. Effectiveness of orthodontic treatment with functional appliances on mandibular growth in the short term. Am J Orthod Dentofacial Orthop. 2011;139(1):24-36.
5. Wahl N. Orthodontics in 3 millennia. Chapter 9: functional appliances to midcentury. Am J Orthod Dentofacial Orthop. 2006;129(6):829-33.
6. Bishara S, Ziaja R. Functional appliances: a review. Am J Orthod Dentofacial Orthop. 1989;95(3):250-8.
7. Rutter R, Witt E. Correction of Class II, Division 2 malocclusions through the use of the Bionator appliance. Am J Orthod Dentofacial Orthop. 1990;97(2):106-12.
8. Barton S, Cook P. Predicting functional appliance treatment outcome in Class II malocclusions-a review. Am J Orthod Dentofacial Orthop. 1997;112:282-6.
9. Aggarwal P, Kharbanda OP, Mathur R, Duggal R, Parkash H. Muscle response to the Twin-block appliance: an electromyographic study of the masseter and anterior temporal muscles. Am J Orthod Dentofacial Orthop. 1999;116(4):405-14.
10. Rudzki-Janson I, Noachtar R. Functional appliance therapy with the bionator. Semin Orthod. 1998;4(1):33-45.
11. Martins R, Martins J, Martins L, Buschang P. Skeletal and dental components of Class II correction with the bionator and removable headgear splint appliances. Am J Orthod Dentofacial Orthop. 2008;134(6):732-41.
12. Meach C. A cephalometric comparison of bony profile changes in Class II, division 1 patients treated with extraoral force and functional jaw orthopedics. Am J Orthod. 1966;52(5):353-70.
13. McNamara Jr JA. Entrevista. Dental Press J Orthod. 2011;16(3):32-53.
14. Al-Omari IK, Al-Bitar ZB, Sonbol HN, Al-Ahmad HT, Cunningham SJ, Al-Omiri M. Impact of bullying due to dentofacial features on oral health-related quality of life. Am J Orthod Dentofacial Orthop. 2014;146(6):734-9.
15. Tulloch JF, Proffit WR, Phillips C. Outcomes in a 2-phase randomized clinical trial of early Class II treatment. Am J Orthod Dentofacial Orthop 2004;125:657-667.
16. Handa C, Tamaoki S, Narutomi M, Kajii T, Ishikawa H. Evaluation of effects of activator treatment on mandibular growth by analyzing components of condylar growth and mandibular rotation. Orthodontic Waves. 2014;73(1):17-24.

17. DeVincenzo J, Winn M. Orthopedic and orthodontic effects resulting from the use of a functional appliance with different amounts of protrusive activation. Am J Orthod Dentofacial Orthop. 1989;96(3):181-90.
18. Freeman C, McNamara J, Baccetti T, Franchi L, Graffe T. Treatment effects of the bionator and high-pull facebow combination followed by fixed appliances in patients with increased vertical dimensions. Am J Orthod Dentofacial Orthop. 2007;131(2):184-95.
19. Hägg U, Rabie B, Bendeus M, Wong R, Wey M, Du X, et al. Condylar growth and mandibular positioning with stepwise vs maximum advancement. Am J Orthod Dentofacial Orthop. 2008;134:525-36.
20. Toth L, McNamara JA. Treatment effects produced by the Twin-block appliance and the FR-2 appliance of Fränkel compared with an untreated Class II sample. Am J Orthod Dentofacial Orthop. 1999;116:597-609.
21. Gilla D, Lee R. Prospective clinical trial comparing the effects of conventional Twin-block and mini-block appliances: Part 1. Hard tissue changes. Am J Orthod Dentofacial Orthop. 2005;127(4):465-72.
22. Rohidaa N, Bhadb W. Accidental ingestion of a fractured Twin-block appliance. Am J Orthod Dentofacial Orthop. 2011;139(1):123-5.
23. Klammt G. Experiencias con el activador abierto. Rev Assoc Argentina Ortop Func Maxilares. 1965;9:34-36.
24. Klammt G. Der elastisch-offene aktivator. Hanser. 1984:68.
25. Almeida M, Henriques J, Ursi W. Comparative study of the Frankel (FR-2) and bionator appliances in the treatment of Class II malocclusion. Am J Orthod Dentofacial Orthop. 2002;121(5):458-66.
26. Jena A, Duggal R, Parkashc H. Skeletal and dentoalveolar effects of Twinblock and bionator appliances in the treatment of Class II malocclusion: a comparative study. Am J Orthod Dentofacial Orthop. 2006;130(5):594-602.
27. Wong L, Hagg U, Wong G. Correction of extreme overjet in 2 phases. Am J Orthod Dentofacial Orthop. 2006;130(4):540-8.
28. Kreia TB, Bittencourt Neto AC, Retamoso LB, Santos-Pinto A, Tanaka O. Type of facial growth trend in orthodontics and dentofacial orthopedics. RGO. 2011;59:97-102.
29. Basciftci FA, Uysal T, Buyukerkmen A, Sari Z. The effects of activator treatment on the craniofacial structures of Class II division 1 patients. Eur J Orthod. 2003;25(1):87-93.
30. Webster T, Harkness M, Herbison P. Associations between changes in selected facial dimensions and the outcome of orthodontic treatment. Am J Orthod Dentofacial Orthop. 1996;110(1):46-53.
31. Blau F. El método funcional em ortopedia dento-facial. Buenos Aires: Editorial Mundi; 1969. 273 p.
32. Lange DW, Kalra V, Broadbent BH Jr, Powers M, Nelson S. Changes in soft tissue profile following treatment with the bionator. Angle Orthod. 1995;65(6):423-30.

7

Influence of intentional ankylosis of deciduous canines to reinforce the anchorage for maxillary protraction

Luís Fernando Castaldi Tocci[1], Omar Gabriel da Silva Filho[2], Acácio Fuziy[3], José Roberto Pereira Lauris[4]

Introduction: This retrospective cephalometric study analyzed the influence of intentional ankylosis of deciduous canines in patients with Class III malocclusion and anterior crossbite, in the deciduous and early mixed dentition stages, treated by orthopedic maxillary expansion followed by maxillary protraction. **Methods:** Lateral cephalograms of 40 patients were used, divided in 2 groups paired for age and gender. The Ankylosis Group was composed of 20 patients (10 boys and 10 girls) treated with induced ankylosis and presenting initial and final mean ages of 7 years 4 months and 8 years 3 months, respectively, with a mean period of maxillary protraction of 11 months. The Control Group comprised 20 patients (10 boys and 10 girls) treated without induced ankylosis, with initial and final mean ages of 7 years 8 months and 8 years 7 months, respectively, with a mean period of maxillary protraction of 11 months. Two-way analysis of variance and covariance analysis were applied to compare the initial and final cephalometric variables and the treatment changes between groups. **Results:** According to the results, the variables evidencing the significant treatment changes between groups confirmed that the intentional ankylosis enhanced the sagittal response of the apical bases (Pg-NPerp) and increased the facial convexity angles (NAP and ANB). **Conclusions:** The protocol involving intentional ankylosis of deciduous canines enhanced the sagittal response of the apical bases.

Keywords: Malocclusion. Angle Class III. Crossbite. Interceptive orthodontics.

[1] MSc in Orthodontics, UNIMAR.
[2] MSc in Orthodontics, UNESP.
[3] Post-Doc in Dentistry, FOB-USP.
[4] Full Professor, USP. PhD in Human Communication Disturb, University of São Paulo.

» The author reports no commercial, proprietary or financial interest in the products or companies described in this article.

Luís Fernando Castaldi Tocci
Rua Carneiro Lobo, 570 – Conj. 1003 – Batel - Curitiba/PR – Brazil
CEP 80240.240 - E-mail: clinica@tocciortodontia.com.br

INTRODUCTION

Some questions still challenge the scientific community concerning the Class III malocclusion: What will be the behavior of the face, and especially of the mandible, during growth? Will the facial growth perpetuate or worsen the skeletal discrepancy? There are no established responses to these questions, raising controversies among orthodontists concerning the indication of early treatment for the Class III malocclusion.[1] The treatment prognosis and posttreatment stability depend on the skeletal pattern related with this malocclusion.[16,18]

Interceptive orthodontics (mechanics applied in the stages before the permanent dentition) has the general objective to optimize the development of occlusion.[18] The treatment with maxillary protraction is more effective in patients with Class III malocclusion with maxillary retrusion, which account for nearly 60% of the cases,[16] and hypodivergent growth pattern,[13,15] explaining the increased professional interest for maxillary protraction. The orthopedic mechanics acts on the direction of spontaneous facial growth.[16] If the treatment is initiated during the period of eruption of maxillary central incisors, it will contribute to stabilize the anterior relationship.[9,13,15]

Clinical results demonstrate that the utilization of maxillary protraction induces orthopedic and orthodontic effects that provide an important improvement in the occlusion and face (Table 1). The immediate favorable impact, though variable and individual,[15] in the deciduous and mixed dentition stages are related to forward maxillary displacement,[1,2,5,6,9-13,15,17,18,21,23] forward displacement of maxillary teeth,[2,6,8,10,18] clockwise mandibular rotation with corresponding significant increase in the lower anterior facial height,[5,10,18] and lingual tipping of mandibular incisors.[2,3,5,9,16,18]

Orthodontists are aware of the importance to optimize the orthopedic effect of maxillary protraction, rather than the orthodontic effects.[6] Within this context, the orthopedic maxillary expansion before maxillary protraction increases the effect of the face mask on the maxilla[1,2] due to the increase in the transverse width, rupture of maxillary sutures and especially to the strong anchorage provided by the expander[16] (Table 1).

The intentional ankylosis of deciduous canines has also been used with the primary goal to potentiate the orthopedic effects of maxillary protraction.[18,19,20] This led to the need to scientifically analyze its utilization, because though biocompatible and accepted by the patients,[19] it is an invasive procedure.

This study evaluated the immediate effects of maxillary protraction applied in the deciduous and early mixed dentition stages to respond to the null hypotheses if there is difference between the immediate results produced by orthopedic maxillary protraction mechanics, using or not the induced ankylosis to reinforce the anchorage.

Table 1 - Literature on the utilization of maxillary protraction (with facial mask) applied immediately after orthopedic maxillary expansion.

AUTHOR	YEAR	ANCHORAGE	FORCE	USE	EFFECT	CHANGE IN POINT A
Baccetti et al.[1]	1998	Fixed maxillary expander with acrylic occlusal coverage	227-397 g/side	24 h	Orthopedic/Orthodontic	2.6 mm
Baik[2]	1995	Hyrax	300-500 g/side	12 h	Orthopedic/Orthodontic	2 mm
Gallagher et al.[6]	1998	Fixed maxillary expander (slow expansion)	600-800 g/ bilaterally	12-24 h	Orthopedic/Orthodontic	1 to 2 mm
Kapust et al.[10]	1998	–	600-800 g/ bilaterally	–	Orthopedic/Orthodontic	2.3 mm
McNamara Jr.[12]	1987	Fixed maxillary expander with acrylic occlusal coverage	397 g/side	24 h	Orthopedic/Orthodontic	1 to 2 mm
Ngan et al.[14]	1996	Hyrax	380 g/side	12 h	Orthopedic/Orthodontic	2 mm
Ngan et al.[16]	1997	Hyrax	380 g/side	12 h	Orthopedic/Orthodontic	1.9 mm
Saadia, Torres[17]	2000	Hyrax or Haas	395 g/side	8-14 h	Orthopedic/Orthodontic	1.9 mm
Shanker et al.[18]	2003	Hyrax	400 g/side	12 h	Orthopedic/Orthodontic	2.4 mm
Silva Filho et al.[19]	1998	Haas	350 g/side	10-14 h	Orthopedic/Orthodontic	2.5 mm
Silva Filho et al.[20]	2003	Haas / Intentional ankylosis	350 g/side	10-14 h	Orthopedic/Orthodontic	2.5 mm
Sung, Baik[22]	1998	Fixed maxillary expander (rapid expansion)	300-400 g/side	Over 12 h	Orthopedic/Orthodontic	1.7 to 2.8 mm
Turley[24]	1998	Hyrax and mandibular occlusal support	150-600 g/side	14-24 h	Orthopedic/Orthodontic	3.3 mm

MATERIAL AND METHODS

The sample was composed of 40 Brazilian Caucasian children aged 5 years to 8 years 11 months, in the deciduous and early mixed dentition stages, retrospectively selected from the files of the Postgraduate course in Preventive and Interceptive Orthodontics of the Hospital for Rehabilitation of Craniofacial Anomalies of University of São Paulo, at Bauru (HRAC-USP-Bauru), Brazil, among the records of 2,060 registered and treated patients.

The inclusion criteria were the following: 1– Brazilian Caucasian children in the deciduous and early mixed dentition stage; 2 – presenting Class III molar relationship; 3 – anterior crossbite; 4 – maxillary retrognathism with little or no mandibular involvement; and 5 – posterior crossbite in most cases. Patients with isolated mandibular impairment (prognathism) were not included.

The sample was divided into two groups of 20 patients (10 boys and 10 girls) matched for age and gender. The Ankylosis Group was composed of patients treated with induced ankylosis with initial (T_1) and final (T_2) mean ages of 7 years 4 months and 8 years 3 months, respectively, with mean period of maxillary protraction of 11 months. The Control Group was treated without induced ankylosis and presented initial mean age of 7 years 8 months and final mean age 8 years 7 months, with a mean period of maxillary protraction of 11 months.

In the Ankylosis Group, among the 20 patients, 16 presented posterior crossbite, being 9 girls and 7 boys, and in the Control Group 17 out of the 20 patients presented posterior crossbite, being 8 boys and 9 girls.

All 40 children were submitted to the same therapeutic protocol of rapid maxillary expansion with modified fixed Haas expander, with activation of the screw until rupture of the midpalatal suture or up to correction of the posterior crossbite, when present. The therapeutic groups were distinguished by the accomplishment of intentional ankylosis of deciduous canines as anchorage reinforcement. Immediately after completion of the active period of rapid maxillary expansion, the facial mask was placed using elastics delivering an approximate force of 500 g connected to hooks soldered at the anterior portion of the expander and bonded to the deciduous canines with resin. The patients were instructed to wear the facial mask for 16 hours/day.

The lateral cephalograms were obtained in centric occlusion, with the lips in relaxed and passive position. The anatomical tracings and identification of the dentoskeletal points were manually performed by a single examiner and digitized on a UMAX 1220S scanner connected to a computer NB HP Pavillion dv6120BR (3400, HD 60 Gb, memory 512 Mb), with operational system Windows XP and software Radiocef Studio – Radiomemory, version 1 – release 16, Belo Horizonte, MG, Brazil (Fig 1). Data were analyzed on this software, which also corrected the magnification factors of radiographic images, which ranged from 6% to 9.8% according to the X-ray machine employed.

The cephalometric measurements selected are representative of the facial convexity (NAP, ANB), sagittal position of the apical bases (SNA, SNB, SND, SN.ANS, Co-A, A-NPerp, Pg-NPerp), mandibular and occlusal plane rotation (SN.GoGn, SN.Gn, SN.OP) and inclination of maxillary and mandibular incisors (1.NA, 1-NA, 1.SN, 1.PP, 1.NB, 1-NB, IMPA) (Table 4).

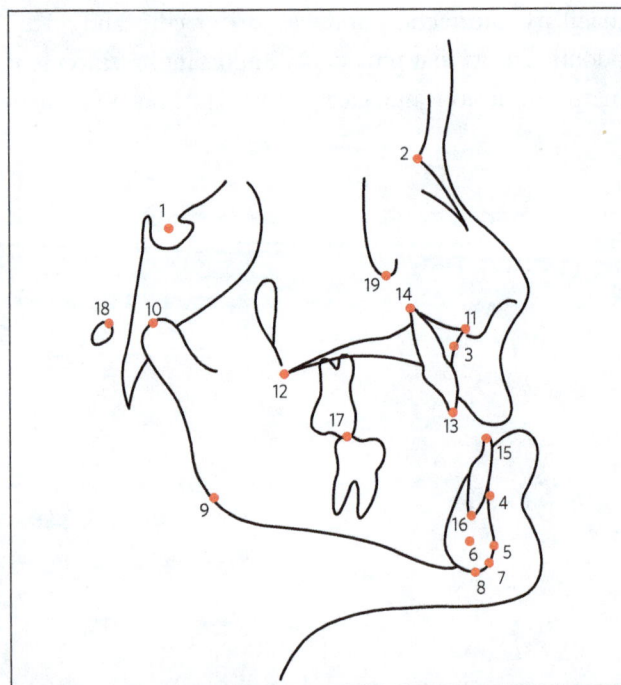

Figure 1 - Cephalometric points used on the lateral tracing: 1) S: sella turcica; 2) N: nasion; 3) A: subspinale; 4) B: supramentale; 5) Pg: pogonion; 6) D: geometric center of the symphysis; 7) Gn: gnathion; 8) Me: menton; 9) Go: gonion; 10) Co: condylion; 11) ANS: anterior nasal spine; 12) PNS: posterior nasal spine; 13) MxIE: incisal edge of maxillary central incisor; 14) MxIA: apex of maxillary central incisor; 15) MdIE: incisal edge of mandibular central incisor; 16) MdIA: apex of mandibular central incisor; 17) OCM1: mean occlusal contact between the maxillary and mandibular first molars; 18) Po: porion; 19) Or: orbitale.

STATISTICAL ANALYSIS
Method error

For calculation of the intraexaminer error, at 20 days after the first tracing, 12 cephalograms of each group (30% of the sample) were randomly selected for achievement of new tracings, identification of points and achievement of linear and angular measurements. The intraexaminer systematic error was evaluated by the paired t test. The casual error was determined according to the Dahlberg formula (error = $(\Sigma d^2/\ 2n)1/2$), in which d represents the difference between the first and second measurements and n indicates the number of retraced cephalograms, according to Houston.[7] The significance level adopted was 5% ($p < 0.05$).

The results of evaluations of systematic errors by the paired t test and by the casual error measured by the Dahlberg formula are presented in Table 4.

STATISTICAL METHODS

Descriptive statistics was performed for all data in the sample: Initial and final ages, treatment time (T_2-T_1) and cephalometric variables analyzed in the study periods. The normality of data distribution was assessed by the Kolmogorov-Smirnov, which revealed that all groups passed the normality criteria.

Two-way analysis of variance was applied for comparison between groups and gender, initial age, treatment time, ANB and A-NPerp, to verify the similarity of data at treatment onset.

Since the groups has different severities (ANB and A-NPerp) at T_1 and the statistical analysis might be influenced by this factor and not only by the difference between groups, comparison between groups was performed by the analysis of covariance (ANCOVA), using the measurements ANB and A-NPerp as co-variables, to take these initial differences into account.

Table 2 - Mean, standard deviation of two measurements, paired t test and Dahlberg formula to evaluate the systematic and casual errors.

measurement	first measurement mean	first measurement SD	second measurement mean	second measurement SD	t	p	Error
NAP	3.77	6.54	3.65	6.41	0.621	0.538 ns	0.79
SNA	81.05	4.70	81.28	4.67	1.816	0.077 ns	0.58
SNB	79.24	4.62	79.41	4.59	1.705	0.097 ns	0.44
ANB	1.80	2.95	1.87	2.83	1.669	0.104 ns	0.53
SND	75.86	4.41	76.27	4.47	1.992	0.054 ns	0.94
SN.ANS	85.75	4.65	86.01	4.62	1.854	0.072 ns	0.63
Co-A	81.09	6.82	81.24	6.73	2.029	0.051 ns	0.33
A-NPerp	1.02	3.27	0.93	3.38	0.967	0.340 ns	0.41
Pg-NPerp	-1.43	6.80	-1.53	6.99	0.620	0.539 ns	0.68
SN.GoGn	36.38	5.99	36.22	6.07	1.667	0.104 ns	0.42
SN.Gn	67.63	4.80	67.52	4.85	1.551	0.129 ns	0.33
SN.OP	22.33	10.41	22.09	10.48	1.603	0.117 ns	0.67
1.NA	24.65	7.85	25.02	7.52	1.966	0.057 ns	0.84
1-NA	2.27	3.33	2.41	3.37	1.907	0.064 ns	0.33
1.SN	105.70	8.12	106.02	8.16	1.514	0.138 ns	0.94
1.PP	111.12	8.01	111.09	8.20	0.158	0.875 ns	0.72
1.NB	23.45	5.60	23.84	5.85	1.557	0.128 ns	1.10
1-NB	3.15	3.00	3.29	3.08	2.489	0.017*	0.28
IMPA	85.39	6.76	85.65	6.77	1.083	0,286 ns	1.03

ns = non significant statistical difference. * = statistically significant difference (p < 0.05).

Table 3 - Dental and skeletal cephalometric variables.

Facial convexity	
1)	NAP: Angle between the NA and AP lines
2)	ANB: Angle between the NA and NB lines
Sagittal position of the apical bases	
3)	SNA: Angle between the SN and NA lines
4)	SNB: Angle between the SN and NB lines
5)	SND: Angle between the SN and ND lines
6)	SN.ANS: Angle between the SN line and the anterior nasal spine point
7)	Co-A: Linear distance between points Co and A
8)	A-NPerp: Linear distance from point A to the nasion-perpendicular
9)	Pg-NPerp: Linear distance from point Pg to the nasion-perpendicular
Mandibular and occlusal plane rotation	
10)	SN.GoGn: Angle between the SN line and the mandibular plane
11)	SN.Gn: Angle between the SN line and point Gn
12)	SN.OP: Angle between the SN line and the mandibular occlusal plane (mandibular occlusal plane – measured from the mean occlusal point on the intercuspation surface of the mandibular first molars to the incisal edge of the mandibular central incisor)
Inclination of maxillary and mandibular incisors	
13)	1.NA: Angle between the long axis of the maxillary incisor and the NA line
14)	1-NA: Distance between the long axis of the maxillary incisor and the NA line
15)	1.SN: Angle between the long axis of the maxillary incisor and the SN line
16)	1.PP: Angle between the long axis of the maxillary incisor and the palatal plane
17)	1.NB: Angle between the long axis of the mandibular incisor and the NB line
18)	1-NB: Distance between the long axis of the mandibular incisor and the NB line
19)	IMPA: Angle between the long axis of the mandibular incisor and the mandibular plane

Therefore, comparison between groups was performed by two-way analysis of variance (Group – Control and Ankylosis, and Gender – Female and Male), fixed model. If the analysis of variance indicated statistically significant difference, the Tukey test for multiple comparisons was applied. A significance level of 5% ($p < 0.05$) was considered for all tests.

All statistical analyses were performed on the software Statistica version 5.1 StatSoft Inc. (Tulsa, USA).

RESULTS

Table 2 presents the analysis of systematic and casual errors, by analysis by the paired t test and the Dahlberg[7] formula applied to all study variables. Only the variable (1-NB) presented statistically significant systematic error, yet with a difference of only 0.14 mm. The casual error ranged from 0.28 mm (1-NB) to 1.10° (1.NB).

Table 5 displays the cephalometric measurements analyzed during the treatment period (T_1 and T_2) for

Table 4 - Comparison of initial and final ages, treatment time, ANB and A-NPerp between groups.

Group	Gender	Initial age Mean	Initial age SD	Treatment time Mean	Treatment time SD	ANB Mean	ANB SD	A-NPerp Mean	A-NPerp SD
Control	M	91.90	9.76	11.60	8.14	2.90	2.86	1.71	4.32
	F	93.00	10.13	9.40	4.45	1.86	1.66	2.44	3.45
Ankylosis	M	87.25	16.02	11.10	4.38	-0.54	3.52	-1.13	3.15
	F	85.38	13.50	10.50	3.21	-0.65	3.00	-0.66	2.79
Anova	p group	0.147 ns		0.861 ns		0.002 *		0.010 *	
	p gender	0.926 ns		0.416 ns		0.524 ns		0.587 ns	
	p interaction	0.721 ns		0.641 ns		0.607 ns		0.906 ns	

ns = statistically non significant difference. * = statistically significant difference ($p < 0.05$).

Table 5 - Mean and standard deviation of cephalometric measurements obtained for the study groups at T_1 and T_2.

Cephalometric measurement	Control female T_1	Control female T_2	Control male T_1	Control male T_2	Ankylosis female T_1	Ankylosis female T_2	Ankylosis male T_1	Ankylosis male T_2
NAP	3.49 ± 4.89	5.22 ± 4.63	5.61 ± 5.98	6.00 ± 5.13	-0.45 ± 7.67	7.07 ± 8.18	-0.54 ± 8.41	6.49 ± 7.44
SNA	80.35 ± 4.81	81.13 ± 5.91	83.2 ± 5.31	83.47 ± 5.44	81.25 ± 5.05	84.19 ± 5.35	80.19 ± 2.87	82.26 ± 3.27
SNB	78.49 ± 4.65	78.35 ± 5.18	80.4 ± 5.49	80.11 ± 4.82	82.13 ± 4.16	81.05 ± 4.04	80.71 ± 3.45	79.25 ± 2.61
ANB	1.86 ± 1.66	2.78 ± 1.80	2.80 ± 2.81	3.36 ± 2.47	-0.65 ± 3.00	3.23 ± 3.61	-0.52 ± 3.55	3.02 ± 3.73
SND	75.23 ± 4.77	75.18 ± 5.24	77.09 ± 5.41	77.18 ± 4.89	77.81 ± 3.31	77.20 ± 3.39	76.65 ± 3.45	75.7 ± 2.59
SN.ANS	85.25 ± 4.41	87.50 ± 6.54	87.30 ± 4.24	88.1 ± 4.82	86.25 ± 4.85	88.20 ± 5.41	84.6 ± 4.01	86.8 ± 4.03
Co-A	79.05 ± 7.80	81.44 ± 7.70	83.20 ± 4.88	86.71 ± 5.4	74.68 ± 3.57	79.15 ± 4.77	76.42 ± 2.26	80.43 ± 4.76
A-NPerp	1.71 ± 4.32	2.90 ± 4.82	2.44 ± 3.45	2.74 ± 3.07	-1.14 ± 3.15	1.40 ± 3.50	-0.66 ± 2.79	0.67 ± 3.12
Pg-NPerp	0.28 ± 8.66	1.12 ± 8.85	-0.39 ± 7.66	-0.12 ± 6.44	-2.16 ± 5.89	-3.46 ± 6.33	-1.28 ± 6.51	-4.13 ± 5.42
SN.GoGn	35.84 ± 5.39	36.44 ± 6.21	35.26 ± 6.81	35.86 ± 5.48	35.80 ± 5.88	37.71 ± 6.17	33.83 ± 5.55	35.5 ± 4.71
SN.Gn	67.76 ± 3.89	68.59 ± 4.23	67.02 ± 6.27	67.50 ± 5.36	65.71 ± 4.05	67.24 ± 3.85	65.00 ± 4.78	66.77 ± 3.85
SN.OP	21.43 ± 5.54	19.18 ± 4.97	23.02 ± 9.76	21.23 ± 9.1	31.63 ± 11.83	21.21 ± 11.77	24.92 ± 11.07	22.19 ± 8.35
1.NA	27.05 ± 6.30	25.97 ± 4.87	18.26 ± 7.51	22.29 ± 3.91	25.42 ± 10.47	27.51 ± 7.6	18.72 ± 9.50	19.83 ± 9.59
1-NA	1.69 ± 2.40	3.47 ± 1.63	0.30 ± 3.77	2.83 ± 1.86	0.04 ± 4.47	2.74 ± 3.61	-1.60 ± 2.26	0.84 ± 3.42
1.SN	107.4 ± 7.09	107.1 ± 4.63	101.46 ± 7.48	105.76 ± 7.61	106.67 ± 10.24	111.63 ± 6.33	98.99 ± 9.29	102.1 ± 8.45
1.PP	116.75 ± 5.66	112.9 ± 6.08	105.95 ± 7.24	109.45 ± 5.01	110.9 ± 7.43	115.2 ± 5.85	104.25 ± 8.93	107.25 ± 9.49
1.NB	28.03 ± 4.69	23.63 ± 7.44	27.00 ± 7.40	26.18 ± 5.38	21.72 ± 6.13	25.29 ± 6.09	19.56 ± 8.21	20.77 ± 5.66
1-NB	3.93 ± 2.04	3.7 ± 2.28	3.82 ± 2.84	3.84 ± 2.7	0.52 ± 3.35	3.78 ± 3.43	1.24 ± 2.83	1.97 ± 3.46
IMPA	91.25 ± 5.73	86.51 ± 8.96	89.11 ± 8.43	87.84 ± 6.33	81.05 ± 7.94	86.61 ± 10.56	82.31 ± 7.42	83.57 ± 5.11

Table 6 - Variation of measurements (mean and standard deviation) during treatment ($T_2 - T_1$), and comparison between groups by Analysis of Covariance and the Tukey test.

| Measure-ments | Female | | Male | | ANCOVA p | | |
	Control mean ± SD	Ankylosis mean ± SD	Control mean ± SD	Ankylosis mean ± SD	Group	Gender	Interaction
Sagittal skeletal measurements							
NAP	1.73 ± 3.87[a]	7.52 ± 5.06[b]	0.39 ± 4.00[a]	7.03 ± 5.33[b]	0.007*	0.651	0.911
SNA	0.78 ± 2.13	2.94 ± 3.07	0.27 ± 2.50	2.08 ± 2.16	0.109	0.459	0.761
SNB	-0.14 ± 1.31	-1.08 ± 1.81	-0.28 ± 1.52	-1.46 ± 1.61	0.083	0.618	0.833
ANB	0.92 ± 1.54[a]	3.88 ± 2.49[b]	0.56 ± 1.81[a]	3.54 ± 2.71[b]	0.005*	0.730	0.898
SND	-0.05 ± 1.48	-0.61 ± 1.39	0.09 ± 1.63	-0.95 ± 1.75	0.368	0.780	0.697
SN.ANS	2.25 ± 4.28	1.95 ± 3.45	0.80 ± 2.73	2.20 ± 2.21	0.700	0.584	0.441
Co-A	2.39 ± 1.62	4.47 ± 3.41	3.51 ± 4.92	4.01 ± 3.43	0.655	0.517	0.351
A-NPerp	1.19 ± 2.58	2.54 ± 2.80	0.30 ± 1.77	1.34 ± 2.60	0.771	0.263	0.747
Pg-NPerp	0.84 ± 3.99[a]	-1.30 ± 2.49[b]	0.26 ± 2.83[a]	-2.85 ± 2.99[b]	<0.001*	0.343	0.607
Vertical skeletal measurements							
SN.GoGn	0.61 ± 1.77	1.91 ± 1.83	0.61 ± 2.63	1.67 ± 1.69	0.447	0.990	0.741
SN.Gn	0.83 ± 1.05	1.53 ± 1.20	0.48 ± 1.81	1.76 ± 1.66	0.378	0.934	0.637
SN.OP	-2.26 ± 1.85[a]	-10.42 ± 6.52[b]	-1.80 ± 3.04[a]	-2.73 ± 6.97[a]	<0.001*	0.005*	0.035*
Dental measurements							
1.NA	-1.08 ± 5.33	2.09 ± 8.82	4.02 ± 6.71	1.11 ± 9.33	0.555	0.475	0.263
1-NA	1.78 ± 2.48	2.70 ± 3.88	2.53 ± 3.17	2.43 ± 2.58	0.253	0.939	0.685
1.SN	-0.31 ± 4.87	4.97 ± 9.87	4.30 ± 7.54	3.11 ± 10.04	0.328	0.665	0.265
1.PP	-3.85 ± 8.48	4.30 ± 4.50	3.50 ± 4.94	3.00 ± 11.37	0.154	0.249	0.107
1.NB	-4.40 ± 3.99[a]	3.57 ± 6.83[b]	-0.82 ± 5.15[a]	1.21 ± 4.44[b]	0.001*	0.855	0.080
1-NB	-0.23 ± 1.14[a]	3.26 ± 3.46[b]	0.02 ± 1.39[a]	0.73 ± 2.74[b]	0.001*	0.076	0.087
IMPA	-4.75 ± 4.48[a]	5.56 ± 10.32[b]	-1.26 ± 5.57[a]	1.26 ± 4.73[b]	0.001*	0.679	0.076

* – statistically significant difference (p < 0.05). Groups with similar letters do not have statistically significant difference to each other.

each study group (female control, female ankylosis, male control, male ankylosis).

The statistical comparison between groups reveals that they were compatible considering the initial age and treatment time. However, there was significant difference in the variables ANB and A-NPerp (Table 4), which led to the utilization of analysis of covariance for comparison between groups.

The statistical analysis revealed that the cephalometric measurements were not influenced by gender, except for the variable SN.OP. The changes in cephalometric measurements occurred in the same direction and magnitude for both genders (Table 6). There was statistically significant difference between groups in the variation of sagittal measurements NAP, ANB and Pg-NPerp, the vertical measurement SN.OP, and the dental measurements 1.NB, 1-NB and IMPA (Table 6).

DISCUSSION

The early treatment of anterior crossbite with Class III malocclusion has the orthopedic goal to promote forward displacement of the maxillary dental arch, with downward and forward advancement of the growth direction of the maxilla.[1,2,5,6,9-13,15-18,21,23] For that purpose, the maxillary protraction after orthopedic maxillary expansion has been used by most orthodontists, with favorable immediate results in 90% of patients treated in the deciduous and mixed dentitions[4] with a relatively short treatment time of nearly 8 months.[18] Regardless of the influence of facial growth on the long-term post-treatment stability, the immediate goal of orthopedic treatment for the Class III malocclusion is to potentiate the skeletal changes rather than the dental compensation, by the utilization of strong anchorage[1] This study addresses the maxillary protraction, more specifically to analyze the influence of intentional ankylosis of deciduous canines to reinforce the anchorage, a protocol established at the Hospital for Rehabilitation of Craniofacial Anomalies of University of São Paulo.[19,20] In this treatment protocol, the deciduous canines are ankylosed before orthopedic expansion and maxillary protraction, in the deciduous or early mixed dentition stages.[19]

This therapeutic possibility was developed to optimize the forward displacement of point A and involves different specialties in addition to Orthodontics, such as Surgery and Endodontics, thus not being promptly accepted by patients and caretakers.[19] For this reason, the cost-benefit relationship of intentional ankylosis should be individually considered, being indicated for cases of anterior crossbite and greater severity of maxillary deficiency, especially when dental anchorage in the maxillary arch is not reliable and satisfactory.[19,21] The ankylosis should be contraindicated in cases of Class III malocclusion assigned only to mandibular prognathism, because of the unpredictable mandibular growth after treatment and the normal maxillary positioning on the face of these patients.[19,21]

The results revealed that the convexity angles, represented by the angular measurements NAP and ANB had a significant impact by the orthopedic mechanics of maxillary protraction (Table 6), which is also observed in studies analyzing the effects of maxillary protraction in the treatment of Class III malocclusion.[3,10,18,20] In addition to the alterations in facial convexity, the soft tissue profile was improved. The intentional ankylosis of deciduous canines increased the facial convexity (Table 6), as an immediate effect of maxillary protraction, which does not depend on facial growth.

The improved facial convexity is assigned to the sagittal change in the maxillary and mandibular apical bases. The literature demonstrated that the maxilla tends to present forward displacement with maxillary protraction.[3,5,6,8,9,10,12,13,17,18,21,22] However, this displacement was not statistically significant for the alveolar portion, represented by the SNA angle and the basal portion, characterized by the SN.ANS angle (Table 6). Even though no statistically significant difference was observed between groups in the SNA angle, this variable presented a greater mean alteration in the Ankylosis Group (2.94 in females and 2.07 in males) than the Control Group (0.78 in males and 0.27 in males), demonstrating that the forward displacement of point A was greater in the

Ankylosis Group (Table 5),explaining the significant increase in facial convexity evaluated by the variables NAP and ANB in the Ankylosis Group compared to the Control Group (Table 6).

The SNB angle presented more posterior positioning, especially in the group with intentional ankylosis of deciduous canines (Table 5). The sagittal improvement in point B is related to the mandibular rotation during maxillary protraction.[13] Indirectly, the increased angle of facial convexity is also influenced by the mandibular rotation. These changes promoted by maxillary protraction have been reported in the literature.[2,3,16,18,20,22,24] In the present study groups, the angles SN.GoGn and NS.Gn demonstrated that the mandible presented clockwise rotation, as mentioned in the literature,[3,4,5,8] yet without statistical significance. This behavior was similar in the two groups, indicating that ankylosis did not influence the mandibular rotation (Table 6).

The occlusal plane in the present study did not follow the mandibular rotation. This occurred in clockwise direction, while the occlusal plane presented counterclockwise rotation (Table 5). Due to the dental age of the sample, in the deciduous and early mixed dentition stages, the references taken to identify the mandibular occlusal plane, (mean occlusal point on the intercuspation surface of maxillary and mandibular first molars to the incisal edge of the permanent mandibular central incisors), were still in the period of eruption, with important variation in vertical direction. The vertical instability of the reference teeth at this period of occlusal development may explain the divergent behavior between the mandibular and occlusal planes. There is concern to maintain the inclination of the occlusal plane during maxillary protraction, by applying the elastic at the region of deciduous canines, directly on the fixed Haas expander.[15] The maxillary protraction from the posterior region is contraindicated in most patients because it lowers the posterior portion of the maxilla,[8] while protraction from the canines region controls this rotation effect during maxillary protraction.[21]

The linear measurements representing the sagittal behavior of the apical bases were defined by the distances Co-A, A-NPerp and Pg-NPerp. The point A presented forward positioning in relation to the cranial base in both groups (Table 5). The displacement of point A reflects the increased maxillary length. The literature has demonstrated that maxillary protraction induces an increase in maxillary length (ANS-PNS) compared to an untreated control group.[21] However, the forward displacement of point A was not influenced by the intentional ankylosis of deciduous canines, even though the maxillary displacement was greater in the group with ankylosis (Tables 5 and 6). Conversely, the point Pog exhibited more posterior positioning in relation to the line NPerp in the group with ankylosis (Table 6). The importance of the behavior of points A and Pog refers to their influence on facial convexity.

The interpretations related to the dental changes should consider that the permanent incisors were still in the period of eruption, since the patients were in the deciduous and early mixed dentition stages. Some changes in the tipping of these teeth occur during occlusion development and thus should be carefully analyzed.

The intentional ankylosis of deciduous canines did not influence the maxillary incisors. The literature unanimously reports the dental effect induced by orthopedic mechanics, with buccal tipping of maxillary incisors,[5,6] regardless of the accomplishment of intentional ankylosis of deciduous canines.[20] No exclusively orthopedic effect may be produced by tooth-supported appliances.[19] The question is if the intentional ankylosis of deciduous canines would reduce the orthodontic effect. Comparison between intentional ankylosis and the control group did not reveal difference between groups, indicating that an-

kylosis did not influence the dental compensation in the maxillary arch (Table 6). This result clearly demonstrates that the intentional ankylosis of deciduous canines may potentiate the orthopedic effect induced by maxillary protraction, yet does not avoid dental compensation in the maxilla, represented by the buccal tipping of maxillary incisors, except for the sample group female control (Table 5).

The mandibular incisors exhibited an unexpected change, with an increase in buccal tipping during orthopedic treatment in the group with intentional ankylosis. In general, reduced tipping of these teeth is expected in the orthopedic treatment for the Class III malocclusion, as part of the compensatory mechanism.[13] This result may be related to the treatment period, in the early mixed dentition stage, when the permanent incisors erupt. Another probable explanation for the behavior of mandibular incisors is the increased overjet provided by the maxillary advancement in the group with intentional ankylosis, providing additional space for buccal tipping of mandibular incisors.

CONCLUSIONS

The null hypothesis was accepted, because it was concluded that intentional ankylosis enhanced the sagittal response of the apical bases, as demonstrated by the alteration in Pg-NPerp and the increase in facial convexity angles (NAP and ANB).

REFERENCES

1. Baccetti T, McGill JS, Franchi L, McNamara JA Jr, Tollaro I. Skeletal effects of early treatment of Class III malocclusion with maxillary expansion and face-mask therapy. Am J Orthod Dentofacial Orthop. 1998;113(3):333-43.

2. Baik HS. Clinical results of the maxillary protraction in Korean children. Am J Orthod Dentofacial Orthop. 1995;108(6):583-92.

3. Chong YH, Ive JC, Artun J. Changes following the use of protraction headgear for early correction of Class III malocclusion. Angle Orthod. 1996;66(5):351-62.

4. Delaire J. Maxillary development revisited: relevance to the orthopedic treatment of Class III malocclusions. Eur J Orthod. 1997;19(3):289-311.

5. Dahlberg G. Statistical methods for medical and biological students. New York: Interscience; 1940.

6. Gallagher RW, Miranda F, Buschang PH. Maxillary protraction: treatment and postreatment effects. Am J Orthod Dentofacial Orthop. 1998;113(6):612-9.

7. Göyenç Y, Ersoy S. The effect of a modified reverse headgear force applied with a facebow on the dentofacial structures. Eur J Orthod. 2004;26(1):51-7.

8. Houston WJ. The analysis of errors in orthodontic measurements. Am J Orthod. 1983;83(5):382-90.

9. Ishii H, Morita S, Takeuchi Y, Nakamura S. Treatment effect of combined maxillary protraction and chincap appliance in severe skeletal Class III cases. Am J Orthod Dentofacial Orthop. 1987;92(4):304-12.

10. Kapust AJ, Sinclair PM, Turley PK. Cephalometric effects of face mask/expansion therapy in Class III children: a comparison of three ages groups. Am J Orthod Dentofacial Orthop. 1998;113(2):204-12.

11. Kiliçoglu H, Kirliç Y. Profile changes in patients with Class III malocclusions after Delaire mask therapy. Am J Orthod Dentofacial Orthop. 1998;113(4):453-62.

12. McNamara JA Jr. An orthopedic approach to the treatment of Class III malocclusion in young patients. J Clin Orthod. 1987;21(9):598-608.

13. Mermigos J, Full CA, Andreasen G. Protraction of the maxillofacial complex. Am J Orthod Dentofacial Orthop. 1990;98(1):47-55.

14. Ngan P, Hägg U, Yiu C, Merwin D, Wei SH. Soft tissue and dentoskeletal profile changes associated with maxillary expansion and protraction headgear treatment. Am J Orthod Dentofacial Orthop. 1996;109(1):38-49.

15. Ngan P, Hägg U, Yiu C, Merwin D, Wei SH. Treatment response to maxillary expansion and protraction. Eur J Orthod. 1996;18(2):151-68.

16. Ngan PW, Hagg U, Yiu C, Wei SH. Treatment response and long-term dentofacial adaptations to maxillary expansion and protraction. Semin Orthod. 1997;3(4):255-64.

17. Saadia M, Torres E. Sagittal changes after maxillary protraction with expansion in Class III patients in the primary, mixed and late mixed dentitions: a longitudinal retrospective study. Am J Orthod Dentofacial Orthop. 2000; 117(6):669-80.

18. Shanker S, Ngan P, Wade D, Beck M, Yiu C, Hägg U, Wei SH. Cephalometric A point changes during and after maxillary protraction and expansion. Am J Orthod Dentofacial Orthop. 1996;110(4):423-30.

19. Silva Filho OG, Magro AC, Capelozza Filho L. Early treatment of the Class III malocclusion with rapid maxillary expansion and maxillary protraction. Am J Orthod Dentofacial Orthop. 1998;113(2):196-203.

20. Silva Filho OG, Ozawa TO, Okada CH, Okada HY, Carvalho RM. Intentional ankylosis of deciduous canines to reinforce maxillary protraction. J Clin Orthod. 2003;37(6):315-20.

21. Silva Filho OG, Ozawa TO, Okada CH, Okada HY, Dahmen L. Anquilose intencional dos caninos decíduos como reforço de ancoragem para a tração reversa da maxila. Estudo cefalométrico prospectivo. Rev Dental Press Ortod Ortop Facial. 2006;11(6):35-44.

22. Sung SJ, Baik HS. Assessment of skeletal and dental changes by maxillary protraction. Am J Orthod Dentofacial Orthop. 1998;114(5):492-502.

23. Takada K, Petdachai S, Sakuda M. Changes in dentofacial morphology in skeletal Class III children treated by a modified maxillary protraction headgear and a chin cup: a longitudinal cephalometric appraisal. Eur J Orthod. 1993;15(3):211-21.

24. Turley PK. Orthopedic correction of Class III malocclusion: Retention and phase II therapy. J Clin Orthod. 1996;30(6):313-24.

8

Compensatory orthodontic treatment of skeletal Class III malocclusion with anterior crossbite

José Valladares Neto[1]

Introduction: This case report describes the orthodontic treatment of an adult patient with skeletal Class III malocclusion and anterior crossbite. A short cranial base led to difficulties in establishing a cephalometric diagnosis. The patient's main complaint comprised esthetics of his smile and difficulties in mastication. **Methods:** The patient did not have the maxillary first premolars and refused orthognathic surgery. Therefore, the treatment chosen was orthodontic camouflage and extraction of mandibular first premolars. For maxillary retraction, the vertical dimension was temporarily increased to avoid obstacles to orthodontic movement. **Results:** At the end of the treatment, ideal overjet and overbite were achieved. **Conclusion:** Examination eight years after orthodontic treatment revealed adequate clinical stability. This case report was submitted to the Brazilian Board of Orthodontics and Facial Orthopedics (BBO) as part of the requirements to become a BBO diplomate.

Keywords: Crossbite. Tooth extraction. Corrective orthodontics.

[1] Adjunct Professor, Department of Orthodontics, Federal University of Goiás.
Certified by the Brazilian Board of Orthodontics and Facial Orthopedics.

» The author reports no commercial, proprietary or financial interest in the products or companies described in this article.

José Valladares Neto
Rua 132, número 113, Setor Sul - Goiânia-GO / Brazil
CEP: 74093-210
E-mail: jvalladares@uol.com.br

INTRODUCTION

A 22-year and 10-month-old male patient arrived for his initial examination in good general health, complaining about his smile, particularly an anterior crossbite and maxillary diastemas, as well as difficulties associated with mastication. His dental history included the extraction of maxillary first premolars at the age of 12, carried out by a clinical dentist due to lack of adequate space for eruption of maxillary canines.

DIAGNOSIS

Facial examination revealed balanced characteristics: mesofacial pattern, symmetric features and adequate lip seal. However, a sagittal maxillomandibular deficiency was also noted. The patient had narrow nostrils, slightly ptotic nasal tip, paranasal deficiency, marked grooves at rest and when smiling, a short mentocervical line and an obtuse mentocervical angle, which confirmed the diagnosis. There was also a discrete predominance of maxillary deficiency (Fig 1).

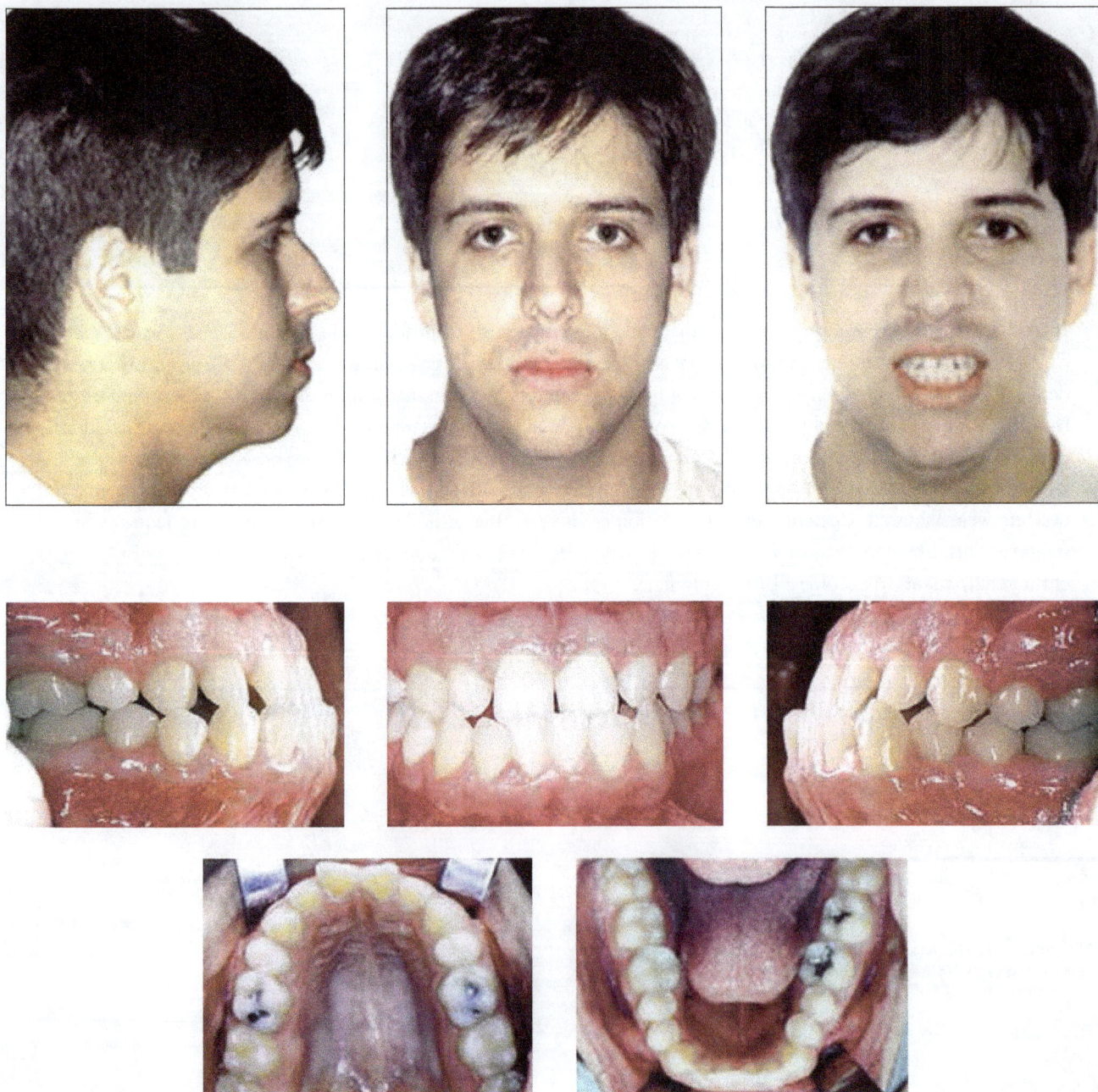

Figure 1 - Initial facial and intraoral photographs.

The examination of temporomandibular joints revealed bilateral clicking at mandibular opening and closing, maximal mouth opening of 43 mm and an irregular path, but no pain.

Intraoral clinical examination revealed adequate oral hygiene. Malocclusion was classified as Angle Class I with anterior crossbite, absence of maxillary first premolars, canines in full Class III relationship, anterior mandibular crowding, rotated maxillary central incisors and anterior diastemas (Figs 1 and 2). There were no differences between usual maximal intercuspation and centric relation. Radiographs showed that the patient had good dental and periodontal health and no endodontic problem or bone loss (Figs 3 and 4).

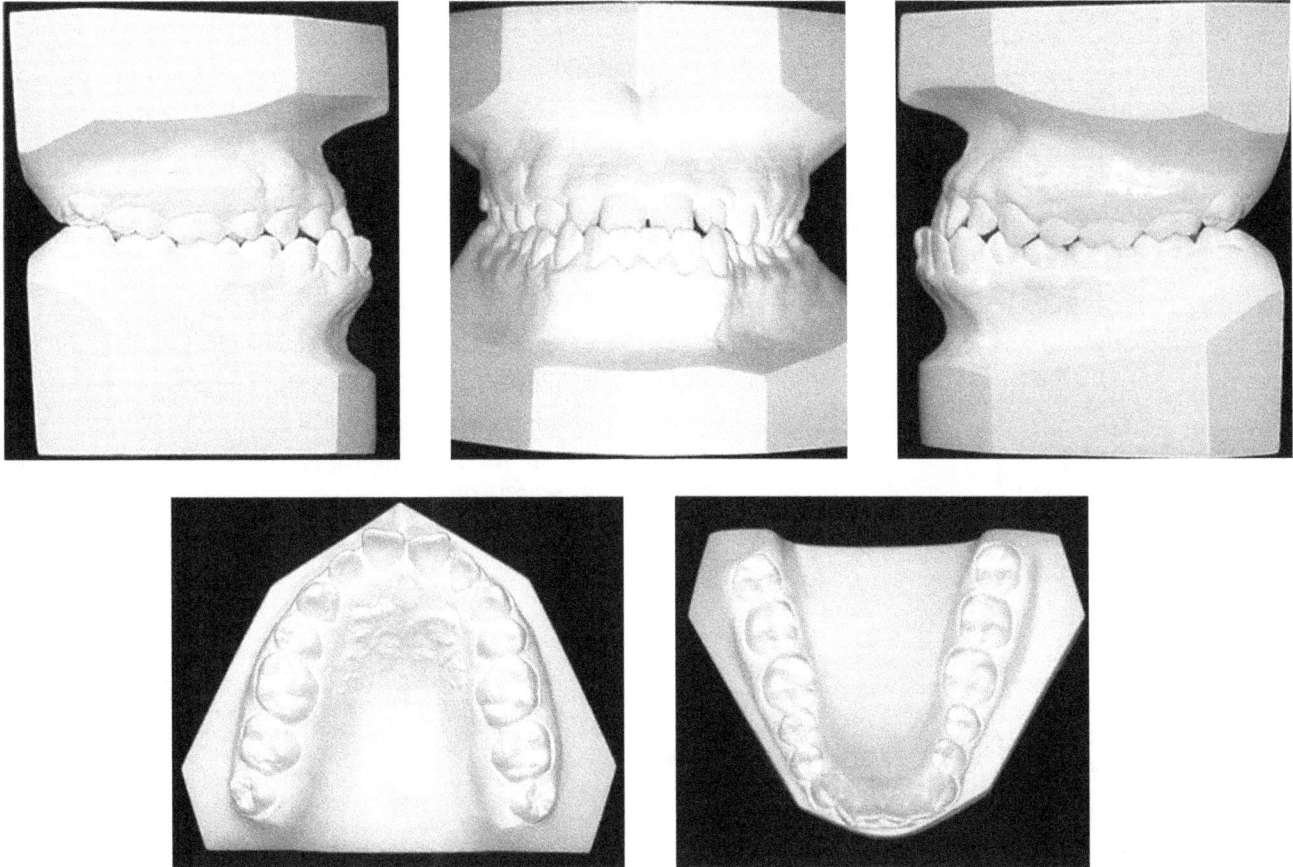

Figure 2 - Initial casts.

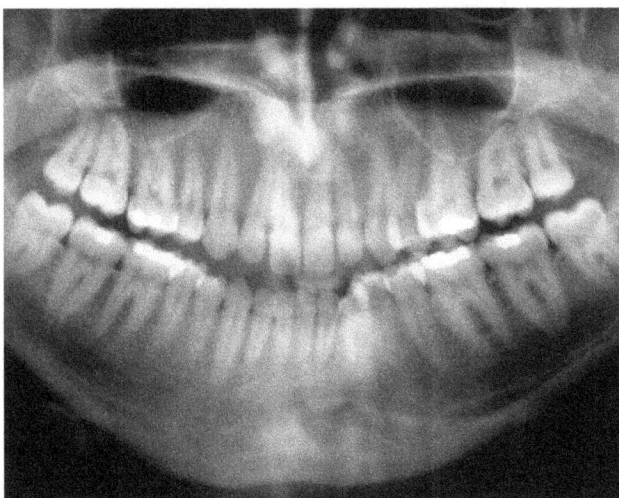

Figure 3 - Initial panoramic radiograph.

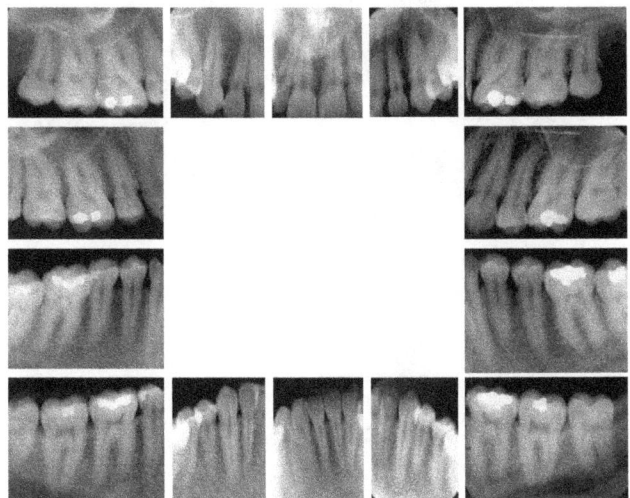

Figure 4 - Initial periapical radiographs.

Cephalometry revealed that the maxillomandibular relationship was apparently normal (ANB = 2°) and that a few angles were slightly greater than normal (Conv. = 5.5°; SNA = 86°; SNB = 84°) (Fig 5). However, the ANB angle is known to be markedly affected by geometrical factors.[1] When the cranial base is short, maxillomandibular discrepancies cannot be evaluated on the sagittal plane using the ANB angle (Fig 6). Other cephalometric parameters (Wits = -8 mm; S-N = 71.5 mm) and particularly facial analysis should be used to elucidate this confounding factor.[2,3]

When evaluated by cephalometry and having the cranial base as reference, maxillary and mandibular incisors showed buccal inclination and marked protrusion (1-NA = 25°, 1-NA = 7 mm) in mandibular teeth (1-NB = 34°, 1-NB = 11 mm). In contrast, the inclination of mandibular incisors in relation to the mandibular plane was good and met the Brazilian standards (IMPA = 94°).[2]

TREATMENT PLAN

The first treatment plan presented to the patient was the orthodontic combined with orthognathic surgery, which the patient promptly refused. For this reason, an alternative plan was suggested. It included orthodontic camouflage with orthodontic appliances in both arches and extraction of mandibular first premolars. The patient had undergone extraction of maxillary first premolars and, therefore, our aim was to achieve normal molar and canine occlusion. Mandibular extractions followed by retraction of anterior teeth should be supported by adequate anchorage control.

The dentist and the patient agreed on the following objectives for the treatment selected: preservation of maxillary and mandibular bones position; alignment and reduction in maxillary diastemas; alignment of mandibular teeth; normal occlusion, correction of negative overjet and functional occlusion; esthetic improvement after lower lip retraction; and achievement of a pleasant smile.

Treatment plan was divided into the following phases: modified Nance lingual arch (away from mandibular incisors); fixed orthodontic appliances in both arches using the straight-wire system and 0.022 x 0.028-in slots; extraction of mandibular first premolars; tooth leveling and alignment with

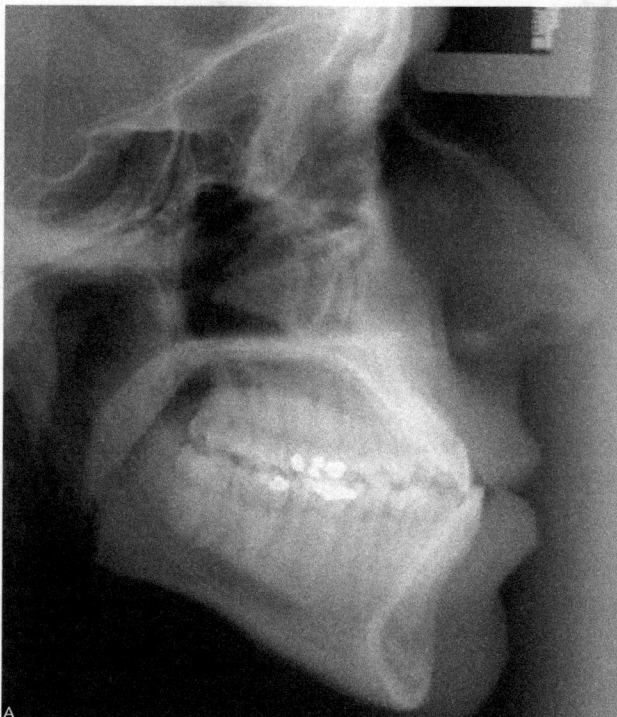

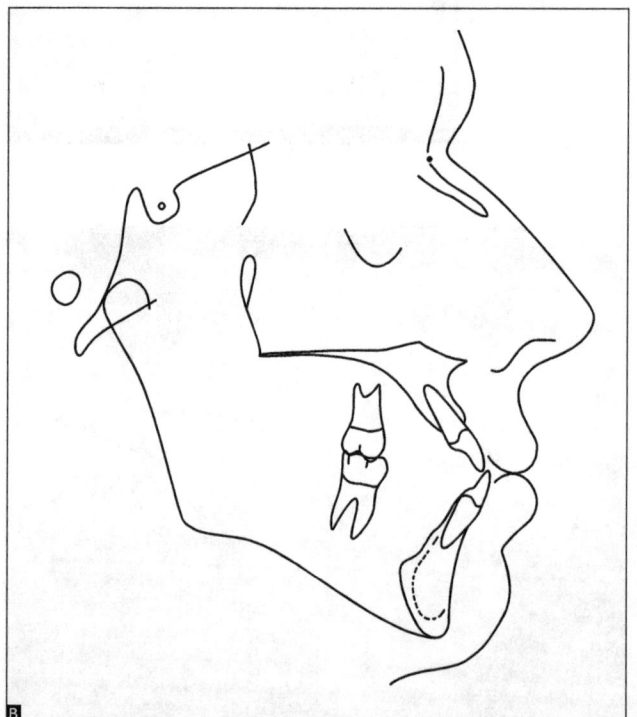

Figure 5 - A) Initial cephalometric profile radiograph and B) cephalometric tracing.

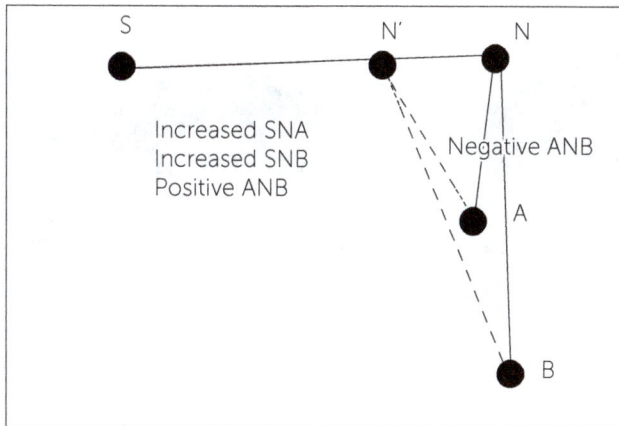

Figure 6 - Diagram illustrating Class III skeletal relationship with short (**N'**) and normal (**N**) anterior cranial bases.

0.012-in, 0.014-in and 0.016-in nickel-titanium wires and 0.018-in, 0.020-in and 0.017 x 0.025-in stainless steel wires; retraction of mandibular anterior teeth using sliding mechanics and 0.019 x 0.025-in stainless steel wire; removal of lingual arch; orthodontic treatment finishing; retention.

TREATMENT PROGRESSION

Treatment progression was in accordance with the plan. Mandibular second molars were included in initial leveling to aggregate an anchorage unit for the retraction of incisors. Maxillary second molars were bonded and included in leveling during orthodontic finishing.

The vertical dimension had to be temporarily increased with glass-ionomer cement built-up on posterior teeth. This procedure was used for retraction of mandibular anterior teeth because anterior crossbite and marked overjet were obstacles to movement (Figs 7A, B and C). Spaces were closed by means of sliding mechanics (0.019 x 0.025-in wire) and hooks were soldered between canines and lateral incisors. Class III intermaxillary elastics (¼-in, medium force) were used to control anchorage together with the lingual arch which was removed after retraction of anterior teeth and closing of extraction spaces. No skeletal anchorage was used. Treatment was completed with 0.018-in archwires, elastic chains in both arches to retain interproximal contacts, and Class II intermaxillary elastics (5/6-in, medium force) to retain the movement achieved (Figs 7D, E and F). After orthodontic completion, intercuspation was good, and canine and molar occlusion relationships, as well as overjet, were normal (Fig 8, 9). Maxillary (2 x 2) and mandibular (4 x 4) V-looped braided bonded lingual archwires were placed for retention.

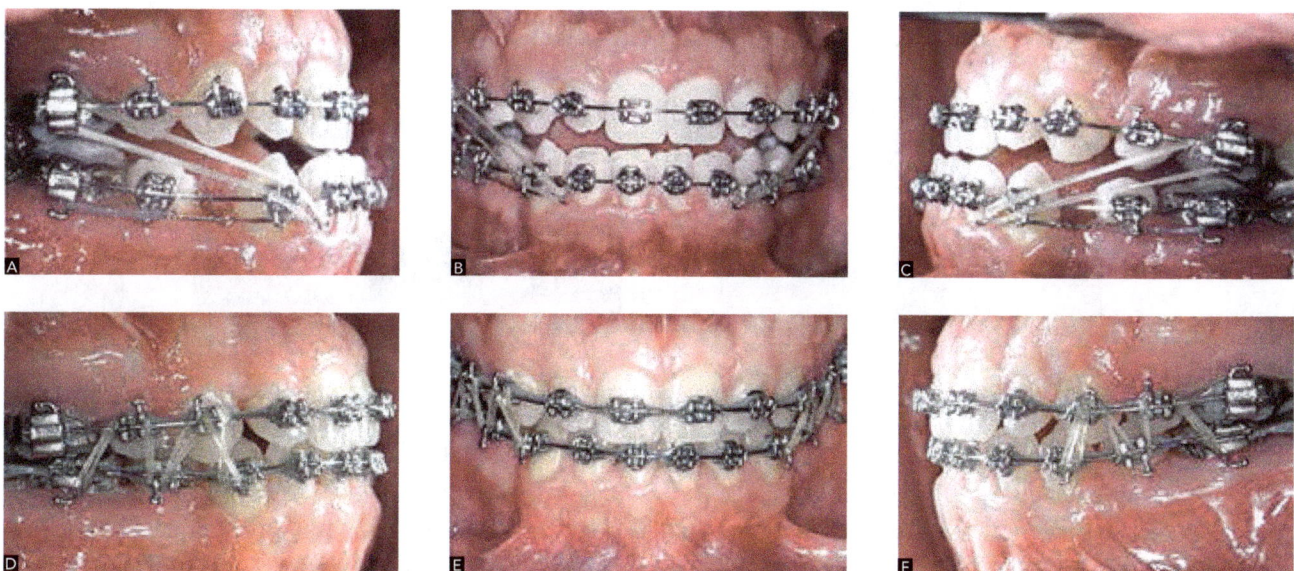

Figure 7 - Increased vertical dimension during retraction of mandibular anterior teeth (**A, B, C**) and treatment completion phase (**D, E, F**).

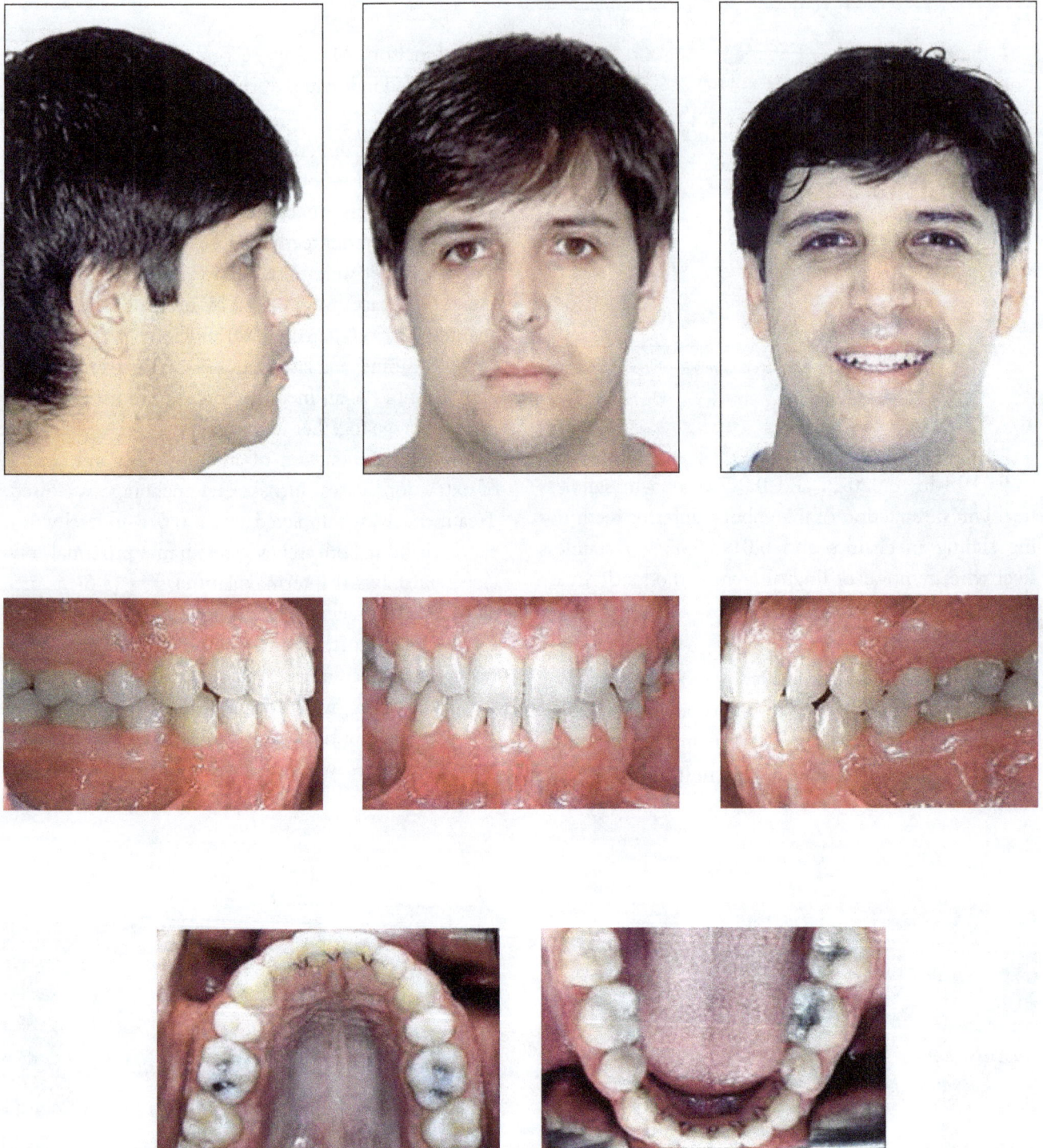

Figure 8 - Final facial and intraoral photographs.

RESULTS

The final radiograph showed that root parallelism was good after space closure and that root size was preserved (Figs 10 and 11).

In the maxillary arch, diastemas were reduced, molars were slightly extruded, intercanine distance (35.5 mm) was preserved and intermolar distance was shortened (from 43.5 mm to 42.0 mm). A marked cephalometric effect was found in the mandibular arch with anterior retraction, intrusion and mesial movement of mandibular molars (Fig 12 and Table 1). However, intercanine (21.5 mm) and intermolar (33.0 mm) distances did not change.

There were no significant changes in the position of the maxilla or the mandible (Fig 13). Facial esthet-

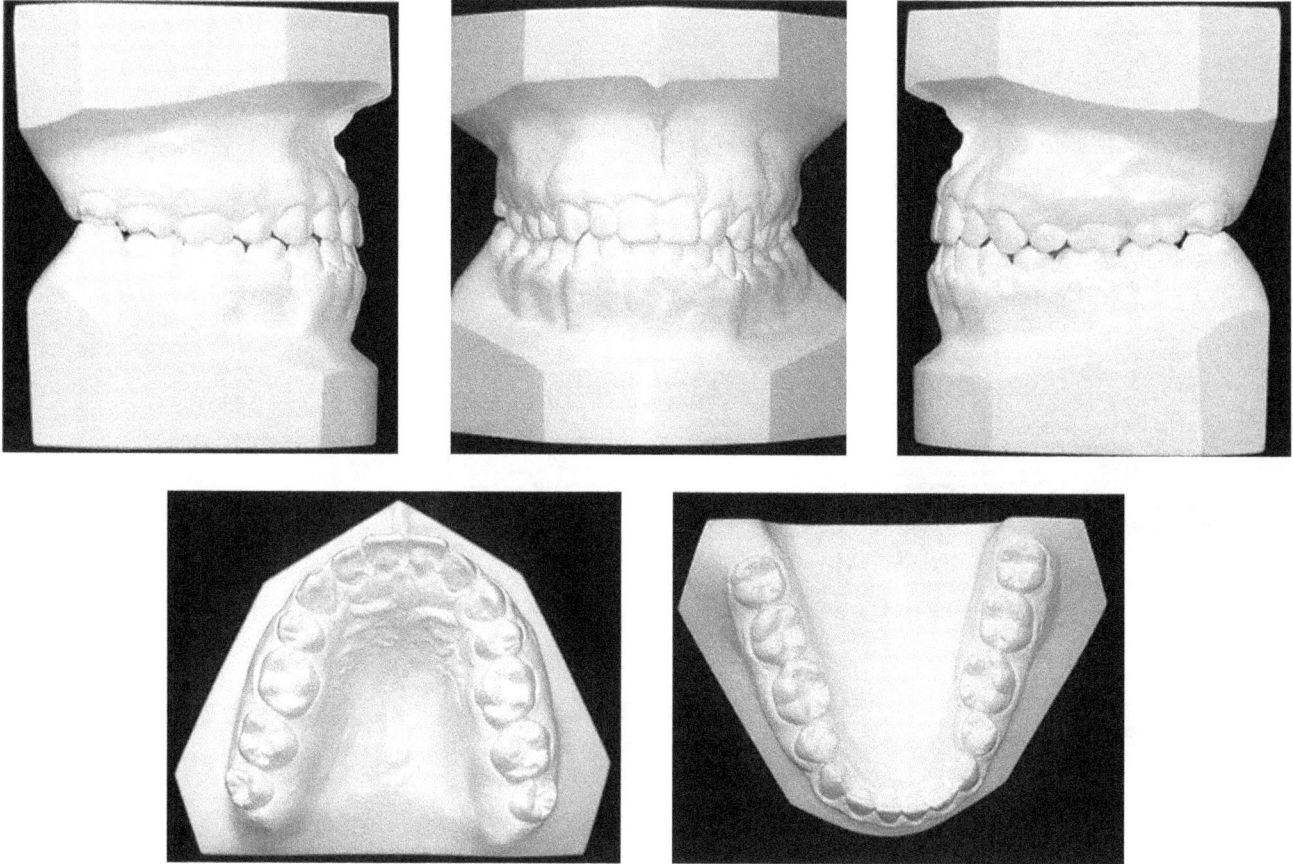

Figure 9 - Final casts.

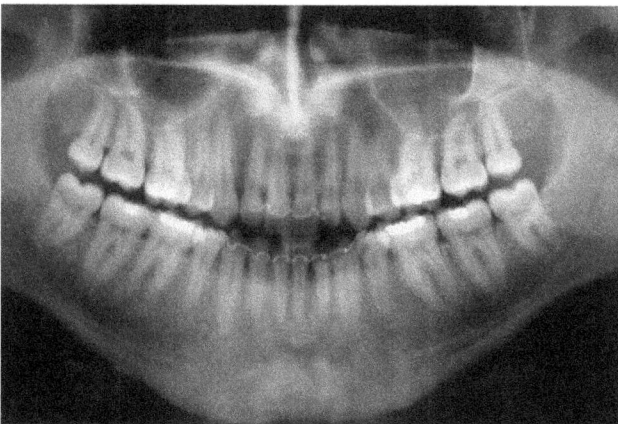

Figure 10 - Final panoramic radiograph.

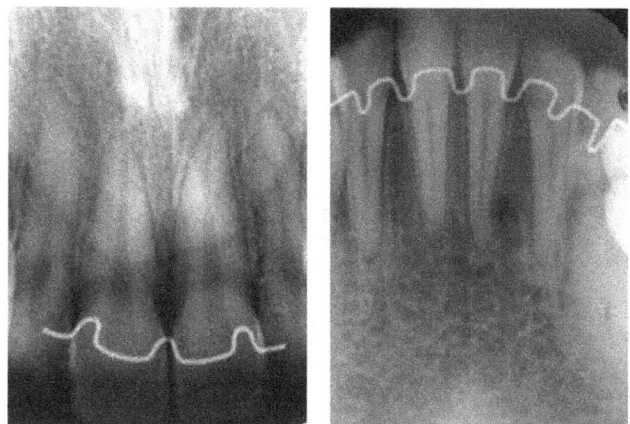

Figure 11 - Final periapical radiographs of maxillary and mandibular incisors.

ics improved due to less marked lower lip protrusion, confirmed by reduction of 2.5 mm in the cephalometric variable that describes the lower lip (S line) (Fig 14 and Table 1).

The relationship between the maxilla and the mandible showed good intercuspation and coordination, although sagittal skeletal discrepancy was camouflaged by dental compensation. Overjet and overbite were fully corrected, and the criteria for ideal functional occlusion were met. The positive results, confirmed by clinical stability eight years after treatment completion, were favored by the lack of remaining facial growth, the use of fixed retention and patient's satisfactory occlusal relationship (Fig 15).

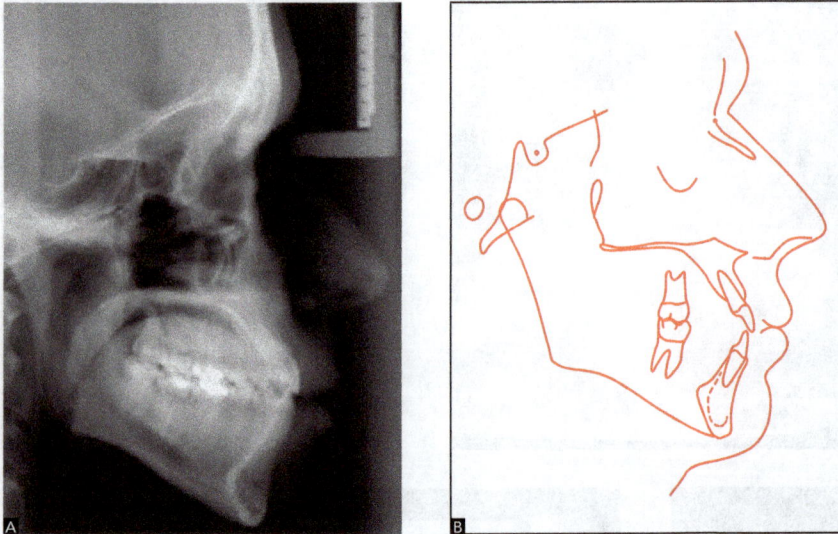

Figure 12 - **A**) Final cephalometric profile radiograph and **B**) cephalometric tracing.

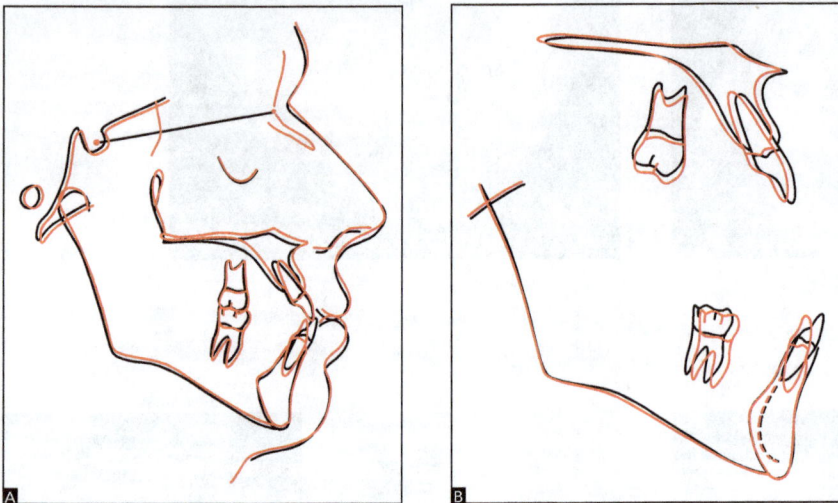

Figure 13 - **A**) Total and **B**) partial superimpositions of initial (black) and final (red) cephalometric tracings.

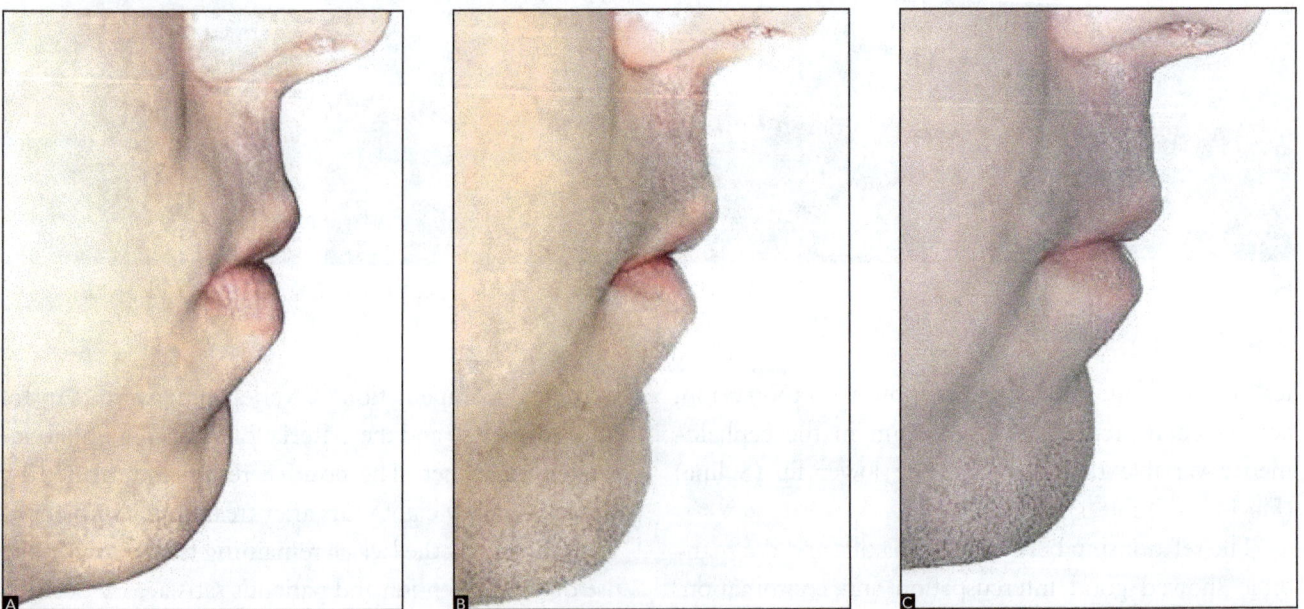

Figure 14 - Comparison of facial profile close-up: **A**) initial, **B**) final and **C**) control eight years later.

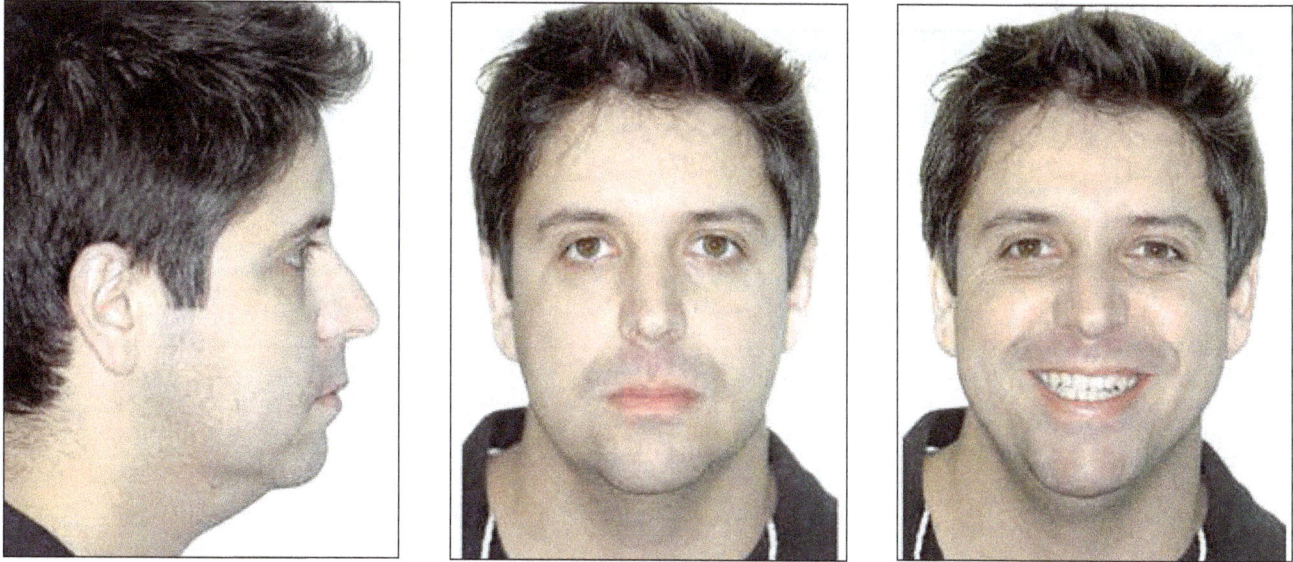

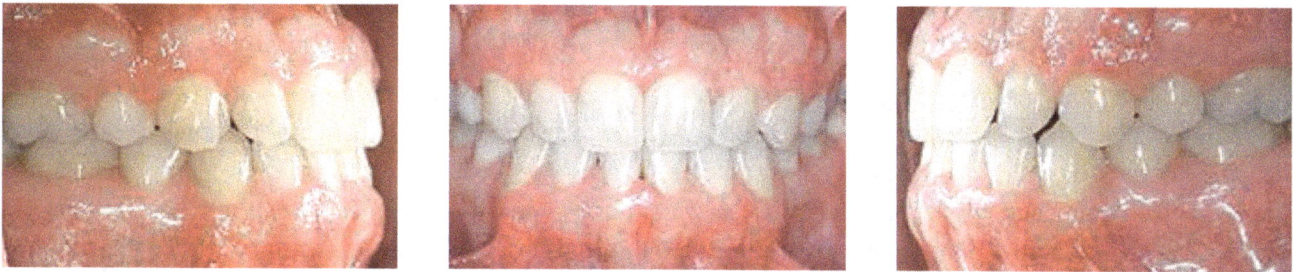

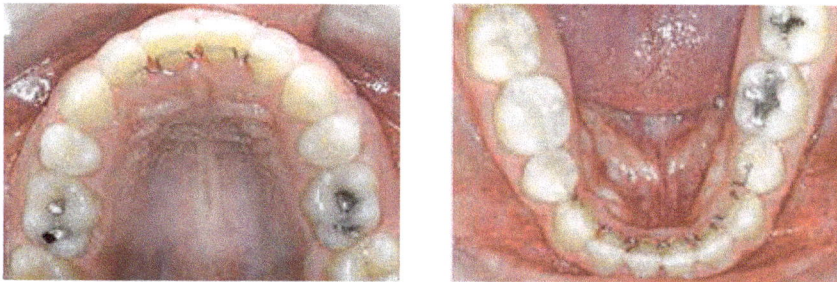

Figure 15 - Facial and intraoral control photographs eight years after treatment completion.

Table 1 - Initial (**A**) and final (**B**) cephalometric values.

	Measures		Normal	A	B	A/B diff.
Skeletal pattern	SNA	(Steiner)	82°	86°	85°	1°
	SNB	(Steiner)	80°	84°	83°	1°
	ANB	(Steiner)	2°	2°	2.5°	-0.5°
	Facial angle	(Downs)	0°	5.5°	6.5°	-1.0°
	Y axis	(Downs)	59°	57°	57°	0°
	Facial angle	(Downs)	87°	93°	92°	1°
	SN-GoGn	(Steiner)	32°	34°	34°	0°
	FMA	(Tweed)	25°	26°	23°	3°
Dental pattern	IMPA	(Tweed)	90°	94°	78°	16°
	1.NA	(Steiner)	22°	26°	25°	1°
	1-NA	(Steiner)	4 mm	7 mm	6 mm	1 mm
	1.NB	(Steiner)	25°	34°	17°	17°
	1-NB	(Steiner)	4 mm	11 mm	4 mm	7 mm
	1.1 – Interincisal angle	(Downs)	130°	115°	135°	-20°
	1-APo	(Ricketts)	1 mm	10 mm	5 mm	5 mm
Profile	Upper lip – S line	(Steiner)	0 mm	0 mm	0 mm	0 mm
	Lower lip – S line	(Steiner)	0 mm	3 mm	0.5 mm	2.5 mm

FINAL CONSIDERATIONS

Cranial base abnormalities strongly affect the interpretation of cephalometric variables in this region, particularly SNA, SNB, ANB and convexity angle. Other cephalometric parameters, correction factors and, above all, facial analysis findings contributed to making the diagnosis and developing a treatment plan. In adults, Class III skeletal patterns may often be treated with either orthodontic camouflage or orthognathic surgery.[4,5] In the case reported here, the treatment chosen was orthodontic camouflage with extraction of mandibular first premolars. Treatment results were satisfactory, and the occlusal objectives were achieved. The final harmonious smile pleased the patient and improved his self-esteem and quality of life.

REFERENCES

1. Hussels W, Nanda RS. Analysis of factors affecting angle ANB. Am J Orthod. 1984;85(5):411-23.

2. Martins DR, Janson GRP, Almeida RR, Pinzan A, Henriques JFC, Freitas MR. Atlas de crescimento craniofacial. 1a ed. São Paulo: Ed. Santos; 1998.

3. Arnett GW, Gunson MJ. Facial planning for orthodontistis and oral surgeons. Am J Orthod Dentofacial Orthop. 2004;126(3):290-5.

4. Benyahia H, Azaroual MF, Garcia C, Hamou E, Abouqal, R, Zaoui F. Treatment of skeletal Class III malocclusions: orthognathic surgery or orthodontic camouflage? How to decide. Int Orthod. 2011;9(2):196-209.

5. Burns NR, Musich DR, Martin C, Razmus T, Gunel E, Ngan P. Class III camouflage treatment: what are the limits? Am J Orthod Dentofacial Orthop. 2010;137(1):9.e1-13; discussion 9-11.

9

Three-dimensional dental arch changes of patients submitted to orthodontic-surgical treatment for correction of Class II malocclusion

Adriano Porto Peixoto[1], Ary dos Santos Pinto[2], Daniela Gamba Garib[3], João Roberto Gonçalves[4]

Introduction: This study assessed the three-dimensional changes in the dental arch of patients submitted to orthodontic-surgical treatment for correction of Class II malocclusions at three different periods. **Methods:** Landmarks previously identified on upper and lower dental casts were digitized on a three-dimensional digitizer MicroScribe-3DX and stored in Excel worksheets in order to assess the width, length and depth of patient's dental arches. **Results:** During orthodontic preparation, the maxillary and mandibular transverse dimensions measured at the premolar regions were increased and maintained throughout the follow-up period. Intercanine width was increased only in the upper arch during orthodontic preparation. Maxillary arch length was reduced during orthodontic finalization, only. Upper and lower arch depths were stable in the study periods. Differences between centroid and gingival changes suggested that upper and lower arch premolars buccaly proclined during the pre-surgical period. **Conclusions:** Maxillary and mandibular dental arches presented transverse expansion at premolar regions during preoperative orthodontic preparation, with a tendency towards buccal tipping. The transverse dimensions were not altered after surgery. No sagittal or vertical changes were observed during the follow-up periods.

Keywords: Orthodontics. Orthognathic surgery. Malocclusion. Dental models.

[1] PhD resident in Oral and Maxillofacial Surgery, School of Dentistry – State University of São Paulo/Araraquara.
[2] Full Professor, Department of Orthodontics, School of Dentistry - State University of São Paulo/Araraquara.
[3] Full Professor, Department of Orthodontics. Hospital of Rehabilitation of Craniofacial Anomalies, School of Dentistry — University of São Paulo/Bauru.
[4] Assistant Professor, Department of Orthodontics, School of Dentistry-State University of São Paulo/Araraquara.

» The authors report no commercial, proprietary or financial interest in the products or companies described in this article.

João Roberto Gonçalves
Rua Humaitá, 1680 - 1º. Andar - 14.801-903 - Araraquara - São Paulo - Brazil
E-mail: joaogonc2002@yahoo.com.br

INTRODUCTION

An increasing number of adult patients seek orthodontic treatment not only for esthetic reasons, but also due to recent improvements in socioeconomic conditions. This new perspective raised the need to investigate skeletal and dental changes in soft tissue morphology occurring in adult individuals, considering the increasing search for orthodontic and orthognathic treatment.[1]

Knowledge on these changes in adulthood may help to determine if changes observed after orthodontic treatment occur primarily due to orthodontic relapse or are part of the natural process of development and maturation.[2]

Harris[3] highlighted that changes in shape and size of the craniofacial dentoskeletal complex do not cease with biological maturity. Adulthood does not necessarily correspond to a period of absence of growth; even though change rates are lower and growth directions may be different than observed in children and adolescents. Therefore, changes occur, especially in the long term.

Long-term studies assessed the postoperative changes of orthodontically treated cases. In general, there is a tendency towards continuous reduction in the width and length of dental arches, with increase in crowding, overbite and overjet. The greatest problem has been the inability to determine whether these changes occur primarily as a result of orthodontic treatment, or if they are part of the natural maturation process.[4]

The stability of surgical changes in transverse dimensions has not been extensively assessed. Few specific studies[5,6] investigated the stability of dental arches. Moreover, these few studies have important limitations because they do not describe the surgical technique employed and do not differentiate orthodontic relapse (dental) from surgical relapse (skeletal). An investigation with good methodology was conducted by Martin[7] to assess the three-dimensional changes occurring in the maxillary dental arch of patients submitted to segmented osteotomy in a long-term follow-up.

In this context, this study aims at assessing the three-dimensional changes occurring in the dental arch morphology of patients submitted to orthognathic surgery for correction of skeletal Class II malocclusions.

MATERIAL AND METHODS

This retrospective study was conducted with 15 patients (10 females and 5 males) with skeletal Class II division 1 malocclusion (Table 1) whose files were obtained from the Center for Research and Treatment of Orofacial Deformities (CEDEFACE, Araraquara, São Paulo, Brazil) and a private maxillofacial surgery practice. Dental casts were obtained at three periods: (T_1) initial, (T_2) immediate preoperative (1 to 15 days before surgery) and (T_3) postoperative (minimum 6 months after the orthodontic appliance was removed). The following inclusion criteria were applied: 1) presence of all permanent teeth erupted and present in the dental arches at least from the maxillary right first molar to the maxillary left first molar; 2) dental casts with good conditions for analysis; 3) absence of anomalies of shape, incisal or occlusal abrasion, coronal fracture, caries or restorations requiring reconstruction during the study period; 4) absence of other craniofacial deformities, syndromes or cleft lip and palate; 5) preoperative and postoperative orthodontic treatment conducted without mechanical expansion or tooth extraction; 6) patients submitted to a single orthognathic surgery on one or both jaws; 7) patients older than 18 years old at surgery.

Patients comprising the sample were operated by means of the following surgical techniques: single-piece Le Fort I osteotomy combined with bilateral sagittal split mandibular osteotomy, or isolated bilateral sagittal split mandibular osteotomy.

The method employed in this retrospective study was similar to that described by Martin[7] who used a three-dimensional digitizer MicroScribe-3DX (3D Digitizer – The Imaging Technology Group, Illinois, USA) for digitization of predetermined landmarks on the dental casts, following the method described by Moyers et al.[8] The software was developed for digitization and automatic storage of captured coordinates by registry in X, Y and Z coordinates on the Excel software (Microsoft Windows - Excel 12.0 - Office 2007).

A total of 54 landmarks were identified on the maxillary arch and 52 on the mandibular arch (Fig 1) from second molar (when present) to te canines at both sides including: mid-distal, mid-buccal, mid-mesial, mid-palatal, and gingival, each individually identified for each tooth. A gingival landmark was also identified between central incisors, the most anterior

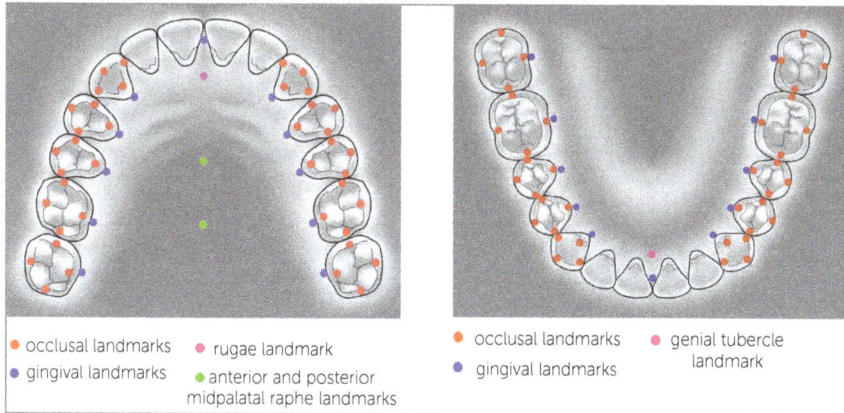

Figure 1 - Landmarks on the maxillary dental cast.

landmark in the dental arches (midline landmark = MP, Fig 1). Additional landmarks were also identified on the maxillary dental arch, namely: the rugae landmark (most posterior landmark on the incisive papilla), two landmarks on the palate (midpalatal raphe), being the first (anterior midpalatal raphe = AMR) between the first and second premolars and the second (posterior midpalatal raphe = PMR) at the mid-region of the first molar, following the position of the gingival landmark. On the mandibular dental arch, a midpoint was identified between the genial tubercles (a small rounded elevation on the lingual surface of the mandible on either side of the midline near the inferior border of the body of the mandible). The gingival landmark was identified on the most convex point of the gingival margin on the lingual aspect of each tooth. This process was repeated for each dental cast at different periods (T_1, T_2 and T_3).

Dental casts were measured by a single examiner who was previously calibrated. Method error was assessed by intraclass correlation coefficient (ICC). For that purpose, all 15 triads of dental casts were digitized at two different periods, with a one-week interval.

At T_2, for digitization of gingival landmarks obtained at the region of first and second molars (when present), the thickness of the band was subtracted, because this situation differs from T_1 and T_3, when the patients were not wearing any fixed appliances. This was performed considering the mean thickness (0.20 mm) of bands of the main brands commercially available in Brazil (Abzil, Morelli).

All landmarks were digitized on each dental cast (T_1, T_2 and T_3) and coordinates were stored in Excel worksheets specifically developed for that purpose.

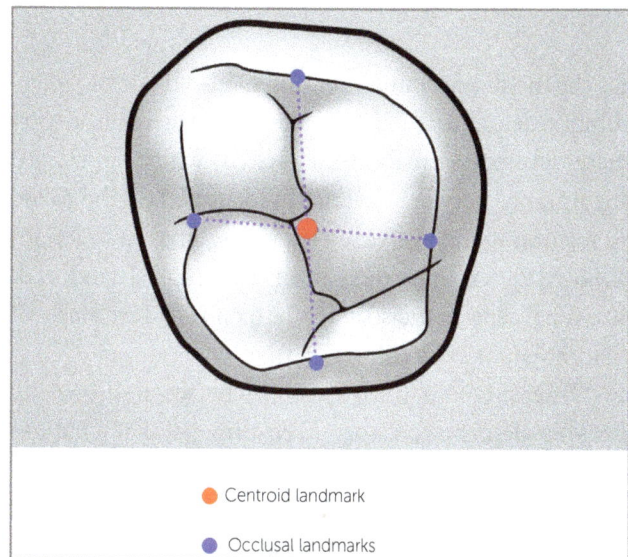

Figure 2 - Identification of the centroid landmark.

After identifying and recording all landmarks, the centroid landmarks were calculated for each tooth (Fig 2) using the values obtained on the X, Y and Z axis between the mid-distal and buccal-palatal landmarks, as described by Moyers et al.[8] As a result, the process obtained measurements that are relatively independent from cusp wear and are sensitive to crown translation and tooth inclination.[5]

Transverse dimensions were calculated between canines (W3-3), first premolars (W4-4), seconds premolars (W5-5), first molars (W6-6) and second molars (W7-7) (when present) at both sides, both on the centroid landmarks (C) of crowns and on gingival margins (G) of teeth.

Arch depths were measured from the gingival landmark between central incisors perpendicular to a line connecting the centroids of canines (D33-RUGAE), premolars (D44-AMR) and first molars (D66-PMR)

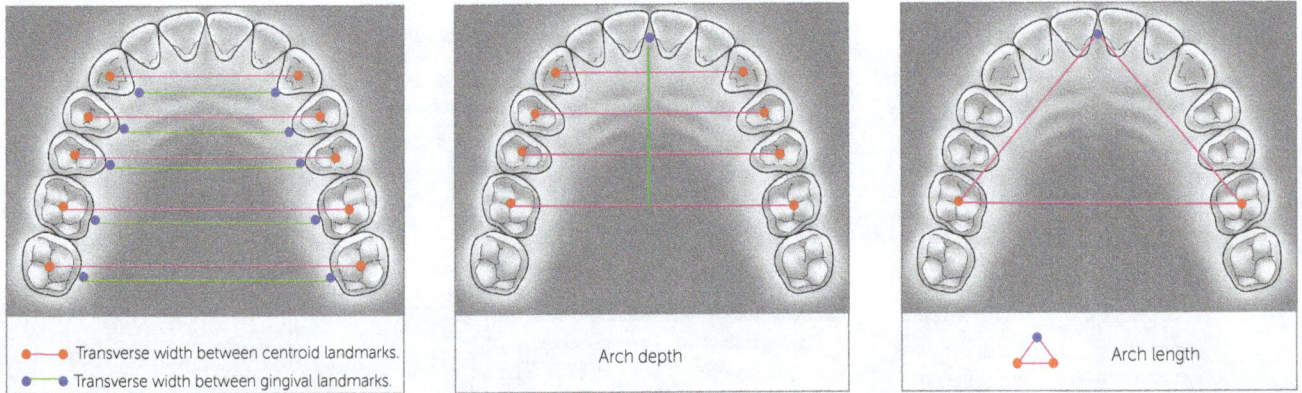

Figure 3 - Width (A), depth (B) and length (C) measurements on maxillary dental cast.

for the maxillary dental arch, and D66-MP for the mandibular dental arch. Values were calculated on a software developed on the Excel system which subtracted the distance between landmarks identified on the palate in relation to a constructed transverse line. Arch length (L66-MP) was measured from the gingival landmark between central incisors to the centroid landmark of first molar on both sides (Fig 3).

Differences in measurements between the study periods determined the three-dimensional changes occurring in the dental arches during preoperative orthodontic treatment (T_2-T_1) and after treatment completion (T_3-T_2). The total differences in treatment were also calculated, including the postoperative period (T_3-T_1).

Data were processed and analyzed on the statistical software SPSS version 15.0 (SPSS Inc, Chicago, Il, USA) for Microsoft Windows. The hypothesis of equality of means at the three periods for each variable was analyzed using the procedure general linear model – repeated measure.

RESULTS

The hypothesis was rejected when the p-value associated with the Hotteling-Lawley Trace was lower than 0.05. The means of variables for which this hypothesis was rejected when compared two by two by Bonferroni test for multiple comparisons of means. Test power is also presented for these variables. The correspondence of tooth movement (centroid) and skeletal movement (gingival) was compared by Student t-test for paired samples and Pearson correlation

coefficient. The sample comprised 10 females and 5 males with mean ages of 27.5 and 20.7 years, respectively, at treatment onset.

Mandibular arch

The transverse dimension between the centroid landmarks of second molars (W7-7) reduced in 0.58 mm after surgery (T_3-T_2). Differences among the measured widths in the centroid landmarks and measured widths in the gingival landmarks (W7-7C x W7-7G), indicative of buccal lingual inclinations, showed an increase of 0.65 mm during the pre-surgical phase (T_2-T_1) and a reduction of 0.54 mm in the post-surgical period (T_3-T_2), returning to the initial dimensions (T_3-T_1).

The difference in width between centroid and gingival landmarks (W6-6C x W6-6G) increased in 0.89 mm during the pre-surgical period (T_2-T_1) and reduced in 1.2 mm after surgery (T_3-T_2), returning to the initial values at the final evaluation, T_3-T_1 (Table 3).

The width between second premolars (W5-5) increased during orthodontic preparation (centroid: +1.69; gingival: +1.29), and remained stable from T_2 to T_3 (Table 2). The differences between centroid and gingival landmarks (W5-5C x W5-5G) increased in 0.4 mm during the pre-surgical period (T_2-T_1) (Table 3).

The width between first premolars (W4-4 C and G) showed similar results, as observed for second premolars at both study periods: T_2-T_1 centroid: +2.41; gingival: +1.81, T_3-T_2: stable. The differences between centroid and gingival landmarks showed great values to centroid landmarks (0.59 mm) during the pre-surgical period (T_2-T_1) and remained stable after surgery, T_3-T_2 (Table 3).

Table 1 - Descriptive sample data.

Variable	Female (n = 10) Mean ± SD	Male (n = 5) Mean ± SD	Total (n = 15) Mean ± SD
Age / onset	27y 5m ± 8y 11m	20y 7m ± 3y 7m	25y 2m ± 8y 1m
Age / surgery	30y 0m ± 8y 11m	25y 7m ± 3y 9m	28y 6m ± 7y 9m
TOrtho	2y 7m ± 1y 5m	4y 12m ± 1y 9m	3y 5m ± 1y 10m
TSurg	1y 1m ± 0y 8m	2y 0m ± 0y 9m	1y 5m ± 0y 9m
Ttotal	3y 8m ± 2y 1m	6y 12m ± 2y 6m	4y 10m ± 2y 7m

Table 2 - Sample size (n), mean, standard deviation of changes between the two study periods, results of tests of equality of repeated measures means (means equals to zero) and multiple comparison of means. Mandibular arch.

Variable	n	T_2-T_1 Mean ± SD	T_3-T_2 Mean ± SD	T_3-T_1 Mean ± SD	Hotteling-Lawley Trace F	DF	p-value	Test power
W7-7C	12	0.78 ± 1.15	-0.58* ± 0.69	0.20 ± 1.16	5.05	2; 10	0.030	0.682
W7-7G	12	0.14 ± 1.09	-0.04 ± 0.84	0.10 ± 0.92	0.09	2; 10	0.911	
W6-6C	14	0.66 ± 1.39	-0.70 ± 1.28	-0.03 ± 1.46	2.41	2; 12	0.132	
W6-6G	14	-0.22 ± 1.01	0.50 ± 0.93	0.28 ± 0.79	2.13	2; 12	0.162	
W5-5C	15	1.69** ± 1.86	-0.47 ± 1.32	1.22* ± 1.69	5.84	2; 13	0.016	0.780
W5-5G	15	1.29* ± 1.59	-0.29 ± 0.96	1.00 ± 1.43	4.64	2; 13	0.030	0.676
W4-4C	15	2.41** ± 2.36	-0.37 ± 1.01	2.04** ± 2.08	7.38	2; 13	0.007	0.871
W4-4G	15	1.81* ± 2.10	-0.26 ± 0.89	1.56* ± 1.73	5.71	2; 13	0.017	0.770
W3-3C	15	0.23 ± 1.83	-0.15 ± 0.64	0.08 ± 1.94	0.51	2; 13	0.612	
W3-3G	15	0.57 ± 1.40	-0.11 ± 0.86	0.46 ± 1.69	1.34	2; 13	0.295	
L66-MP	14	0.85 ± 1.28	-0.34 ± 0.66	0.51 ± 1.14	3.22	2; 12	0.076	
D66-MP	14	0.67* ± 0.81	-0.16 ± 0.75	0.51 ± 1.14	4.73	2; 12	0.031	0.675

*, **, *** account for means of changes statistically different from zero with significance level set at 0.05; 0.01 and 0.001, respectively, detected by Bonferroni's test for multiple comparison of repeated measurements means.

Table 3 - Comparison of mean changes between centroid and gingival landmarks. Means and standard deviation of differences between changes, t—test for the hypothesis that changes are equal and correlation coefficient between changes. Mandibular arch.

Variables	Study period	Differences between changes Mean ± SD	t	DF	T-test p	r
	T_2 - T_1	0.65 ± 0.72	3.10	11	0.010	0.79**
W7-7C x W7-7G	T_3 - T_2	-0.54 ± 0.55	-3.43	11	0.006	0.76**
	T_3 - T_1	0.10 ± 0.82	0.44	11	0.671	0.72**
	T_2 - T_1	0.89 ± 0.71	4.69	13	0.000	0.87***
W6-6C x W6-6G	T_3 - T_2	-1.20 ± 0.98	-4.57	13	0.001	0.65*
	T_3 - T_1	-0.31 ± 0.95	-1.23	13	0.241	0.80***
	T_2 - T_1	0.40 ± 0.45	3.44	14	0.004	0.98***
W5-5C x W5-5G	T_3 - T_2	-0.18 ± 0.55	-1.24	14	0.235	0.93***
	T_3 - T_1	0.22 ± 0.59	1.45	14	0.168	0.94***
	T_2 - T_1	0.59 ± 0.64	3.58	14	0.003	0.97***
W4-4C x W4-4G	T_3 - T_2	-0.11 ± 0.57	-0.78	14	0.451	0.83***
	T_3 - T_1	0.48 ± 0.80	2.32	14	0.036	0.93***
	T_2 - T_1	-0.34 ± 0.93	-1.43	14	0.175	0.87***
W3-3C x W3-3G	T_3 - T_2	-0.04 ± 0.44	-0.36	14	0.725	0.87***
	T_3 - T_1	-0.38 ± 0.91	-1.64	14	0.123	0.88***

*, **, *** Statistically significant correlation coefficient with significance level set at 0.05; 0.01 and 0.001, respectively.

Dental arch length (L66-MP) and depth (D66- MP) were stable during the study periods, except for the depth assessed during orthodontic preparation which increased in 0.67 mm (Table 2).

Maxillary arch

W6-6G remained stable during orthodontic preparation and increased in 0.86 mm after surgery (T_3-T_2). Comparison between T_3-T_1 revealed an increase of 1.11 mm in W6-6C. The difference between centroid and gingival landmarks (W6-6C x W6-6G) increased in 1.18 mm during the pre-surgical period (T_2-T_1) (Table 5).

W5-5G (+0.96) and C (+2.51) distances increased during orthodontic preparation and remained stable from T_2 to T_3 (Table 4). Differences between centroid and gingival landmarks (W5-5C x W5-5G) increased in 1.54 mm during pre-surgical orthodontic preparation (T_2-T_1) (Table 5).

The same behavior was observed for W4-4 C (+3.29 mm) and W4-4 G (+2.25 mm) distances that increased during the pre-surgical period. Differences between centroid and gingival landmarks (W4-4C x W4-4G) increased in 1.04 mm during the pre-surgical period and remained stable after surgery.

At the region 3-3, there was an increase of 1.72 mm between centroids and 1.23 mm in the gingival landmark between T_1 and T_2. Differences between centroid and gingival landmarks (W3-3C x W3-3G) decreased in 0.23 mm in the post-surgical period (Table 5).

Arch length (L66-MP) remained stable during orthodontic preparation (T_2-T_1) and reduced in -0.74 mm from T_2 to T_3. Arch depth remained stable at all study periods (Table 4).

DISCUSSION

This study analyzed the three-dimensional changes occurring in the maxillary and mandibular dental arches of patients submitted to orthognathic surgery at two different periods: during preoperative orthodontic preparation and in the postoperative follow-up. The postoperative period included patients monitored for at least 6 months after the orthodontic appliance was removed with a mean period of postoperative evaluation of 1.1 years for females and 2 years for males (Table 1). Patients used retainers after removal of fixed appliances for an average period of 6 months. This period was adequate for assessing the most critical period of stability. No long-term

Table 4 - Sample size (n), mean, standard deviation of changes between the two study periods, results of tests of equality of repeated measures means (means equals to zero) and multiple comparison of means. Maxillary arch.

Variable	n	T_2-T_1 Mean ± SD	T_3-T_2 Mean ± SD	T_3-T_1 Mean ± SD	F	DF	p-value	Test power
W7-7C	13	0.26 ± 1.60	0.20 ± 2.34	0.46 ± 1.72	0.59	2; 11	0.573	
W7-7G	13	-0.15 ± 1.65	0.31 ± 1.94	0.16 ± 1.40	0.16	2; 11	0.856	
W6-6C	15	0.52 ± 1.90	0.59 ± 1.32	1.11* ± 1.46	5.12	2; 13	0.023	0.721
W6-6G	15	-0.66 ± 1.56	0.86* ± 1.18	0.20 ± 0.82	4.74	2; 13	0.029	0.686
W5-5C	15	2.51** ± 2.19	0.11 ± 1.02	2.61*** ± 1.86	14.10	2; 13	0.001	0.991
W5-5G	15	0.96* ± 1.34	0.23 ± 1.02	1.20** ± 1.32	5.84	2; 13	0.016	0.780
W4-4C	15	3.29*** ± 2.50	-0.14 ± 1.29	3.15*** ± 2.28	13.75	2; 13	0.001	0.990
W4-4G	15	2.25*** ± 1.67	-0.18 ± 1.04	2.07*** ± 1.59	13.65	2; 13	0.001	0.990
W3-3C	15	1.72* ± 2.11	-0.52 ± 1.11	1.19 ± 2.04	4.95	2; 13	0.025	0.706
W3-3G	15	1.23* ± 1.48	-0.29 ± 1.02	0.94 ± 1.53	4.85	2; 13	0.027	0.697
L66-MP	15	-0.07 ± 2.25	-0.74** ± 0.80	-0.81 ± 2.14	6.69	2; 13	0.010	0.836
D33-RUGAE	15	-0.09 ± 0.83	-0.01 ± 0.39	-0.10 ± 0.81	0.11	2; 13	0.845	
D44-AMR	15	-0.12 ± 1.36	-0.54 ± 1.43	-0.66 ± 1.26	2.03	2; 13	0.171	
D66-PMR	15	-0.20 ± 0.65	0.26 ± 0.59	0.06 ± 0.72	1.53	2; 13	0.253	

*, **, *** Account for means of changes statistically different from zero with significance level set at 0.05; 0.01 and 0.001, respectively, detected by Bonferroni's test for multiple comparison of repeated measurements means.

Table 5 - Means and standard deviation of differences between centroid and gingival landmarks, means and standard deviation of differences of changes, t—test for the hypothesis that changes are equal and correlation coefficient between changes. Maxillary arch.

Variables	Difference between changes		T-test			r
	Study period	Mean ± SD	t	DF	p	
W7-7C x W7-7G	$T_2 - T_1$	0.41 ± 1.01	1.46	12	0.169	0.81***
	$T_3 - T_2$	-0.11 ± 0.58	-0.70	12	0.496	0.98***
	$T_3 - T_1$	0.30 ± 0.89	1.20	12	0.252	0.86***
W6-6C x W6-6G	$T_2 - T_1$	1.18 ± 0.77	5.93	14	0.000	0.92***
	$T_3 - T_2$	-0.27 ± 0.72	-1.45	14	0.169	0.84***
	$T_3 - T_1$	0.91 ± 0.81	4.35	14	0.001	0.90***
W5-5C x W5-5G	$T_2 - T_1$	1.54 ± 1.36	4.38	14	0.001	0.81***
	$T_3 - T_2$	-0.13 ± 0.71	-0.69	14	0.501	0.76**
	$T_3 - T_1$	1.42 ± 1.25	4.38	14	0.001	0.74**
W4-4C x W4-4G	$T_2 - T_1$	1.04 ± 1.20	3.36	14	0.005	0.91***
	$T_3 - T_2$	0.04 ± 0.76	0.18	14	0.857	0.80***
	$T_3 - T_1$	1.08 ± 1.00	4.18	14	0.001	0.93***
W3-3C x W3-3G	$T_2 - T_1$	0.49 ± 0.97	1.94	14	0.072	0.91***
	$T_3 - T_2$	-0.23 ± 0.34	-2.60	14	0.021	0.95***
	$T_3 - T_1$	0.25 ± 1.01	0.98	14	0.343	0.88***

*, **, *** Statistically significant correlation coefficient with significance level set at 0.05; 0.01 and 0.001, respectively.

evaluations were included to reduce the chance of influence from slight dental arches changes after growth completion, as described in the literature,[2,3,9,10,11] since these changes were observed in 10-year to 34-year longitudinal studies.

Comparison with an untreated group would be valuable, since dimensional changes in the dental arches continue to occur even after post-pubertal growth.[2,3,11,12,13] Description of changes that naturally occur in untreated individuals may be taken as gold standard to assess the changes caused by orthodontic treatment.[13] The difficulty to achieve a paired group in terms of age, sex and type of malocclusion, as well as the ethical aspect concerning the impossibility to offer treatment during the study period (58 months) led to the decision to include a single group in this study.

Dimensional changes in the dental arches of untreated individuals are known, yet some divergences still persist among authors. Nevertheless, the described changes are of small magnitude (smaller than 1 mm) for a study period of 10 to 34 years, with a tendency towards narrowing and shortening of maxillary and mandibular dental arches over time. Bondevik[14] reported different results, with changes slightly greater than 1 mm and in opposite direction of what was reported by other studies. In the present study, assessment was conducted for a mean period of 4 years and 10 months, which reduces the interference of

potential changes in the maturation of occlusion on the present results. However, dimensional changes smaller than 1 mm should be carefully considered to avoid confusion with occasional changes inherent to sample aging.

The methods employed in this study, which included the use of the three-dimensional digitizer Micro-Scribe-3DX, a tool with proven efficacy,[15] allowed assessment of three-dimensional changes of dental arches and possible influences caused by orthodontic treatment and surgical therapy.

Sample size was calculated based on data available in the literature,[7] and was used to assess the hypothesis that the mean changes of a measurement between two study periods would be equal to zero. That is to say, the hypothesis that treatment performed between the two periods did not cause any average changes at a maximum significance level of 5%, minimum power of 80%, and under the condition that the mean was different from zero for at least half standard deviation. In these conditions, the minimum sample size was established at 25 patients. During the study, we decided to separate patients with Class II and Class III malocclusions in order to allow better homogenization of the sample. This resulted in two groups of 15, one of each class of patients. Power at these new conditions was calculated to confirm that they did not significantly reduce the power of the tests employed (Tables 2 and 4).

The preoperative period (T_2-T_1) revealed the role orthodontic treatment plays to prepare the dental arches in order to achieve normal occlusion after surgery. In general, maxillary and mandibular dental arches exhibited similar features at this period (Tables 2 and 4). Inter-premolar widths were increased at this period (from 1.69 mm to 3.29 mm) and buccal tipping, demonstrated by differences between the centroid and gingival landmarks, was very important (Tables 3 and 5). A study with similar methodology[7] revealed that, during orthodontic preparation, W4-4 (1.5 ± 2.0) and W5-5 (1.4 ± 2.0) measured by the centroid were expanded, revealing the clear orthodontic tendency towards eliminating the natural compensation established.

The idea that mandibular inter-canine width is basically unchangeable has been repeatedly supported in the literature. Burke et al[16] assessed stability in the mandibular inter-canine width of cases orthodontically treated with and without extractions. Their results revealed that, regardless of diagnosis and type of treatment, mandibular inter-canine width presents a tendency towards expansion in 1 to 2 mm during treatment, returning to the initial dimensions after the retention period. Our results revealed that inter-canine width remained stable for the mandibular arch at the three study periods. Conversely, the maxillary arch increased in the orthodontic period (centroid 1.72 mm and gingival 1.23 mm) with stability in the postoperative period. Similar results were described by Martin[7] who observed an increase in the maxillary W3-3 of 0.7 ± 2.1 from the centroid landmark, during the orthodontic period. Ward et al[17] observed that, from 20 to 31 years of age, small increases occur in maxillary and mandibular intercanine widths (+0.22 and +0.05, respectively).

In the mandibular arch, the distance between second molars measured from the centroid landmark reduced during orthodontic finalization (T_3-T_2). Despite such reduction, measurements obtained between the centroid and gingival landmarks (Table 3) at T_2-T_1 revealed greater movement of the centroid landmark, with opposite movement at T_3-T_2.

Martin[7] observed that, during orthodontic preparation, W6-6 and W7-7 measured from the centroid landmark remained stable, differently from what was observed when measurement was performed from the gingival landmark, which revealed a reduction in W6-6 (-2.1 ± 3.0) and W7-7 (-1.6 ± 2.2). A possible explanation

for this finding might be related to the presence of bands at T_2 when measurements comparing the initial treatment period were obtained, thus impairing the correct identification of gingival landmarks and giving rise to smaller preoperative measurements . In the present study, 0.2 mm were decreased from T_2 measurement on each side of the arch in order to avoid this interference.

The use of preformed archwires may be related to an increase in inter-premolar width, since patients with Class II division 1 malocclusion often present triangular-shaped dental arches. The greater increase observed in the maxillary arch may be related to the need to coordinate maxillary and mandibular archwires in transverse direction, since the dental arches of patients with Class II relationship tend to present posterior crossbite when changed to a Class I relationship at surgery. The surgeries performed did not include dentoalveolar segmentation so as to allow surgical correction of transverse discrepancies in three or four pieces. Even though this study did not include individuals treated with mechanical expansions, the coordination of archwires with the use of diagrams is very common during the preoperative period. Surprisingly, no transverse relapse was observed in the postoperative period (T_3-T_2). Considering that potentially unstable movements should be avoided during the preoperative orthodontic period,[18] widening of dental arches in the transverse direction by expansion and buccal tipping may be an unadvisable procedure. However, the preoperative changes observed in the present study did not cause contraction of dental arches after removal of the orthodontic appliance. Conversely, solid transverse stability was observed both in the maxillary and mandibular arches. During T_3-T_1, three out of four measurements in the mandibular arch indicating arch expansion at period T_2 remained positive and higher than what was observed at the onset of assessment at T_1 (Table 2). In the maxillary dental arch, four out of six measurements indicating transverse expansion observed in preoperative orthodontics were still increased by the end of the assessment period (Table 4).

The clinical application of these findings is very important. Transverse expansions during preoperative orthodontic treatment allow adequacy of dental arch dimensions and prevent the need for maxillary segmentation, commonly used for that purpose. This would reduce the period of surgical intervention and inherent morbidity of the additional procedure.

Moreover, expansion of dental arches favors the resolution of tooth crowding without affecting the incisors inclination.

These findings should be carefully interpreted. In the mandibular arch, except for first premolars, all measurements indicating inclination of posterior teeth at T_3-T_1, which compared the first and last evaluations of the present study, were non-significant, revealing that buccal tipping observed at T_2 was not present at T_3 (Table 3). In the maxillary dental arch, both transverse dimensions and buccal tipping of posterior teeth achieved by preoperative orthodontic treatment presented a tendency towards maintenance at the final study period (Tables 4 and 5). The length and depth of maxillary and mandibular dental arches remained unchanged in the study periods. This may be assigned to transverse expansion of dental arches, which was maintained throughout treatment. The only exception observed was a slight decrease (0.74 mm) in the length of the maxillary dental arch at the postoperative period (Table 4).

Future studies with longer follow-ups after the retention period, conducted with larger samples and with paired control groups, may contribute to confirm the present findings.

CONCLUSIONS

Maxillary and mandibular dental arches presented transverse expansion with buccal tipping of maxillary and mandibular premolars and maxillary canines during preoperative orthodontic preparation of patients with Class II division 1 malocclusion. This expansion remained throughout the study period. With regards to inclination of posterior teeth, the maxillary arch presented greater stability than the mandibular arch. Further studies are necessary to confirm the present findings.

REFERENCES

1. Bishara SE, Treder JE, Damon P, Olsen M. Changes in the dental arches and dentition between 25 and 45 years of age. Angle Orthod. 1996;66(6):417-22.
2. Akgül AA, Toygar TU. Natural craniofacial changes in the third decade of life: a longitudinal study. Am J Orthod Dentofacial Orthop. 2002;122(5):512-22.
3. Harris EF. A longitudinal study of arch size and form in untreated adults. Am J Orthod Dentofacial Orthop. 1997;111(4):419-27.
4. Sinclair PM, Little RM. Maturation of untreated normal occlusions. Am J Orthod Dentofacial Orthop. 1983;83(2):114-23.
5. Phillips C, Medland WH, Fields HW Jr, Proffit WR, White RP Jr. Stability of surgical maxillary expansion. Int J Adult Orthod Orthog Surg. 1992;7(3):139-46.
6. Hoppenreijs TJ, Van Der Linden FP, Freihofer HP, Stoelinga PJ, Tuinzing DB, Jacobs BT, et al. Stability of transverse maxillary dental arch dimensions following orthodontic-surgical correction of anterior open bites. Int J Adult Orthod Orthog Surg. 1998;13(1):7-22.
7. Martin DL. Transverse stability of multi-segment LeFort I expansion procedures [Thesis]. Dallas (TX): Baylor College of Dentistry; 1998.
8. Moyers RE, Van Der Linden FPGM, Riolo ML. Method and Sample. In: Moyers RE, van der Linden FPGM, Riolo ML, McNamara JA Jr. Standarts of human occlusal development. Michigan: Center for Human Grownth and Development; 1976. cap. 2, p. 5-26.
9. Bishara SE, Jakobsen JR, Treder J, Nowak A. Arch width changes from 6 weeks to 45 years of age. Am J Orthod Dentofacial Orthop. 1997;111(4):401-9.
10. Bishara SE, Jakobsen JR, Treder J, Nowak A. Arch length changes from 6 weeks to 45 years. Angle Orthod. 1998;68(1):69-74.
11. Harris EF, Behrents RG. The intrinsic stability of Class I molar relationship: a longitudinal study of untreated cases. Am J Orthod Dentofacial Orthop. 1988;94(1):63-7.
12. Bishara SE, Treder JE, Jakobsen JR. Facial and dental changes in adulthood. Am J Orthod Dentofacial Orthop. 1994;106(2):175-86.
13. Carter GA, McNamara JA. Longitudinal dental arch changes in adults. Am J Orthod Dentofacial Orthop. 1998;114(1):88-99.
14. Bondevik O. Changes in occlusion between 23 and 34 years. Angle Orthod. 1998;68(1):75-80.
15. Hayasaki H, Martins RP, Gandini Jr LG, Saitoh I, Nonakae K. A new way of analyzing occlusion 3 dimensionally. Am J Orthod Dentofacial Orthop. 2005;128(1):128-32.
16. Burke SP, Silveira AM, Goldsmith LJ, Yancey MA, Stewart AV, Scarfe WC. A meta-analysis of mandibular intercanine width in treatment and postretention. Angle Orthod. 1997;68(1):53-60.
17. Ward DE, Workman J, Brown R, Richmond S. Changes in Arch Width. A 20-year Longitudinal study of orthodontic treatment. Angle Orthod. 2006;76(1):6-13.
18. Wolford LM, Stevao ELL, Alexander CM, Goncalves JR. Orthodontics for orthognathic surgery. In: Miloro M, editor. Peterson´s principles of oral and maxillofacial surgery. 2nd ed. Hamilton; 2004. v. 1.

10

Factors associated with the prevalence of anterior open bite among preschool children

Daniella Borges Machado[1], Valéria Silva Cândido Brizon[1], Gláucia Maria Bovi Ambrosano[2], Davidson Fróis Madureira[3], Viviane Elisângela Gomes[4], Ana Cristina Borges de Oliveira[4]

Introduction: The aim of this study was to identify factors associated with the prevalence of anterior open bite among five-year-old Brazilian children. **Methods:** A cross-sectional study was undertaken using data from the National Survey of Oral Health (SB Brazil 2010). The outcome variable was anterior open bite classified as present or absent. The independent variables were classified by individual, sociodemographic and clinical factors. Data were analyzed through bivariate and multivariate analysis using SPSS statistical software (version 18.0) with a 95% level of significance. **Results:** The prevalence of anterior open bite was 12.1%. Multivariate analysis showed that preschool children living in Southern Brazil had an increased chance of 1.8 more times of having anterior open bite (CI 95%: 1.16-3.02). Children identified with alterations in overjet had 14.6 times greater chances of having anterior open bite (CI 95%: 8.98-24.03). **Conclusion:** There was a significant association between anterior open bite and the region of Brazil where the children lived, the presence of altered overjet and the prevalence of posterior crossbite.

Keywords: Oral health surveys. Open bite. Preschool child.

[1] MSc in Dentistry, Federal University of Minas Gerais (UFMG).
[2] Professor, School of Dentistry — State University of Campinas (UNICAMP).
[3] PhD resident, Biological Sciences Institute of UFMG.
[4] Professor, School of Dentistry — UFMG.

Ana Cristina Borges de Oliveira
Faculdade de Odontologia da UFMG, Av. Antônio Carlos, 6627
Campus Pampulha CEP: 31270-901 Belo Horizonte, MG — Brazil
E-mail: anacboliveira@yahoo.com.br

» The authors report no commercial, proprietary or financial interest in the products or companies described in this article.

INTRODUCTION

With worldwide reduction in dental caries prevalence, other oral problems have become more common.[1,2] Malocclusion is among them and may be associated with genetic, environmental and behavioral factors, thereby resulting in morphological, functional and esthetic problems.[3]

Anterior open bite (AOB) and posterior crossbite have been identified as the most common occlusal abnormalities in primary dentition.[4,5] AOB is characterized by lack of occlusal contact in the anterior region, while the remaining teeth are in occlusion.[6,7] AOB is more prevalent in primary dentition, with a prevalence between 6.2% and 50.0% worldwide, varying according to the population group studied.[3,4,5,8-11] This is most likely to be associated with an increase in overbite during the mixed dentition period, and the self-correcting nature of the majority of cases of anterior open bite in primary dentition.[5,12]

When non-nutritive sucking habits are no longer present in children, AOB tends to disappear.[3,5,8,10,12,13] Góis et al[13] showed that 70.1% of AOB present in primary dentition were self-corrected during the transition from primary to mixed dentition. Early treatment of AOB, during the primary or mixed dentition, usually reaches better results and reduces indices of relapse;[14,15,16] thus, spontaneous correction of AOB during the initial stages might be, in part, result of individual's face and dentition development process.[12,16]

In this context, primary dentition directly influences the development of permanent occlusion. A number of anomalies and occlusal characteristics present in the primary dentition remain or even deteriorate in permanent dentition.[13] It is important to advise parents that these habits should be eliminated before eruption of upper permanent incisors in order to allow further self-correction of this malocclusion.[3,5,8,10,12,13] AOB is considered one of the most difficult occlusal abnormalities to be corrected in the permanent dentition, especially with respect to stability.[3-10,12-20] Due to functional and esthetic abnormalities, AOB may cause negative psychosocial impact in many cases, predisposing individuals to low self-esteem, social alienation due to bullying, and behavioral disorders, with potential negative impact on their quality of life.[13]

The aim of this study was to identify factors associated with the prevalence of AOB among five–year-old children in Brazil.

MATERIAL AND METHODS

Study design

A cross-sectional analytical study was performed. Data from the Epidemiological Survey of the Oral Health Conditions of the Brazilian Population, known as "SB Brasil 2010", was used.[2]

Ethical considerations

The Brazilian Oral Health Project was submitted to and approved by the National Council on Ethics and Human Research. An informed consent form was signed by all individuals participating in the study.[2]

Sample population

The population of Brazil comprises approximately 190.7 million people, with 2.9 million children under the age of five.[21]

The epidemiological survey SB Brasil 2010 assessed the oral health conditions of the Brazilian population in urban and rural areas, classifying it into different age ranges. The study surveyed 37, 519 individuals living in 26 state capitals in the Federal District and in 150 municipal districts of varying population sizes located in the countryside.[2]

The database created by this study is of public domain and freely accessible on the website of the Brazilian Ministry of Health.[2]

Data collection

Data were collected in each participant's home. Data collection included an oral examination and a questionnaire. Dental teams comprised an examiner and an assistant who performed clinical data collection using instruments (oral mirror and periodontal probe), as recommended by the World Health Organization (WHO).[22]

The presence of AOB or any other form of malocclusion was registered using the Foster and Hamilton index (Table 1).[23]

Sample calculation

A conglomerate sampling technique was used with three stratifications. The first used domains and primary sampling units: Capitals and municipal districts from the countryside, according to each macroregion. The second was a subdivision of municipal districts: 27 capitals plus 30 municipal districts from the countryside of each region of Brazil. The third used lottery to

Table 1 - Foster and Hamilton index.

Diagnosis	Diagnostic criteria
Canine relationship	» Class I: Tip of upper canine in the same vertical plane as the distal surface of lower canine when in centric occlusion. » Class II: Tip of upper canine in anterior relationship to the distal surface of lower canine when in centric occlusion. » Class III: Tip of upper canine in posterior relationship to the distal surface of lower canine when in centric occlusion.
Overjet	Normal: Primary upper central incisor overjet ≤ 2 mm. With alteration: » Increased: Primary upper central incisor overjet > 2 mm. » Edge-to-edge: Upper and lower primary central incisors in edge-to-edge position. » Anterior crossbite: Lower primary central incisors in anterior relationship to upper primary central incisors in occlusion.
Overbite	Normal: Incisal tips of primary lower central incisors contacting the palatal surfaces of upper primary central incisors when in centric occlusion. With alteration: » Reduced: Incisal tips of primary lower central incisors not contacting the palatal or incisal surfaces of upper primary central incisors when in centric occlusion. » Anterior open bite: Incisal tips of lower primary central incisors below the level of the incisal tips of upper primary central incisors when in centric occlusion. » Deep bite: Incisal tips of lower primary central incisors touching the palate when in centric occlusion.
Posterior crossbite	Present: Upper primary molars occluding in lingual relationship with lower primary molars when in centric occlusion. Absent

Source: Adapted from Foster and Hamilton[23].

guarantee representativeness in the municipal districts, census sectors, and residences.

A maximum of 250 volunteers were assessed for anterior open bite in each one of the 172 cities in Brazil, thereby resulting in a total sample of 5,622 five-year-old children. The following parameters were used to calculate sample size: Values of z, variance, mean DEFT, acceptable margin of error, effect of design and non-reply rate. These data were taken from *SB Brasil 2003*.[1]

Calibration

Each fieldwork team was properly trained in work-shops of 20 hours (6 classes). Training was divided into phases as follows: 4 hours of theory, 2 hours of practical training, 8 hours for calibration, 2 hours of final discussion and 4 hours of fieldwork strategy. The technique of consensus was used to calculate the correlation between each examiner and the results obtained by consensus of the team. The model proposed by the WHO was used as reference. Kappa coefficient was calculated, weighted for each examiner, age-group and medical complaint with a value of 0.65 adopted as the minimal acceptable limit.[2]

Study variables

The dependent variable was AOB. Table 2 describes the independent variables.

Data analysis

Data were analyzed using the Statistical Package for Social Sciences (SPSS for Windows, version 18.0, SPSS Inc, Chicago, IL, USA) software. First, bivariate data analysis was performed. Chi-square test was used to investigate the association between the dependent variable (AOB) and the independent variables (child's city of residence, region of Brazil, sex, family income, dental caries, need for treatment of dental caries, canine relationship, overjet, posterior crossbite) (P < 0.05). In order to identify the independent impact of each variable, multiple logistic regression was performed. The independent variables were inserted into logistic model on a decreasing scale according to their statistical significance (P < 0.25, stepwise backward procedure).

RESULTS

Table 1 displays the results of bivariate analysis. The variables statistically associated with the prevalence of AOB among five-year-old children were: Region of Brazil in which the child lived, canine relationship, overjet and posterior crossbite (P < 0.001).

The results of multivariate analysis are shown in Table 2. Regardless of the other variables analyzed, five-year-old children from Southern Brazil were two times more likely to be identified with AOB than children in the Southeastern region of the country (OR = 1.87 [CI 95%: 1.16 – 3.02]). Preschool children diagnosed with alterations in overjet had 14.7 times greater chances of suffering from AOB (OR = 14.69 [CI 95%: 8.98 – 24.03]).

Table 2 - Independent variables and respective categories.

Independent variables	Category						
Age	State capital				Other city		
Region of Brazil	North		Northeast	Southeast	South		Midwest
Sex	Male				Female		
Family income[a]	< 250	251 - 500	501 - 1500[b]	1501 - 2500	2501 - 4500	4500 - 9500	> 9501
Tooth caries	deft = 0				deft > 1		
Need for treatment	Absent				Present		
Canine relationship	Class I			Class II		Class III	
Overjet	Normal			With alteration			
Posterior crossbite	Absent			Present			

[a]R$ (R$ 1,00 = US$ 0,49) / [b]population family income.

DISCUSSION

The prevalence of AOB in the studied population of five-year-old children was 12.1%.[2] However, there is considerable variation in such epidemiological data in worldwide literature (6.2 to 50.0%), even when the same regions of Brazil are compared.[3,4,5,8,9,10,24] A direct comparison of the results yielded by different studies is difficult due to variation in diagnostic and classification criteria from an epidemiological perspective. Variations in study design, sample criteria and methods of analyzing results can also result in data discrepancy.

Multivariate data analysis confirmed the prevalence of AOB statistically associated with the region in which the child lived and also with the prevalence of posterior crossbite and alterations in overjet. The chances of children resident in the Southern of Brazil being diagnosed with AOB was nearly twice greater than that of children living in other regions of the country. This variation can be possibly explained by different cultural habits that may result in greater or less exposure to risk factors associated with AOB, such as time spent in breast-feeding, diet and variations in non-nutritive sucking habits in different regions of Brazil.[9,13,24] These data corroborate the findings in the literature. Another study conducted in Southern Brazil also found a higher percentage of AOB in primary dentition when compared with studies undertaken in the Southeastern and Northeast regions.[3,4,9,10]

Regional, cultural and socioeconomic variations of each city should be considered and are the most probable explanation for the different prevalence of AOB found in other studies. A survey undertaken in the Southeastern of Brazil found a prevalence of AOB of 7.9% among 1,069 preschool children from Belo Horizonte,[4] whereas in São Paulo there was a prevalence of 22.4% among 309 children.[3] In Southern Brazil, particularly in Pelotas, 46.3% of 359 children had AOB in primary dentition.[19] In the Northeastern Brazil, particularly in Recife, 30.2% of 1,308 five-year-old children had AOB.[10] Moreover, studies outside Brazil also demonstrate a range of different results, with a prevalence of AOB among preschool children varying from 13.0% in Italy to 50.0% in Sweden.[5,8] In addition, racial characteristics may influence the occurrence of AOB. Thus, there was significant difference in the prevalence of malocclusion between Caucasian and Afro American children aged from 3 to 5 years old, with no differences between males and females.[19] In the present study, the statistical significance found between prevalence of AOB and the region of children's residence can also be related to diverse racial, economic and sociodemographic characteristics in Brazil. The Brazilian population is one of the most diverse in the world, with bi or trihybrid miscegenation prevailing in some regions. The country is of continental extension; thus, its population reveals great complexity and diversity, especially in terms of physical and cultural characteristics. Although the present study did not investigate the racial composition of the Brazilian population, the Brazilian Census of 2010 demonstrates that racial characteristics, which were self-declared, among children between 0-14 years old considerably vary according to each region of Brazil.[21] The Brazilian Census of 2010 also demonstrates that higher median income and lower illiteracy indices were seen in Midwestern, Southeastern and Southern Brazil, while lower median income and higher illiteracy indices were present in Northern and Northeastern Brazil.[21] However, family income did not influence the occurrence of AOB.

Table 1 - Sample distribution according to the prevalence of anterior open bite and associated factors. (n = 5,622).

Independent variables	n (total)	Prevalence of anterior open bite		P value*
		n (%)	Gross OR (CI 95%)	
Age				
State capital	4,272	543 (16.6)	1	0.472
Other city	1,350	163 (13.7)	0.93 (0.77-1.13)	
Region of Brazil				
North	1,476	127 (9.41)	0.53 (0.41-0.69)	
Northeast	1,567	214 (15.8)	0.97 (0.77-1.22)	
Southeast	1,009	141 (16.2)	1	<0.001
South	751	152 (25.3)	1.75 (1.36-2.27)	
Midwest	819	72 (9.6)	0.55 (0.41-0.74)	
Sex				
Male	2,803	337 (13.6)	1	0.163
Female	2,819	369 (15.0)	1.12 (0.96-1.31)	
Family income*				
< 250[a]	270	37 (15.8)	1.05 (0.73-1.52)	
251 to 500	894	97 (12.1)	0.77 (0.61-0.98)	
501 to 1,500[b]	2,917	386 (15.2)	1	
1,501 to 2,500	808	104 (14.7)	0.96 (0.76-1.22)	0.335
2,501 to 4,500	309	43 (16.1)	1.07 (0.76-1.51)	
4,501 to 9,500	112	11 (10.8)	0.68 (0.36-1.28)	
> 9,500	48	5 (11.6)	0.73 (0.29-1.87)	
Tooth caries				
deft = 0	2,571	303 (13.3)	1	0.062
deft = > 1	3,051	403 (15.2)	1.16 (0.99-1.37)	
Need for treatment of tooth caries				
Absent	2,764	335 (13.7)	1	0.263
Present	2,858	371 (14.9)	1.10 (0.93-1.29)	
Canine relationship*				
Class I	4,308	385 (9.81)	1	
Class II	941	228 (31.98)	4.32 (3.58-5.22)	< 0.001
Class III	361	92 (34.20)	4.78 (3.64-6.28)	
Overjet*				
Normal	3,842	157 (4.26)	1	< 0.001
With alteration	138	44 (46.81)	19.78 (12.79-30.57)	
Posterior crossbite*				
Absent	1,142	194 (20.46)	1	< 0.001
Present	4,447	509 (12.93)	0.58 (0.48-0.69)	

OR: Odds ratio; CI 95%: Confidence interval.
* χ^2 test/ ** missing values / [a] R$ (R$ 1,00 = US$ 0,49) / [b] population family income.

Table 2 - Multiple logistic regression models explaining the prevalence of anterior open bite in five-year-old children in Brazil.

Categories	Adjusted OR [CI]	P value*
Southern Brazil	1.87 (1.16-3.02)	< 0.001
Overjet with alteration	14.69 (8.98-24.03)	< 0.001
Posterior crossbite present	0.62 (0.44-0.87)	0.006

OR: Odds ratio; CI 95%: Confidence interval.

Therefore, differences in race and sociodemographic characteristics may influence the prevalence of malocclusion among the population.[24]

Preschool children identified with alterations in overjet (increased edge-to-edge bite or anterior crossbite) had greater chances of having AOB.[5,23-26] Non-nutritive sucking habits and tongue posture are included as environmental factors.[4,5] Such transversal and sagittal abnormalities, which share the same etiological factors, may be associated with AOB. Considering that AOB is directly related to non-nutritive sucking habits, the increased prevalence of malocclusion at a younger age can be associated with an increased incidence of this habit among younger children. A longitudinal study of 386 children (aged 3 years old at study onset and examined again at 7 years of age) performed in Sweden found that the prevalence of non-nutritive sucking habits decreased from 66.0% to 4.0% between 3 and 7 years of age, which might have influenced the reduction of AOB incidence from 50% to 10% at the age of seven.[5] In addition, oral respiration may also significantly contribute to the etiology of dentofacial abnormalities in children during growth.[28] Furthermore, a study of schoolchildren from Lithuania aged between 7 and 15 years old found a significant association between nasal obstruction and increased overjet, open bite and maxillary growth.[27] A study performed among preschool children in Brazil showed that children who had the habit of sucking a pacifier after two years of age and those who were oral breathers had a greater chance of developing malocclusion.[19] While the design of the present study is robust, some limitations should be observed. Data assessed the presence or

absence of AOB without differentiating its extension, severity and dental or skeletal impairment. Other factors such as the presence of harmful habits, facial and respiratory patterns, which are etiological factors of this malocclusion, were not investigated either. This is most probably due to the comprehensive character of the other variables studied, as well as the need for collecting brief data because of the large sample comprising 5.622 children. Data provided, however, is an accurate indicator of the prevalence of AOB in the different regions of Brazil. Such data are important for the strategic planning of government programs aimed at prevention, interception and treatment of AOB.

The present study alerts oral health care programs to the need for preventive measures that can deter or at least reduce the prevalence of this and other malocclusions among the infant population. In Brazil, the road towards an universal dental care for the general population, especially infants, is long. Orthodontic treatment is not just a matter of vanity. The more severe the problem, the greater the functional and psychological impact of anterior open bite. Child may often become target of bullying which can result in behavioral disorders and personality maladjustments. Additional studies are needed to clarify the etiology and severity of AOB according to each region of Brazil.

CONCLUSION

Children living in Southern Brazil showed greater chances of being diagnosed with anterior open bite.

Children identified with alterations in overjet showed greater chances of having anterior open bite.

REFERENCES

1. Brasil. Ministério da Saúde. Secretaria de Atenção à Saúde. Projeto SB Brasil 2003: condições de saúde bucal da população brasileira 2002-2003. Resultados principais. Brasília, DF: Ministério da Saúde; 2004. [Acesso em: 2012 Jul. 12]. Disponível em: http://portalweb02.saude.gov.br/portal/arquivos/pdf/relatorio_brasil_sorridente.pdf.
2. Brasil. Ministério da Saúde. Secretaria de Vigilância em Saúde. Secretaria de Atenção à Saúde. Coordenação Nacional de Saúde Bucal. SB2010. Pesquisa Nacional de Saúde Bucal. Resultados principais. Brasília, DF: MS, 2011. [Acesso: 2012 Jul. 12]. Disponível em: http://dab.saude.gov.br/cnsb/sbbrasil/download.htm.
3. Romero CC, Scavone-Junior H, Garib DG, Cotrim-Ferreira FA, Ferreira RI. Breastfeeding and non-nutritive sucking patterns related to the prevalence of anterior open bite in primary dentition. J Appl Oral Sci. 2011;19(2):161-8.
4. Carvalho AC, Paiva SM, Scarpelli AC, Viegas CM, Ferreira FM, Pordeus IA. Prevalence of malocclusion in primary dentition in a population-based sample of Brazilian preschool children. Eur J Paediatr Dent. 2011;12(2):107-11.
5. Dimberg L, Lennartsson B, Söderfeldt B, Bondemark L. Malocclusions in children at 3 and 7 years of age: a longitudinal study. Eur J Orthod. 2011;33(3):1-7.
6. Fränkel R, Fränkel C. A functional approach to treatment of skeletal open bite. Am J Orthod. 1983;84(1):54-68.
7. Artese A, Drummond S, Nascimento JM, Artese F. Criteria for diagnosing and treating anterior open bite with stability. Dental Press J Orthod. 2011;16(3):136-61.
8. Viggiano D, Fasano D, Monaco G, Strohmenger L. Breast feeding, bottle feeding, and non-nutritive sucking; effects on occlusion in deciduous dentition. Arch Dis Child. 2004;89(12):1121-3.
9. Peres KG, Latorre MR, Sheiham A, Peres MA, Victora CG, Barros FC. Social and biological early life influences on the prevalence of open bite in Brazilian 6-year-olds. Int J Paediatr Dent. 2007;17(1):41-9.
10. Vasconcelos FM, Massoni AC, Heimer MV, Ferreira AM, Katz CR, Rosenblatt A. Non-nutritive sucking habits, anterior open bite and associated factors in Brazilian children aged 30-59 months. Braz Dent J. 2011;22(2):140-5.

11. Proffit WR, Fields HW Jr, Moray LJ. Prevalence of malocclusion and orthodontic treatment need in the United States: estimates from the NHANES III survey. Int J Adult Orthodon Orthognath Surg. 1998;13(2):97-106.

12. Klocke A, Nanda RS, Kahl-Nieke B. Anterior open bite in the deciduous dentition: longitudinal follow-up and craniofacial growth considerations. Am J Orthod Dentofacial Orthop. 2002;122(4):353-8.

13. Góis EG, Vale MP, Paiva SM, Abreu MH, Serra-Negra JM, Pordeus IA. Incidence of malocclusion between primary and mixed dentitions among Brazilian children: a 5-year longitudinal study. Angle Orthod. 2012;82(3):495-500.

14. Huang GJ, Justus R, Kennedy DB, Kokich VG. Stability of anterior openbite treated with crib therapy. Angle Orthod. 1990;60(1):17-26.

15. Ngan P, Fields HW. Open bite: a review of etiology and management. Pediatr Dent. 1997;19(2):91-8.

16. Janson G, Valarelli FP, Beltrão RT, Freitas MR, Henriques JF. Stability of anterior open-bite extraction and nonextraction treatment in the permanent dentition. Am J Orthod Dentofacial Orthop. 2006;129(6):768-74.

17. Trottman A, Elsbach HG. Comparison of malocclusion in preschool black and white children. Am J Orthod Dentofacial Orthop. 1996;110(1):69-72.

18. Katz CR, Rosenblatt A, Gondim PP. Nonnutritive sucking habits in Brazilian children: effects on deciduous dentition and relationship with facial morphology. Am J Orthod Dentofacial Orthop. 2004;126(1):53-7.

19. Peres KG, Barros AJ, Peres MA, Victora CG. Effects of breastfeeding and sucking habits on malocclusion in a birth cohort study. Rev Saúde Pública. 2007;41(3):343-50.

20. Onyeaso CO, Isiekwe MC. Occlusal changes from primary to mixed dentitions in Nigerian children. Angle Orthod. 2008;78(1):64-9.

21. Instituto Brasileiro de Geografia e Estatística. Censo demográfico 2010. Rio de Janeiro, 2010. [Acesso em : 2012 Jul. 12]. Disponível em: ftp://ftp.ibge. gov.br/Censos/Censo_Demografico_2010/Caracteristicas_Gerais_Religiao_ Deficiencia/tab1_1.pdf.

22. World Health Organization. Oral Health Surveys: basic methods. 4th ed. Geneva, Switzerland: World Health Organization; 1997.

23. Foster TD, Hamilton MC. Occlusion in the primary dentition. Study of children at 2 and one-half to 3 years of age. Br Dent J. 1969;126(2):76-9.

24. Tomita NE, Bijella VT, Franco LJ. The relationship between oral habits and malocclusion in preschool children. Rev Saúde Pública. 2000;34(3):299-303.

25. Greenlee GM, Huang GJ, Chen SS, Chen J, Koepsell T, Hujoel P. Stability of treatment for anterior open-bite malocclusion: a meta-analysis. Am J Orthod Dentofacial Orthop. 2011;139(2):154-69.

26. Cuccia AM, Eotti M, Caradonna D. Oral breathing and head posture. Angle Orthod. 2008;78(1):77-82.

27. Lopatienė K, Babarskas A. Malocclusion and upper airway obstruction. Medicina. 2002;38(3):277-83.

11

Orthodontic camouflage of skeletal Class III malocclusion with miniplate

Marcel Marchiori Farret[1], Milton M. Benitez Farret[2], Alessandro Marchiori Farret[3]

Introduction: Skeletal Class III malocclusion is often referred for orthodontic treatment combined with orthognathic surgery. However, with the aid of miniplates, some moderate discrepancies become feasible to be treated without surgery. **Objective:** To report the case of a 24-year-old man with severe skeletal Angle Class III malocclusion with anterior cross-bite and a consequent concave facial profile. **Methods:** The patient refused to undergo orthognathic surgery; therefore, orthodontic camouflage treatment with the aid of miniplates placed on the mandibular arch was proposed. **Results:** After 18 months of treatment, a Class I molar and canine relationship was achieved, while anterior crossbite was corrected by retraction of mandibular teeth. The consequent decrease in lower lip fullness and increased exposure of maxillary incisors at smiling resulted in a remarkable improvement of patient's facial profile, in addition to an esthetically pleasing smile, respectively. One year later, follow-up revealed good stability of results.

Keywords: Angle Class III malocclusion. Orthodontic anchorage procedures. Orthodontic appliance design.

[1] Professor, Centro de Estudos Odontológicos Meridional (CEOM), Graduate Program in Orthodontics, Passo Fundo/RS, Brazil; and Fundação para Reabilitação das Deformidades Crânio-faciais (FUNDEF), Lajeado/RS, Brazil.
[2] Professor, Universidade Federal de Santa Maria (UFSM), Santa Maria/RS, Brazil.
[3] Private practice, Santa Maria/RS, Brazil.

» The authors report no commercial, proprietary or financial interest in the products or companies described in this article.

Marcel Marchiori Farret
E-mail: marcelfarret@yahoo.com.br

INTRODUCTION

Skeletal Class III malocclusion is one of the biggest challenges faced by orthodontists.[1,2] If patients consent to orthognathic surgery, subsequent mechanical orthodontic treatment becomes simple with superior functional and esthetic results.[3,4,5] However, several patients refuse surgery. In such situations, orthodontic camouflage treatment may be an alternative, particularly if discrepancy is slight or moderate.[3,4,6]

The introduction of skeletal anchorage has increased the number of patients with skeletal problems who can be treated by mechanical orthodontic treatment only, thereby avoiding the need for complementary orthognathic surgery.[2,7] Mini-implants are preferred for patients with slight discrepancies because of less invasive insertion and removal procedures.[8,9] However, in patients with moderate skeletal and dental discrepancies, miniplates are the treatment of choice to improve anchorage and eliminate the possibility of contact between implant screws and tooth roots during tooth movement, as it can occur with mini-implants.[2,8,10,11]

In the present study, we report the case of a 24-year-old man with severe skeletal Angle Class III malocclusion who was treated by orthodontic camouflage treatment with miniplate anchorage.

CASE REPORT
Diagnosis and etiology

A 24-year-old man presented for orthodontic treatment with the chief complaint of an unesthetic smile. Undesired appearance was caused by protrusion of anterior teeth and decreased visibility of maxillary anterior teeth at smiling. Extraoral examination revealed a concave facial profile (Fig 1). Clinical manipulation in centric relation demonstrated that there was no mandibular anterior deviation during bite closing. Intraoral examination and analysis of dental casts revealed Angle Class III malocclusion, Class III canine relationship, anterior crossbite, and maxillary incisor crowding, with a negative discrepancy of 4 mm (Figs 2 and 3). Furthermore, Bolton analysis revealed 1-mm excess for maxillary posterior teeth and 2-mm excess for mandibular anterior teeth. Cephalometric analysis revealed skeletal Class III (ANB = −5°) malocclusion, a hypodivergent facial pattern (SN-GoGn = 20°, FMA = 9° and Y-axis = 44°), severe maxillary incisor proclination, and uprighted mandibular incisors (Fig 4).

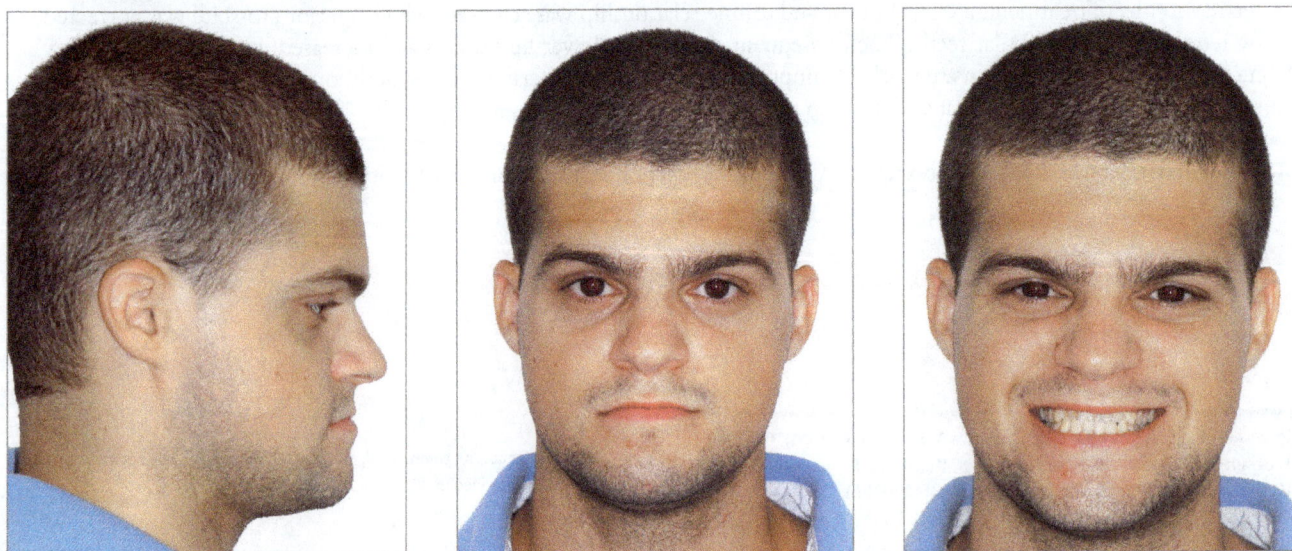

Figure 1 - Pretreatment facial photographs.

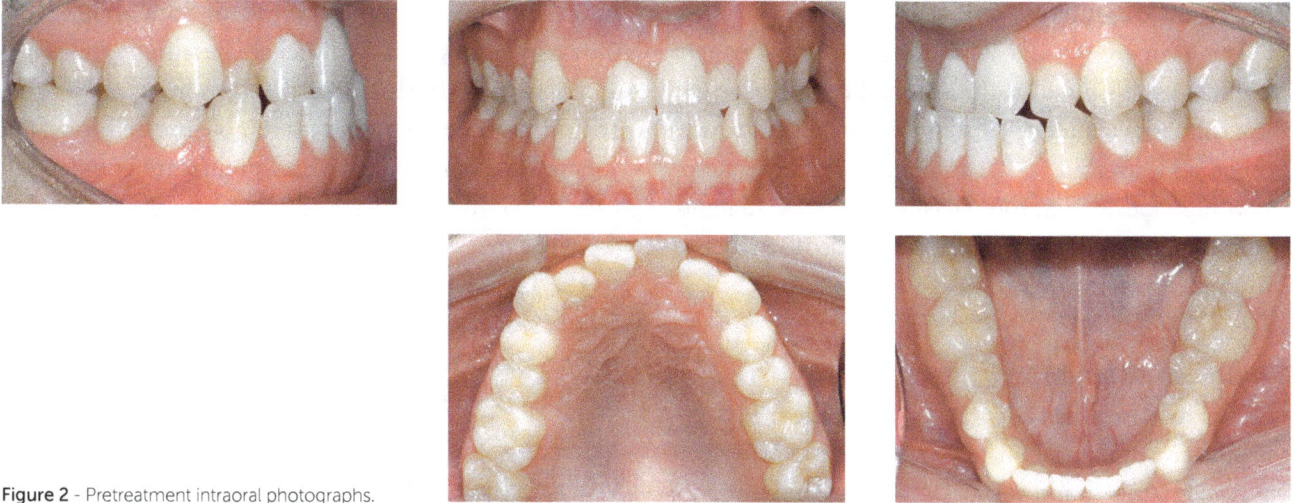

Figure 2 - Pretreatment intraoral photographs.

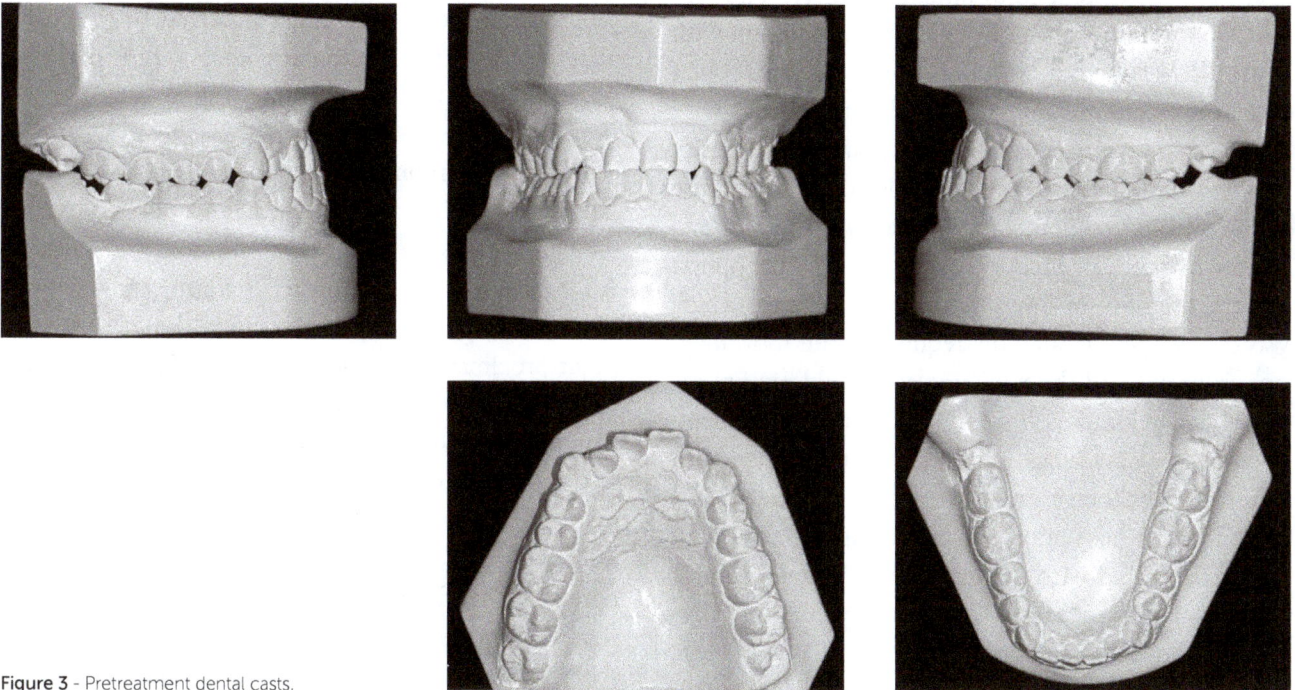

Figure 3 - Pretreatment dental casts.

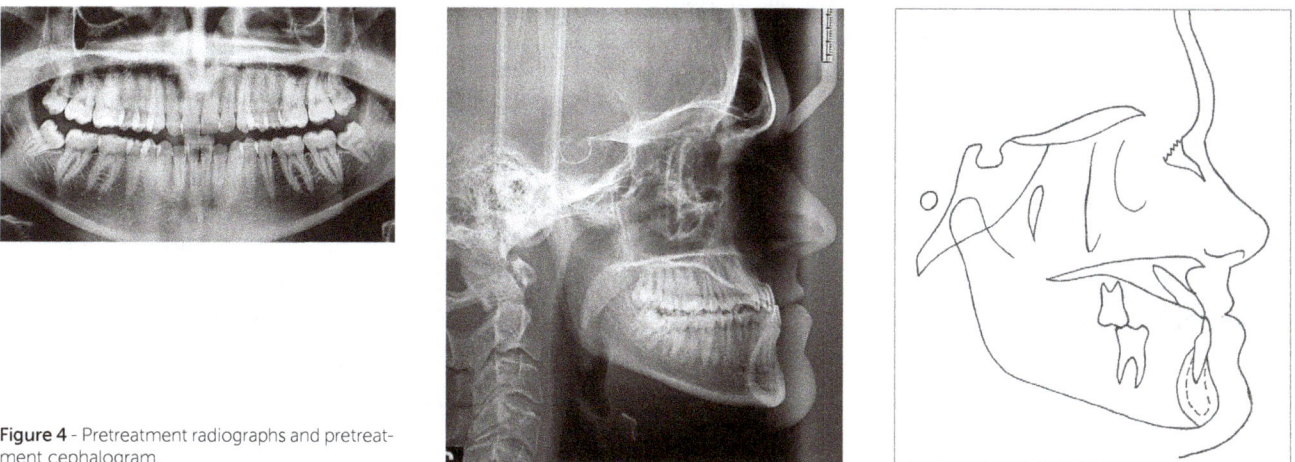

Figure 4 - Pretreatment radiographs and pretreatment cephalogram.

Treatment objectives

The primary treatment objectives for this patient were: (1) establish a Class I molar and canine relationship; (2) correct anterior crossbite and achieve adequate overjet and overbite; (3) eliminate maxillary incisor crowding; and (4) improve facial esthetics by straightening the facial profile and increasing maxillary incisor exposure at smiling.

Treatment alternatives

The first treatment option for this patient was orthognathic surgery for maxillary advancement, which would certainly improve facial esthetics and simplify subsequent mechanical orthodontic treatment; however, the patient refused to undergo surgery. The second option was mechanical orthodontic treatment with Class III elastics and a sliding jig on the mandibular arch. This would require prolonged use of elastics with extremely good patient compliance and could result in some undesirable effects, such as counterclockwise occlusal plane rotation, with less maxillary incisor and greater mandibular incisor exposure. The third option was the use of mini-implants as anchorage unit; which was disregarded because the required tooth movement was extensive and the mini-implant would require removal and relocation at some point during treatment. Eventually, camouflage orthodontic treatment with miniplate anchorage was proposed and the patient agreed with this option. In this planning, treatment would be started with alignment and leveling of lower and upper arches, except for maxillary incisors, thus avoiding further proclination. After alignment and leveling of the upper arch, stripping was considered from second molar to first premolar on each side, so as to gain space for incisors alignment. On the lower arch, after alignment and leveling, miniplates would be inserted on each side of the posterior mandible, so to be used as the anchorage unit to retract all mandibular teeth. During anterior crossbite correction, a posterior bite plate was also planned to be used, so as to avoid interferences between maxillary and mandibular incisors.

Treatment progress

Treatment was initiated by bonding 0.022 × 0.028-in Edgewise standard brackets followed by alignment and leveling of both arches with 0.014-in and 0.016-in Nickel–Titanium archwires and 0.016-in, 0.018-in, and 0.020-in stainless steel archwires. The archwires were not inserted for incisors to avoid proclination and premature contact between maxillary and mandibular incisors. Stripping from the mesial surface of the maxillary second molar to the mesial surface of the maxillary first premolar was performed on both sides, followed by distalization of all maxillary posterior teeth. Mandibular posterior teeth were aligned and leveled up to a 0.020-in stainless steel archwire, and at this point in treatment, miniplates were placed on the external oblique ridge. Subsequently, a 0.019 × 0.025-in stainless steel archwire was set with hooks between the canine and first premolar on both sides and connected to the miniplates by means of elastomeric chains, thus resulting in a load of 400 g/f on each side (Fig 5).

After two months, an improved anteroposterior (AP) relationship was achieved, and maxillary and mandibular incisors were included in treatment (Fig 6). An overlayed 0.012-in nickel–titanium archwire was placed in the maxillary arch to align the incisors with slight proclination, while a 0.019 × 0.025-in stainless steel archwire was set with bull loops and placed in the mandibular arch to retract the incisors. This archwire was activated on the miniplates, and another elastomeric chain was connected to the mandibular first premolar on each side to maintain mandibular dentition retraction. To facilitate anterior crossbite correction, a removable posterior bite plate was used for two months. After 14 months, anterior crossbite was completely corrected and a Class I molar and canine relationship was achieved. At this point, upper and lower 0.019 × 0.025-in stainless steel archwires were placed to achieve the appropriate torque, with elastomeric chains connected only on the left miniplate, so as to correct slight midline deviation (Fig 7).

Treatment results

Patient's treatment was complete after 18 months. His facial profile remarkably improved with an esthetically pleasing smile (Fig 8). Intraoral examination and dental casts analysis revealed a Class I molar and canine relationship on both sides, with excel-

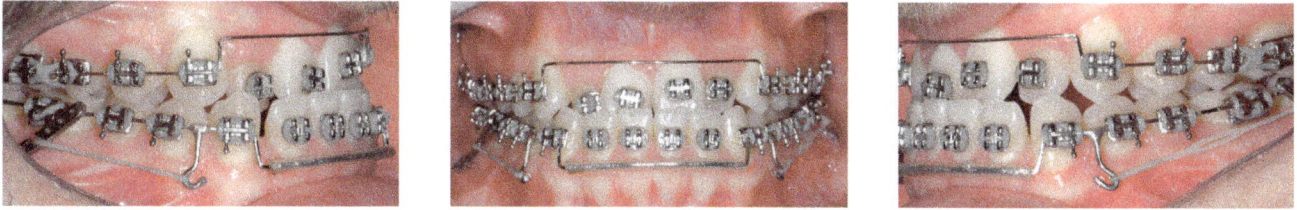

Figure 5 - Intraoral photographs at the beginning of mandibular dentition distalization.

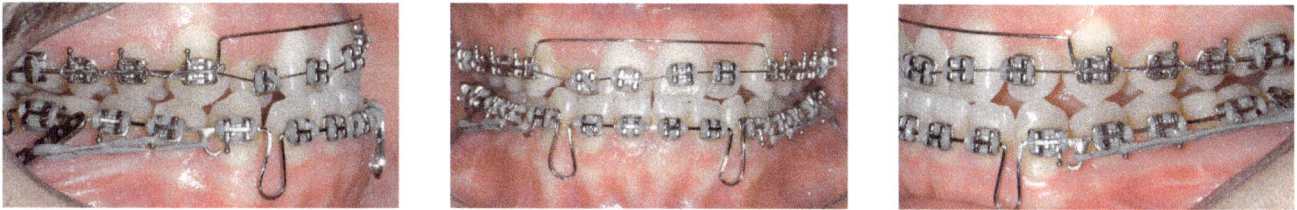

Figure 6 - Intraoral photographs when maxillary and mandibular incisors were included on the mechanics to correct anterior crossbite.

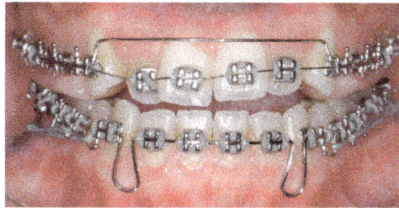

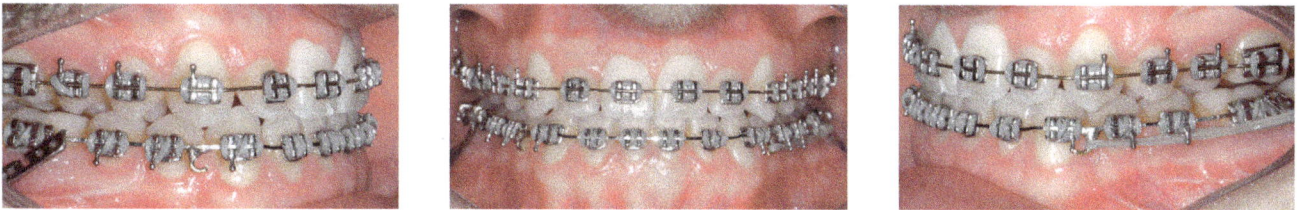

Figure 7 - Intraoral photographs after anterior crossbite correction.

lent intercuspation (Figs 9 and 10). Due to anterior Bolton discrepancy, spaces were kept unchanged between maxillary lateral incisors and canines, which would be filled with composite resin. Anterior crossbite was successfully corrected and adequate overjet and overbite were achieved. Panoramic radiograph showed good parallelism among tooth roots, and eephalometric analysis with superimpositions re

vealed that maxillary incisors remained nearly at the same position, with mandibular molar uprighting and distalization and high mandibular incisors retraction, with a consequent decrease in lower lip fullness (Fig 11). Fortunately, one year after treatment follow-up showed that the occlusion remained stable, with molar and canine in Class I relationship and good intercuspation (Figs 12 and 13).

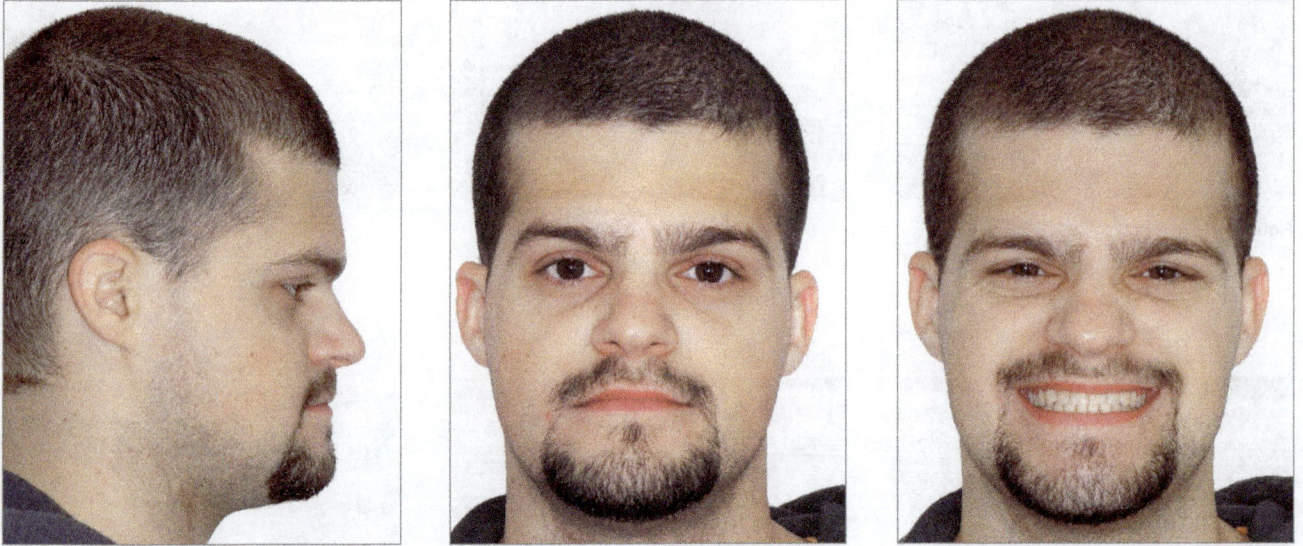

Figure 8 - Post-treatment facial photographs.

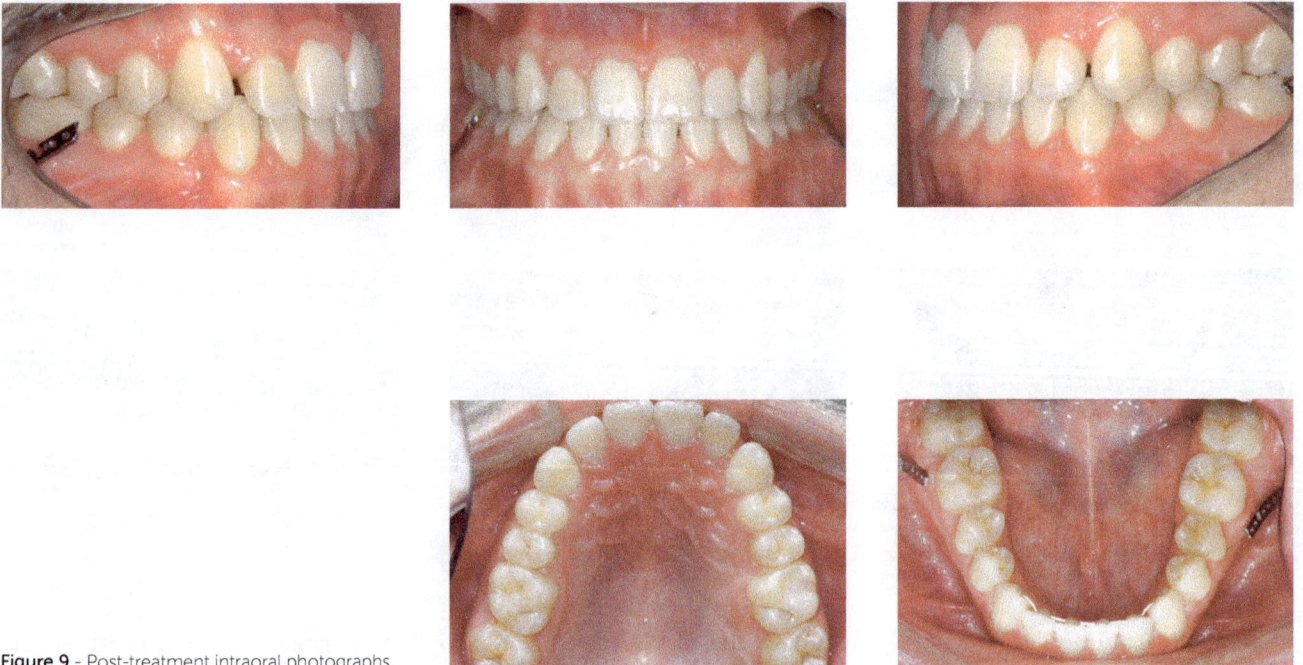

Figure 9 - Post-treatment intraoral photographs.

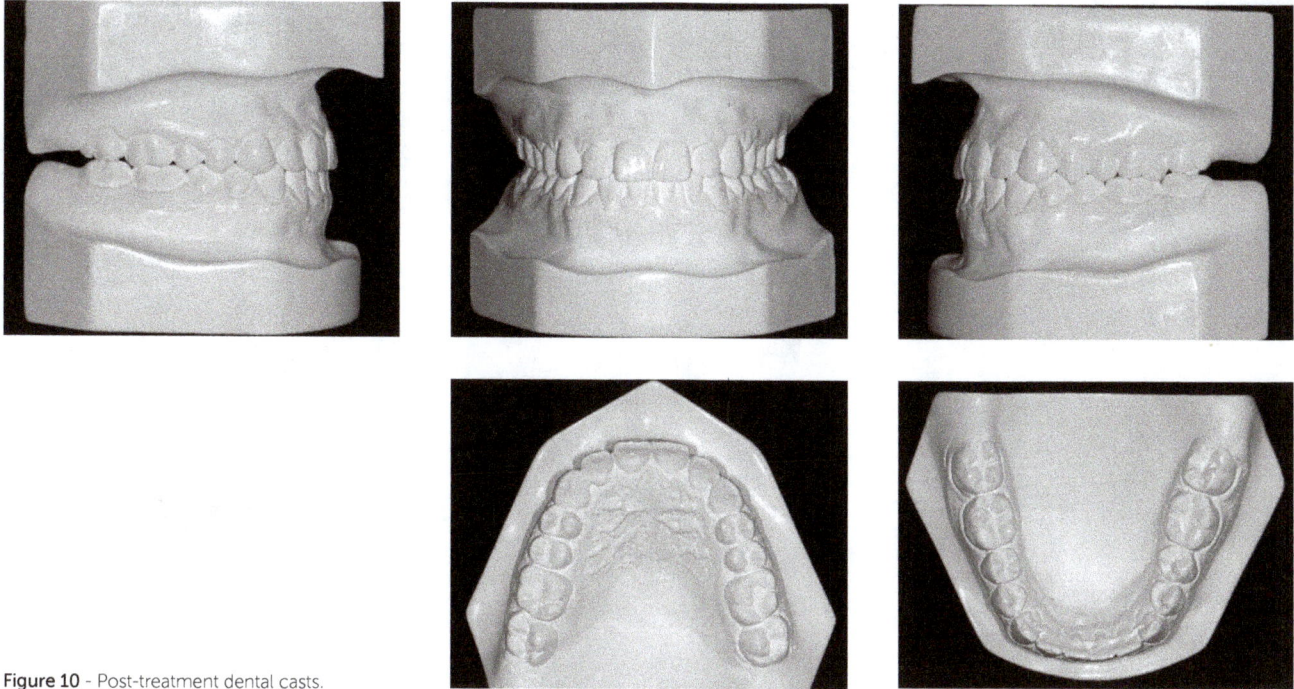

Figure 10 - Post-treatment dental casts.

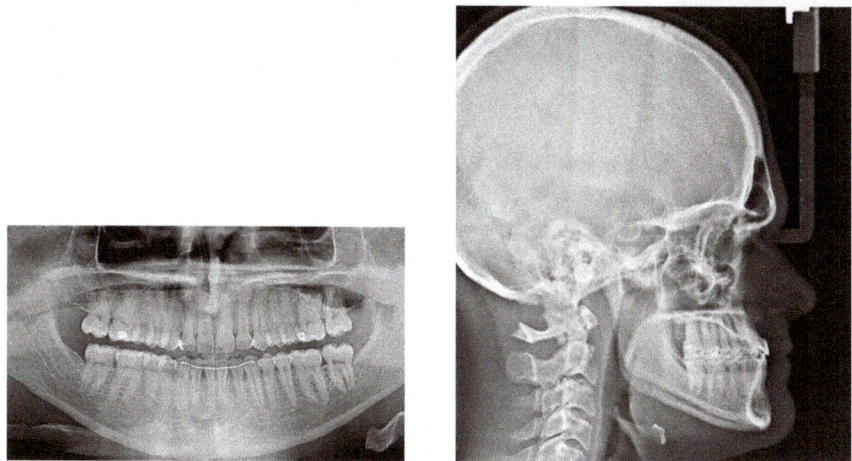

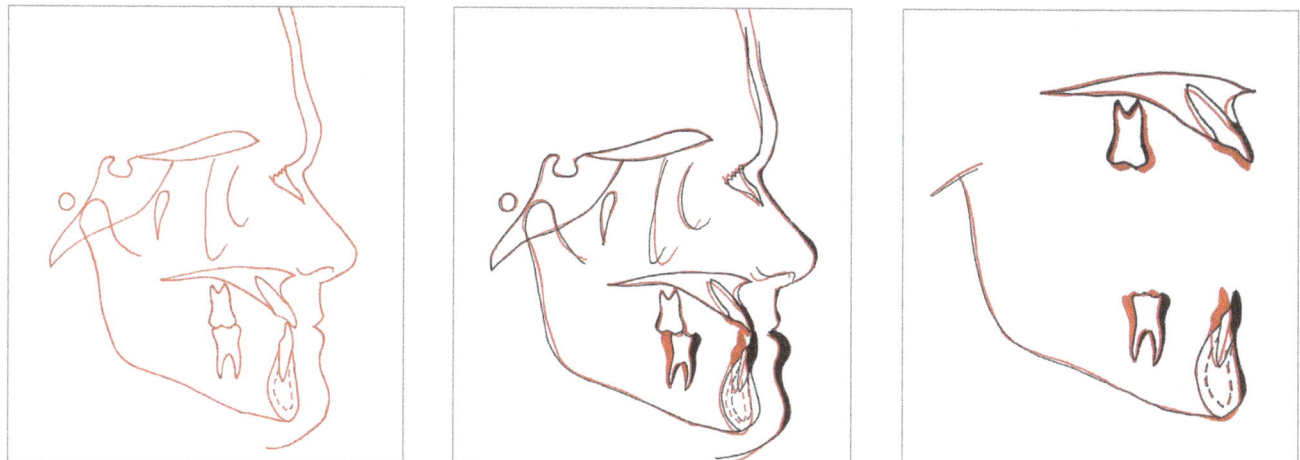

Figure 11 - Post-treatment radiographs, post-treatment cephalogram, total superimposition and partial superimpositions.

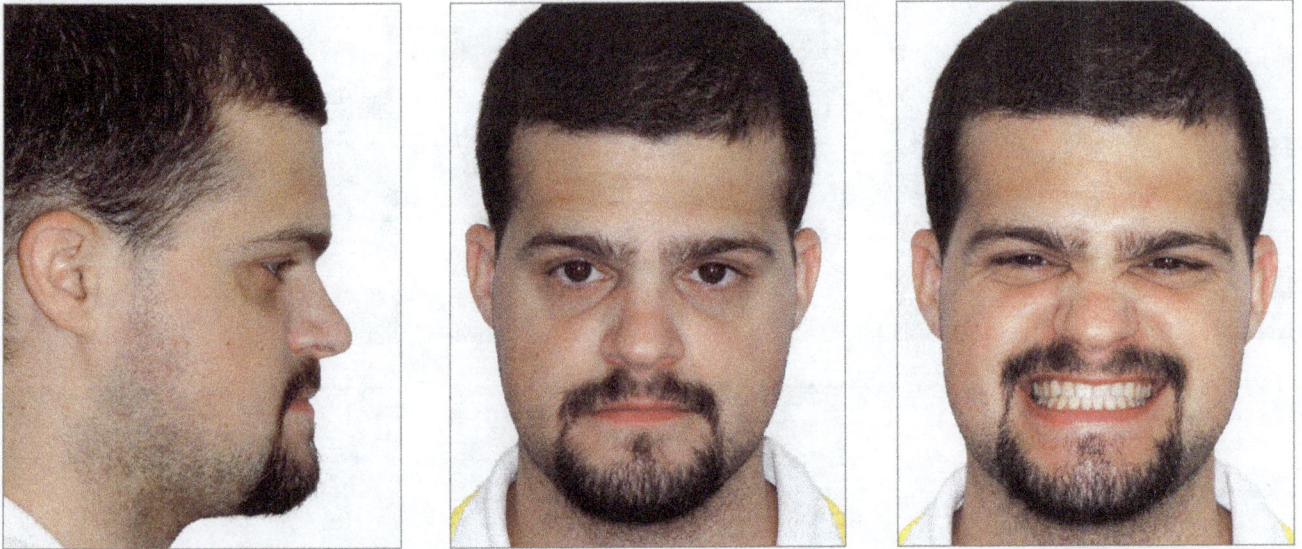

Figure 12 - 1-year post treatment facial photographs.

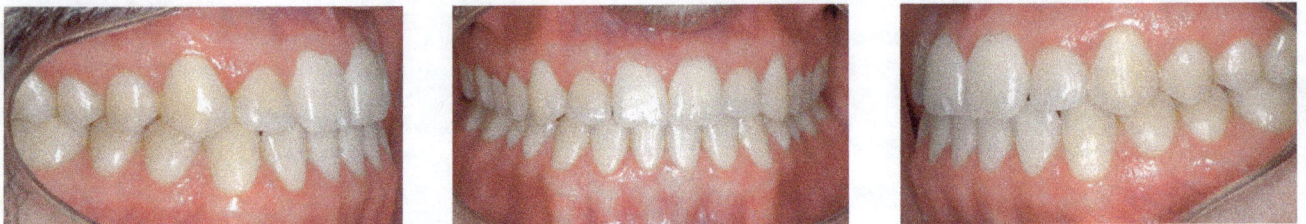

Figure 13 - 1-year post-treatment intraoral photographs.

Table 1 - Cephalometric measurements.

Measurements	Norms (SD)	Initial	Post-treatment
SNA	82° (3)	86	85
SNB	80° (3)	91	90
ANB	2° (2)	-5	-5
Facial convexity (NA.APog)	0° (2)	-13	-14
Facial angle (PoOr.NPog)	87° (3)	103	102
Y-axis	59° (6)	44	45
SN.GoGn	32° (3)	20	21
1-NA (°)	22°	44	41
1-NA (mm)	5 mm	6	8
1-NB (°)	25°	13	5
1-NB (mm)	5 mm	3	0
Inter-incisal angle	131° (5)	126	139
Ul-S line	0 mm (2)	-5	-4
Ll-S line	0 mm (2)	-1	-3
IMPA	90° (4)	85	74
FMA	25° (3)	9	11
FMIA	65° (4)	86	95

DISCUSSION

The present article reported the case of a 24-year-old man with severe skeletal Angle Class III malocclusion. The patient was treated by orthodontic camouflage treatment with miniplate anchorage. In the last few years, only slight skeletal discrepancies in adult patients were usually treated without orthognathic surgery.[9] Treatment options included the use of Class III elastics alone or in combination with a sliding jig or even headgears, stripping, and tooth extraction.[3,6,10] Unfortunately, all these options were associated with complications, such as counterclockwise rotation of the occlusal plane,[2,4,12,13] patient's noncompliance with elastics or headgears,[14,15] patient's refusal to undergo extraction, and the creation of Bolton discrepancy in cases of stripping. The advent of skeletal anchorage increased the reliability of results because it does not require patient compliance and it is associated with minimal or no side effects. In this context, miniplates represent the best option for simultaneous multiple tooth movement because of the increased stability generated by multiple screws instead of a single screw as with mini-implants. Conventionally, miniplates are inserted at two sites in Class III patients: on the external oblique ridge with the active end positioned at the mesial or distal surface of the first molar or on the lower border of the mandible with the active end positioned at the mesial surface of the first molar.[10] For the presented case, the surgeon faced some difficulty during the procedure and had to fix right and left miniplates with their active ends around the mesial and distal surfaces of the first molar, respectively, with no mechanical issues thereafter.

In patients with moderate skeletal Class III malocclusion, one question must always be addressed by orthodontists: is it possible to camouflage this malocclusion? There are several parameters influencing this decision. First, the extent of compromise on facial esthetics, and whether compromise is a big concern for the patient must be judged.[4,5,13] In the present study, the patient was not hugely concerned about his facial esthetics, and profile concavity was moderate. Certainly, if the patient's chief complaint was facial esthetics, orthognathic surgery, and not camouflage treatment alone, would be necessary. The second parameter is the anteroposterior position and angulation of maxillary and mandibular incisors. In patients with an edge-to-edge anterior bite or a slight anterior crossbite, correction can be achieved after judging the extent of maxillary incisor proclination and mandibular incisor retroclination. Our patient showed severe maxillary incisor proclination; however, mandibular incisors were not retroclined, thereby facilitating orthodontic camouflage by means of incisor retraction. The third parameter is thickness of mandibular symphysis, which should be adequate to allow extensive incisor retraction.[3] Fortunately, in our patient, the anteroposterior dimension of the symphysis was adequate. Finally, the last parameter is the degree of anteroposterior discrepancy. Even if facial esthetics is acceptable, the symphysis is thick enough, and mandibular incisors are slightly proclined, camouflage is not possible if anteroposterior discrepancy is too severe. Considering that anteroposterior discrepancy was moderate in the patient reported herein, orthodontic camouflage was selected.

One major concern for orthodontists is stability of camouflage treatment after mandibular incisor retraction in patients with Class III malocclusion.[5,14] Considering that the entire arch is retracted by 4–5 mm, the tongue has less space after treatment, thus resulting in extreme tongue pressure on mandibular incisors and consequent relapse with premature contact between incisors and abnormal spacing between mandibular teeth.[10,16] Some alternatives to improve stability in such cases include achieving an ideal overjet, overbite, and intercuspation;[2,5] maintenance of mandibular posterior teeth in an upright position after distalization because distal tipping tends cause them to return to their original position according to their root apices;[10,14,15] using a 3 × 3 bonded mandibular retainer for an undetermined period of time;[13] myofunctional therapy to eliminate tongue interposition during swallowing and rest; and to position the tip of the tongue at the incisive papilla during swallowing and in the posterior region of the oral cavity at rest.[17]

Superimpositions at follow-up revealed excessive remodeling of the symphysis because of mandibular incisor retraction. Incisors centered on the symphysis at the beginning of treatment maintained the centers at the end of treatment, thus avoiding gingival recession in the long-term and improving stability.[5] In the case presented herein, analysis one year after treatment revealed excellent stability of results. The patient will remain under post-treatment follow-up once a year.

CONCLUSION

In the case reported herein, miniplates proved to be reliable as anchorage unit for mandibular dentition distalization and camouflage of skeletal Class III, thus avoiding orthognathic surgery.

REFERENCES

1. Antoszewska J, Kosior M, Antoszewska N. Treatment approaches in Class III malocclusion with emphasis on maximum skeletal anchorage: review of literature. J Stomatol. 2011;64:667-83.

2. Farret MM, Benitez Farret MM. Skeletal Class III malocclusion treated using a non-surgical approach supplemented with mini-implants: a case report. J Orthod. 2013 Sept;40(3):256-63.

3. Choi JY, Lim WH, Chun YS. Class III nonsurgical treatment using indirect skeletal anchorage: A case report. Korean J Orthod. 2008;38(1):60-7.

4. Lin J, Gu Y. Preliminary investigation of nonsurgical treatment of severe skeletal Class III malocclusion in the permanent dentition. Angle Orthod. 2003 Aug;73(4):401-10.

5. Moullas AT, Palomo JM, Gass JR, Amberman BD, White J, Gustovich D. Nonsurgical treatment of a patient with a Class III malocclusion. Am J Orthod Dentofacial Orthop. 2006;129(4 Suppl):S111-8.

6. Kuroda Y, Kuroda S, Alexander RG, Tanaka E. Adult Class III treatment using a J-hook headgear to the mandibular arch. Angle Orthod. 2010 Mar;80(2):336-43.

7. Freire-Maia B, Pereira TJ, Ribeiro MP. Distalization of impacted mandibular second molar using miniplates for skeletal anchorage: case report. Dent Press J Orthod. 2011;16(4):132-6.

8. Kuroda S, Tanaka E. Application of temporary anchorage devices for the treatment of adult Class III malocclusions. Semin Orthod. 2011;17(2):91-7.

9. Sugawara Y, Kuroda S, Tamamura N, Takano-Yamamoto T. Adult patient with mandibular protrusion and unstable occlusion treated with titanium screw anchorage. Am J Orthod Dentofacial Orthop. 2008 Jan;133(1):102-11.

10. Sugawara J, Daimaruya T, Umemori M, Nagasaka H, Takahashi I, Kawamura H, et al. Distal movement of mandibular molars in adult patients with the skeletal anchorage system. Am J Orthod Dentofacial Orthop. 2004 Feb;125(2):130-8.

11. Consolaro A. Mini-implants and miniplates generate sub-absolute and absolute anchorage. Dental Press J Orthod. 2014 May-Jun;19(3):20-3.

12. Baek S-H, Yang I-H, Kim K-W, Ahn H-W. Treatment of Class III malocclusions using miniplate and mini-implant anchorage. Semin Orthod. 2011;17(2):98-107.

13. Sobral MC, Habib FA, Nascimento AC. Vertical control in the Class III compensatory treatment. Dental Press J Orthod. 2013 Mar-Apr;18(2):141-59.

14. Chung KR, Kim SH, Choo H, Kook YA, Cope JB. Distalization of the mandibular dentition with mini-implants to correct a Class III malocclusion with a midline deviation. Am J Orthod Dentofacial Orthop. 2010 Jan;137(1):135-46.

15. Sakai Y, Kuroda S, Murshid SA, Takano-Yamamoto T. Skeletal Class III severe openbite treatment using implant anchorage. Angle Orthod. 2008 Jan;78(1):157-66.

16. Saito I, Yamaki M, Hanada K. Nonsurgical treatment of adult open bite using edgewise appliance combined with high-pull headgear and Class III elastics. Angle Orthod. 2005 Mar;75(2):277-83.

17. Farret MM, Farret MM, Farret AM. Skeletal Class III and anterior open bite treatment with different retention protocols: a report of three cases. J Orthod. 2012 Sept;39(3):212-23.

12

Fixed Lingual Mandibular Growth Modificator: A new appliance for Class II correction

Osama Hasan Alali[1]

Introduction: This article demonstrates the description and use of a new appliance for Class II correction. **Material and Methods:** A case report of a 10-year 5 month-old girl who presented with a skeletally-based Class II division 1 malocclusion (ANB = 6.5°) on a slightly low-angle pattern, with ML-NSL angle of 30° and ML-NL angle of 22.5°. Overjet was increased (7 mm) and associated with a deep bite. **Results:** Overjet and overbite reduction was undertaken with the new appliance, Fixed Lingual Mandibular Growth Modificator (FLMGM). **Conclusion:** FLMGM may be effective in stimulating the growth of the mandible and correcting skeletal Class II malocclusions. Clinicians can benefit from the unique clinical advantages that FLMGM provides, such as easy handling and full integration with bracketed appliance at any phase.

Keywords: Orthodontic appliance design. Functional orthodontic appliances. Angle Class II malocclusion.

[1] MDS in Orthodontics, Teaching Assistant, Graduate-PhD.

Osama Hasan Alali
P.O.box: 10256 – Aleppo, Syrian Arab Republic
E-mail: osama-alali@hotmail.com

INTRODUCTION

Many different appliances are now available for correcting skeletal Class II malocclusions. Some are removable[1] such as activator and double-plate; and others are fixed[2] such as Herbst appliance and MARA.

Double plate system, that was introduced for the first time by Schwarz in the early 1940s,[3] is a reliable means for treating Angle Class II, Division 1 malocclusions[4]. Sander et al.[5,6,7] have verified the effectiveness of this system in a number of studies, providing detailed information on the biomechanics and thus on the working principles. This effectiveness prompted the author to develop a fixed double-plate system, Fixed Lingual Mandibular Growth Modificator (FLMGM), that would not require patient compliance; especially because several studies[8-11] have proven that fixed functional appliances are much more efficient in stimulating skeletal mandibular growth than removable ones.

From a clinical perspective, the FLMGM offers the following advantages:

1) Permanent effect, independent of patient compliance, as it is fixed.
2) Esthetics, as it is small and lingually located.
3) Eliminates the need for two separate treatment phases, as it is suitable for use in parallel with complete multibracket appliance in both arches.
4) Flexibility in treatment timing, as it can be used anytime during the mixed and permanent dentition.
5) No interference with occlusal development.
6) Wide and comfortable range of mastication movements, as the appliance consists of two separate parts with no permanent and physical intermaxillary connection.

7) Construction bite is unnecessary because of the easy and quick chairside reactivation and progressive advancement of the mandible in small increments.
8) Easy to handle because its insertion, clipping, and removal are very simple.
9) Economic and cost effective, because it does not involve ready-made components, and only one appliance is necessary for entire orthopedic phase.

APPLIANCE DESIGN

The FLMGM consists of two separate and fixed parts. The upper one is palatally positioned but bucally clipped to traditional upper molars bands (Fig 1A), while the lower is lingually welded to traditional lower molars bands (Fig 1B).

Maxillary part

It has the following components (Fig 2):

1) Acrylic button: it is similar to Nance button, and designed to connect wire elements of the maxillary part, preventing them from embedding into the mucosa. This button is seated on the anterior area of the palate as anterior as possible with no contact with front teeth (1-2 mm away from the gingival margin). Its dimensions should be as small as possible to allow mucosal and periodontal hygiene.

2) Two retention wires: one in each side, specifically designed by the author to give excellent retention, facilitate dealing with the appliance, and to enhance oral hygiene condition. They are fabricated with round 1 mm thick stainless steel orthodontic wire. The wires are anteriorly embedded into the acrylic button, run posteriorly without any contact with palatal mucosa, and each one contains an "U" loop with coil (giving some flexibility

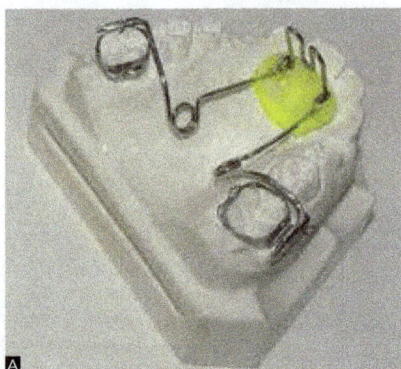

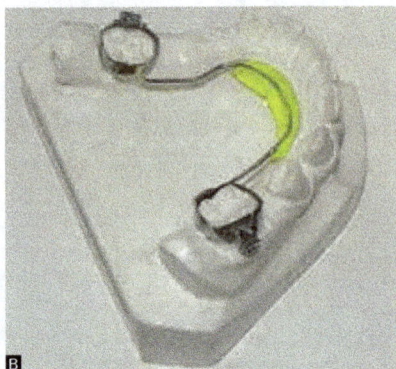

Figure 1 - Fixed lingual mandibular growth modificator (FLMGM). No physical attachment between maxillary (**A**) and mandibular (**B**) parts.

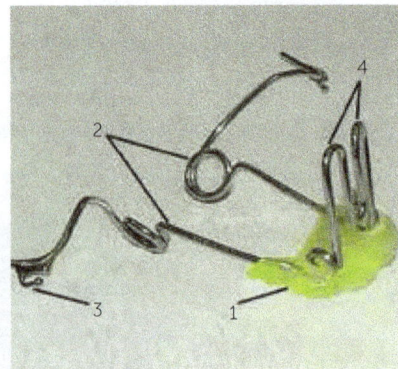

Figure 2 - Components of maxillary part: acrylic button (**1**); retention wires (**2**); retention hooks (**3**) and advancement loops (**4**).

to help in easy insertion and removal) at the level of second upper premolar. After the coils, the wires should run perpendicular to the midline towards the vestibule at the level of the mesial surface of upper first molar through the interdental space. Then, in the vestibule, the wires should run posteriorly to enter into the headgear tube.

3) Two retention hooks: one in each side, have a ball end to avoid irritation, and are directed anteriorly and welded to the retention wire before entering the headgear tube.

4) Advancement loops: wire projection embedded in the acrylic button and extended towards the mandible. They consist of two consecutive long "U" loops, contain small protection coils where the wire exits the acrylic button, and are fabricated with round 1 mm thick hard stainless steel wire. The inclination of this advancing loops to the occlusal plane is about 70°, measured posteriorly.[12]

Mandibular part

It is made in a similar manner to a standard lingual arch with 1.0 mm stainless steel hard wire welded to the lingual aspect of first molars bands (Fig 3), and has the following features:

1) Its level in the anterior region must be 3-4 mm below the gingival margins of the incisors (Fig 4).

2) It includes an inclined guiding plane, made of acrylic resin, fixed on the anterior part of lingual arch, seated on the lingual alveolar mucosa below the level of incisors necks till the level of mouth floor, and it is smooth to allow sliding against the advancement loops during mandibular closing movement to reach its anterior position.

CLINICAL PROCEDURE

Separators are placed mesial and distal to the lower first molars. Subsequently, bands are selected and placed in position (Fig 5A and C). Optionally, construction bite can be taken in an edge-to-edge mandible position. Upper and lower good alginate impressions are taken over the bands, with a good extension in the lingual sulcus. Bands are removed from the mouth and seated accurately in the impressions (Fig 5B and D). The impressions are sent to the laboratory for appliance fabrication. In the sequence, upper molar bands are cemented in position (Fig 6A). The inclined plane supported by lingual arch must be checked for stability, then the lower molar bands are cemented (Fig 6B). On the next day, maxillary part of corrector is attached to the upper molar bands (Fig 7A) by inserting the posterior ends of the retention wires into the headgear tubes. To ensure good stabilization of the maxillary part, an elastomeric ligature is used to tie the band hook and the retention hook together (Fig 7B).

Reactivation visits

Reactivation is generally required about every 2-3 months, and is carried out at the chairside, intra- or extraorally, by bending the advancement loops using orthodontic pliers.

CASE REPORT
Diagnosis

A 10-year 5-month-old girl presented with the chief complaints of the appearance of proclined upper incisors, retro-positioned chin, and dissatisfaction with her gingival smile. The family was concerned about the

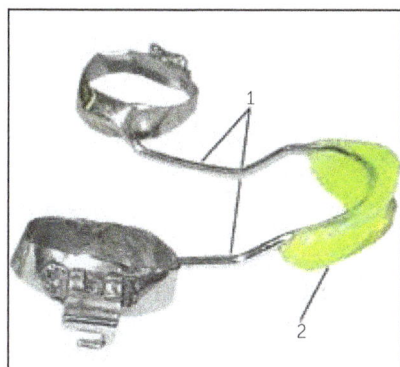

Figure 3 - Components of mandibular part: lingual arch (**1**) and inclined guiding plane (**2**).

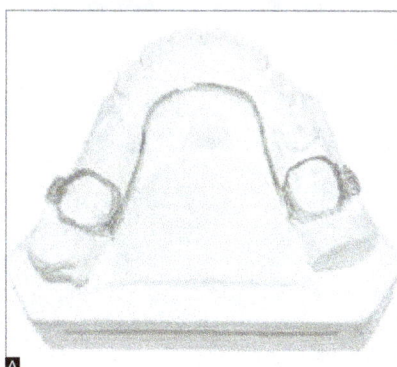

Figure 4 - Level of the lingual arch 3-4 mm below the gingival margin.

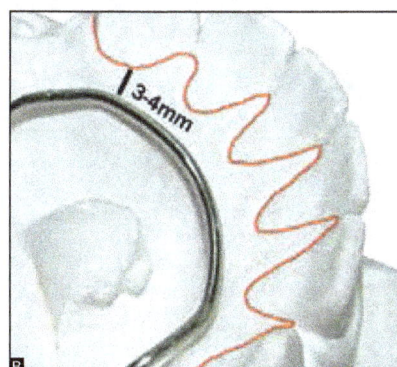

lack of facial harmony and anxious for its improvement. The patient reported a history of bad oral habit, lower-lip sucking, many years ago and an early loss of four lower primary molars.

On examination, she presented with a Class II division 1 incisor relationship on a moderate Skeletal II bases. Clinical examination showed a convex-type facial profile with a decreased anterior lower facial height and obviously obtuse nasolabial angle (Fig 8A to C). Pretreatment intraoral examination of her dentition (Fig 8D to I) revealed that the pattern of oral hygiene was good and that she was in the late mixed dentition. The upper and lower labial segments were well aligned

and slightly protrusive in appearance. There was some tipping of the lower right canine, first premolar and first permanent molar into the second primary molar extraction site. Apart from this slight constriction in the lower right buccal segment, the lower arch had a good form. In occlusion, the incisor relationship was Class II division I with an increased overjet of 7 mm and a traumatic deep bite of 5 mm (Fig 8E and H). The upper dental midline was coincident with the facial midline, whilst the lower centerline was displaced 1 mm to the right. The molar relationship was an end-on (half unit) Class II on the left side and Class I on the right (Fig 8G and I).

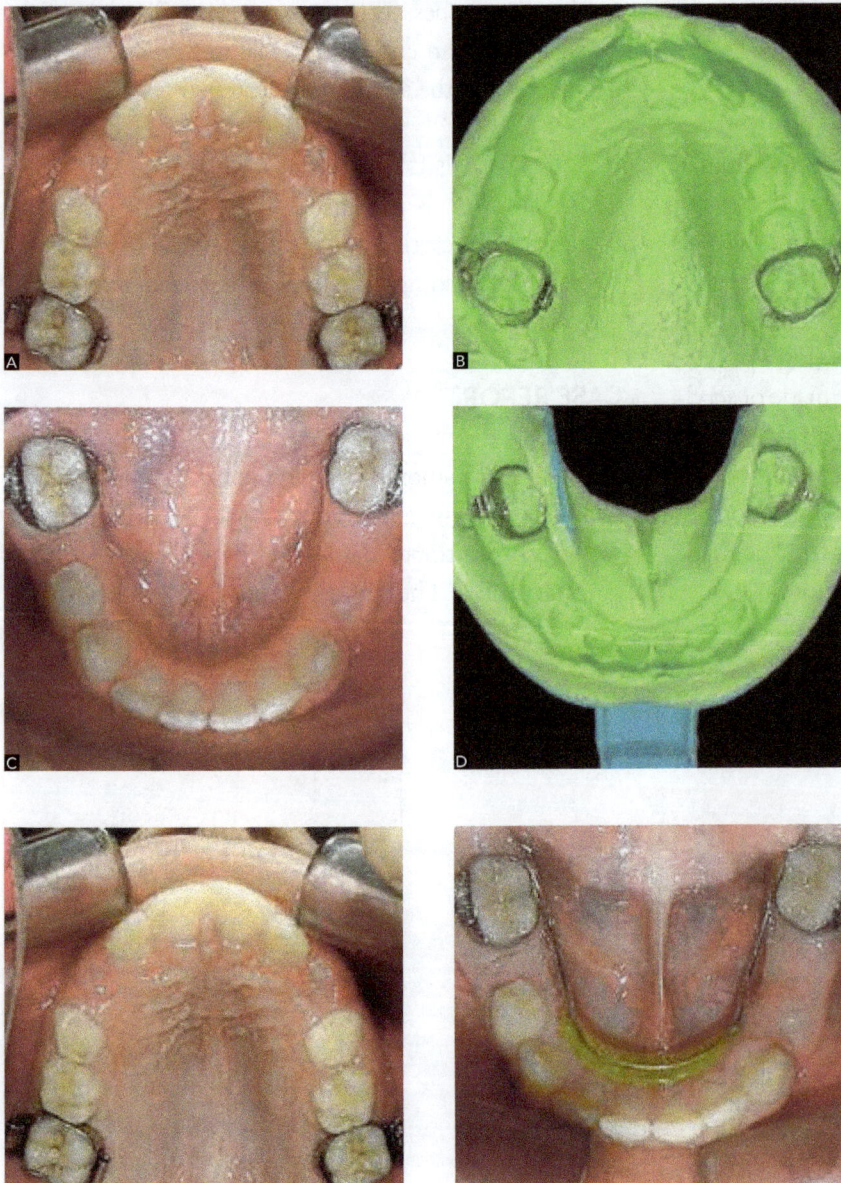

Figure 5 - Molar bands placed in situ (**A** and **C**), and repositioned in alginate impressions (**B** and **D**).

Figure 6 - The upper bands and the mandibular part cemented in place.

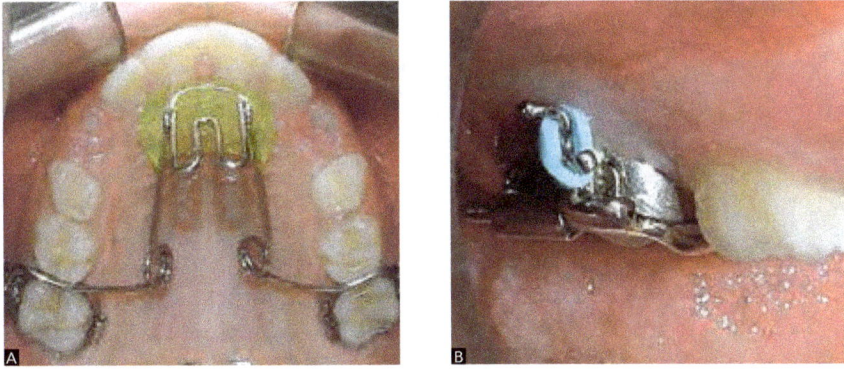

Figure 7 - Maxillary part inserted into headgear tubes (**A**) and an elastomeric ligature placed between the band hook and the retention hook to clip the maxillary part (**B**).

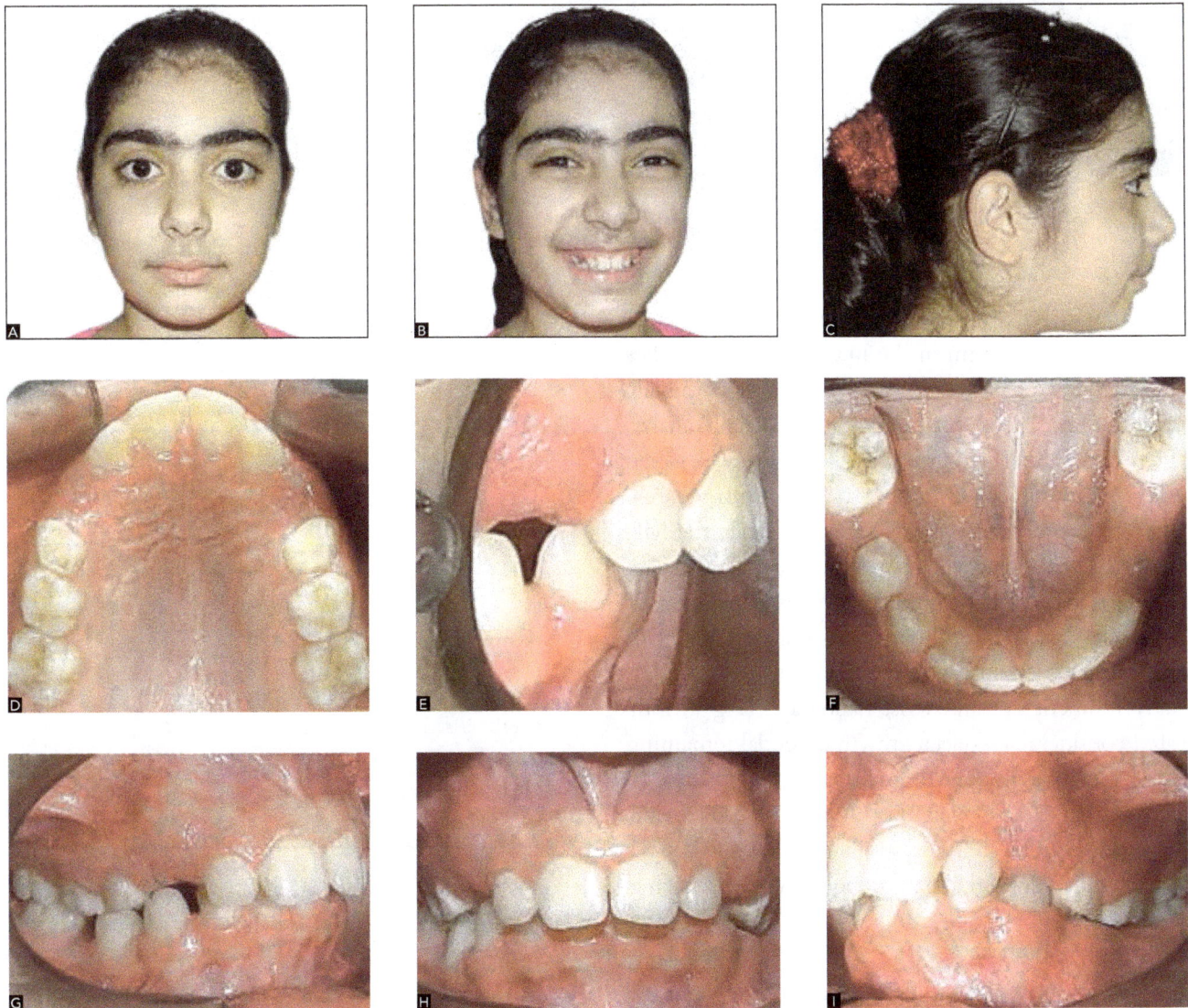

Figure 8 - Pretreatment facial and intraoral photographs (age 10 years and 5 months). Increased overjet and overbite.

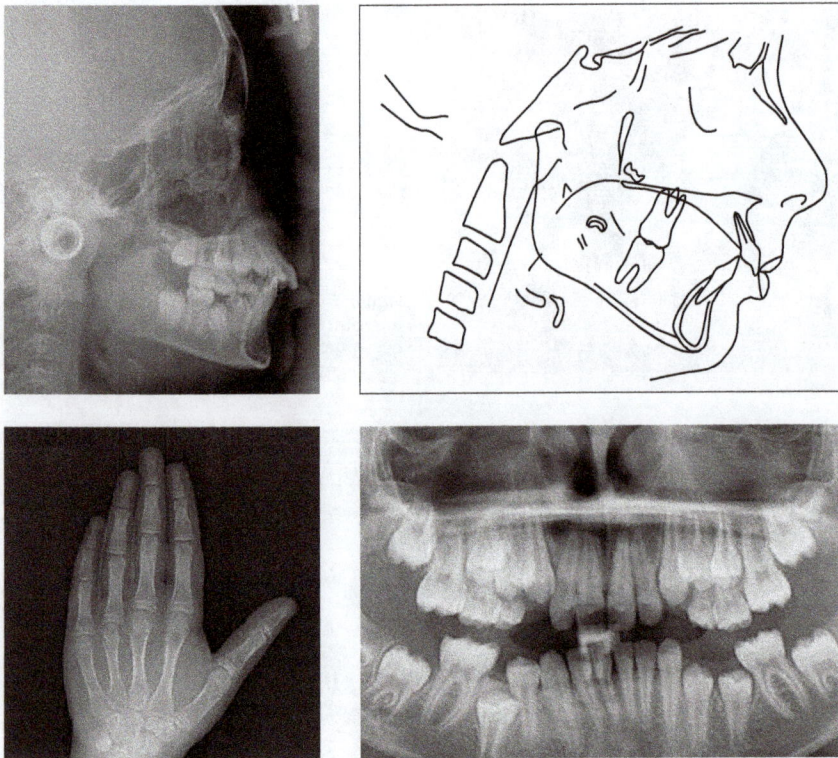

Figure 9 - Pretreatment radiographs and cephalometric tracing.

Cast analysis revealed arch-length discrepancies of +3 mm and -3 mm in the upper and lower arches, respectively. The lower right first molar was mesially drifted. The lateral cephalometric radiograph analysis (Fig 9 and Table 1) confirmed that, skeletally, the patient had a moderate Class II jaw relationship, ANB was 6.5°, and a reduced maxillomandibular plane angle, the ML-NL was 22.5°. Dentally, there was a degree of bimaxillary proclination and the interincisal angle was 120.5°. Soft tissue profile showed that the upper lip was slightly behind 'E' line, and the nasolabial angle was obviously obtuse (124°).

Assessment of hand-wrist radiograph (Fig 9) indicated considerable skeletal growth potential remaining. The patient was in the MP3cap stage.

Panoramic radiograph (Fig 9) revealed no obvious pathology present. The lower right second premolar was impacted. In addition, the third molars were developing.

Treatment objectives

The objectives of nonextraction treatment for the patient were identified as follows: (1) Reduce the anteroposterior skeletal disharmony; (2) Establish ideal overjet and overbite relationship; and (3) Achieve a functional occlusion with good interdigitation.

Table 1 - Cephalometric summary.

variables	T_0	T_1	Δ (T_1-T_0)
SNA (degrees)	84	83	-1
SNB (degrees)	77.5	80	+2.5
ANB (degrees)	6.5	3	-3.5
NSAr (degrees)	128.5	126	-1.5
SNL.NL (degrees)	7.5	7	-0.5
SNL.ML (degrees)	30	31	+1
NL.ML (degrees)	22.5	24	+1.5
U1.SNL (degrees)	108	104.5	-3.5
U1.NL (degrees)	116	111.5	-4.5
L1.ML (degrees)	101.5	98.5	-3
Interincisal angle (degrees)	120.5	126	+5.5
Upper lip (mm)	-1	-2	-1
Lower lip (mm)	1	1	0
Nasolabial angle (degrees)	124	127.5	+3.5

T_0: Pre-treatment records (Fig 9),
T_1: after 8 months and 1 week of orthopedic correction (Fig 13).

Treatment plan

Two-phase nonextraction approach was planned. For the first phase (orthopedic), treatment goal was to stimulate mandibular growth, improving facial appearance and profile, and reduce the overjet and overbite to an acceptable level (with re-evaluation after 8 months). During the second phase (orthodontic), the goal would be to maintain the improvement achieved in the orthopedic phase, and to obtain a functional occlusion with a Class I molar and canine relationships. Retainers would be placed immediately after appliances were removed for retention purposes.

Treatment progress

At 10 years and 5 months, FLMGM was used to improve skeletal Class II by stimulating mandibular growth.

The patient was very motivated with the treatment. An additional motivating factor is the noticeable improvement of facial appearance when FLMGM is fitted. The patient was instructed to bite in an edge-to-edge position and to keep her lips in touch as much as possible (Fig 11). The patient was seen regularly at 6 weeks intervals, and at each visit, the occlusion was checked. The lip seal was maintained throughout treatment. At 11 years and 3 months, to assess the orthopedic changes, only the maxillary part was removed, and a set of facial and intraoral photographs was taken (Fig 12); and radiographs were requested (Fig 13).

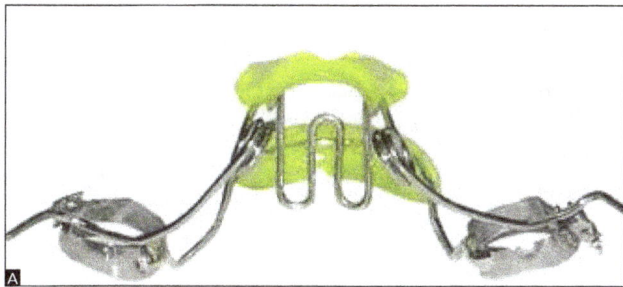

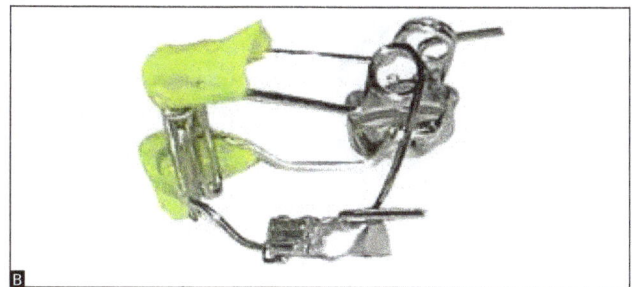

Figure 10 - Design of FLMGM: Posterior (**A**) and lateral (**B**) views.

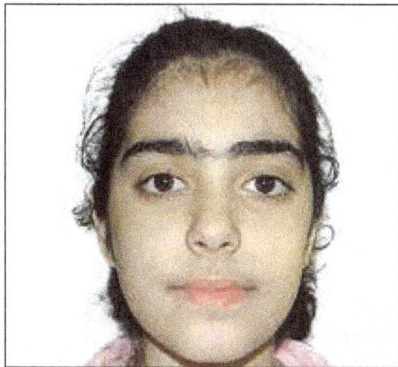

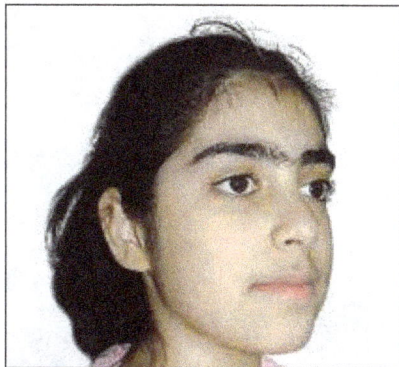

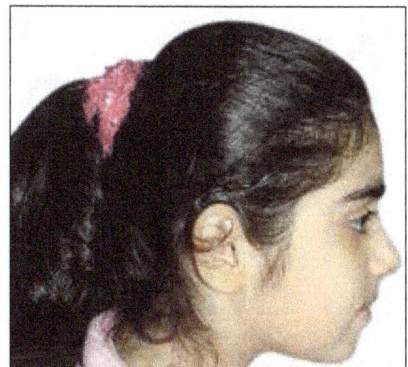

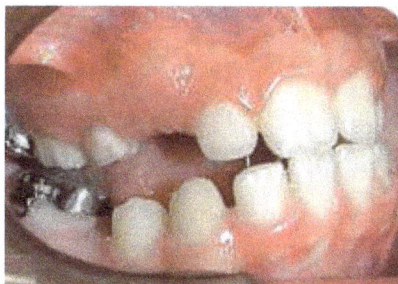

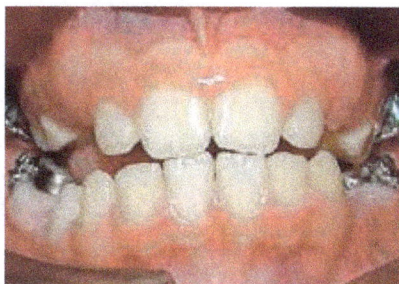

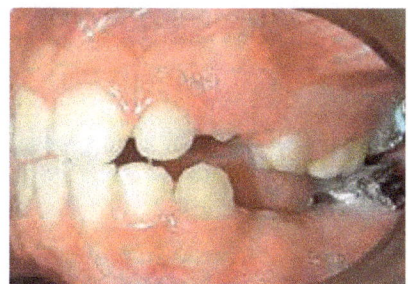

Figure 11 - Beginning of treatment, the FLMGM in place. Facial and intraoral photographs. The incisors were in an edge-to-edge bite and the lips touching.

Results achieved

Through the course of FLMGM correction, about 8 months, the overjet was reduced from 7 mm to approximately 2 mm, normal incisor and canine relationships were established, vertical eruption of lateral segments was enhanced, the lower midline coincided with the soft tissue midline, and a nice improvement in the facial esthetics and balance were achieved (Fig 12).

Data derived from cephalometric analysis (Fig 13 and Table 1) and superimpositions (Fig 14) reveal that there was continued vertical growth with valuable change in the anteroposterior relationship. Skeletally, ANB angle decreased from 6.5° to 3°, indicating that FLMGM caused skeletal change. Anteroposterior growth of the maxilla was held, although A point still came forward. SNB angle increased by 2.5°, and significant growth of the mandible occurred. ML–NSL angle increased by 1°. Dentally, even with no brackets, the tipped-out upper incisors underwent 4.5° of uprighting, and the lower incisors were extruded and slightly uprighted by 3°, which is considered quite surprising. Eventually, interincisal angle increased to a good value, 130°. In addition to vertical movement, the maxillary first molars also moved distally (Headgear effect) as shown in Figure 14.

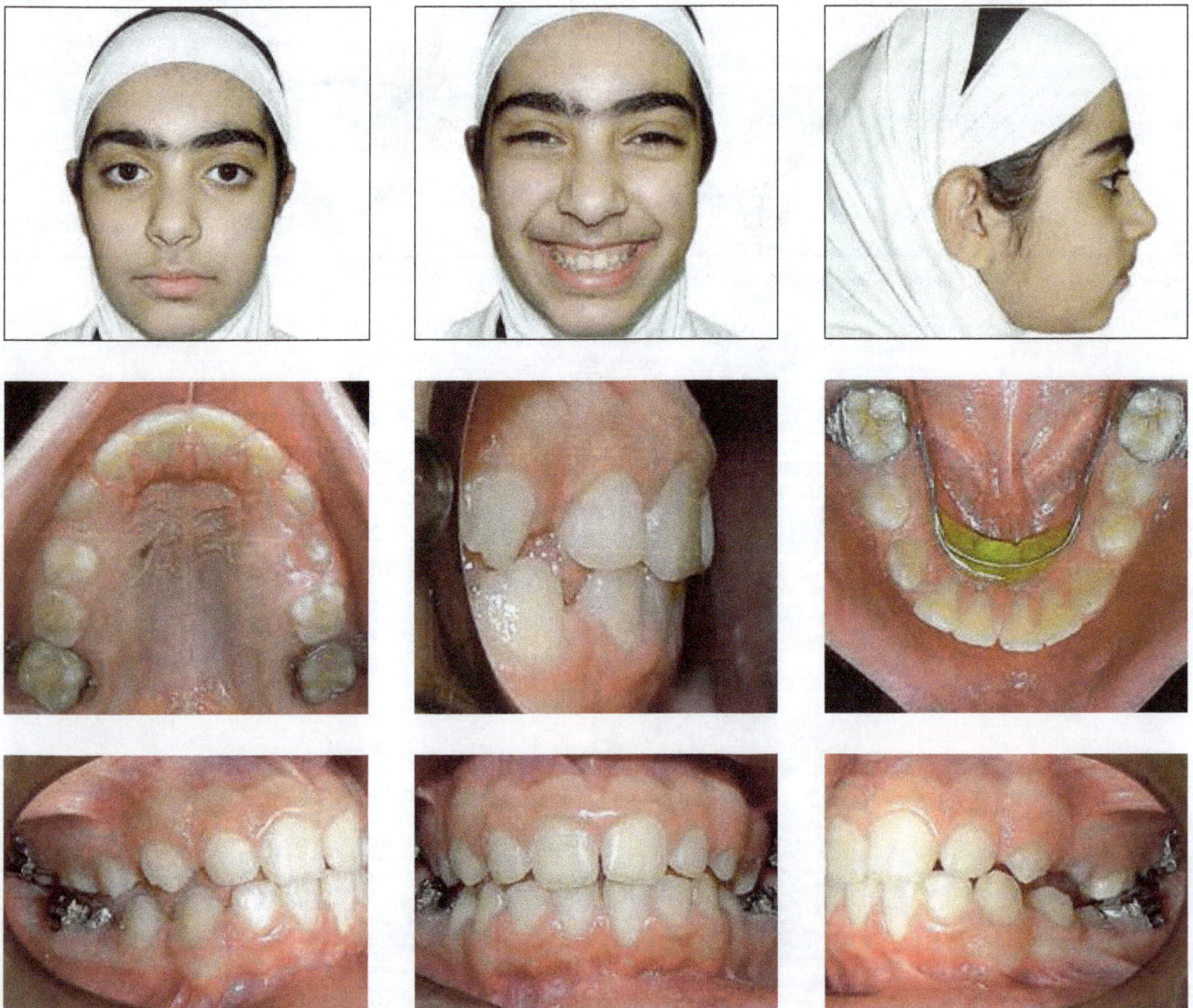

Figure 12 - Facial and intraoral photographs immediately after removal of the maxillary part, promoting a normal incisor relationship, with buccal segments partially out of occlusion.

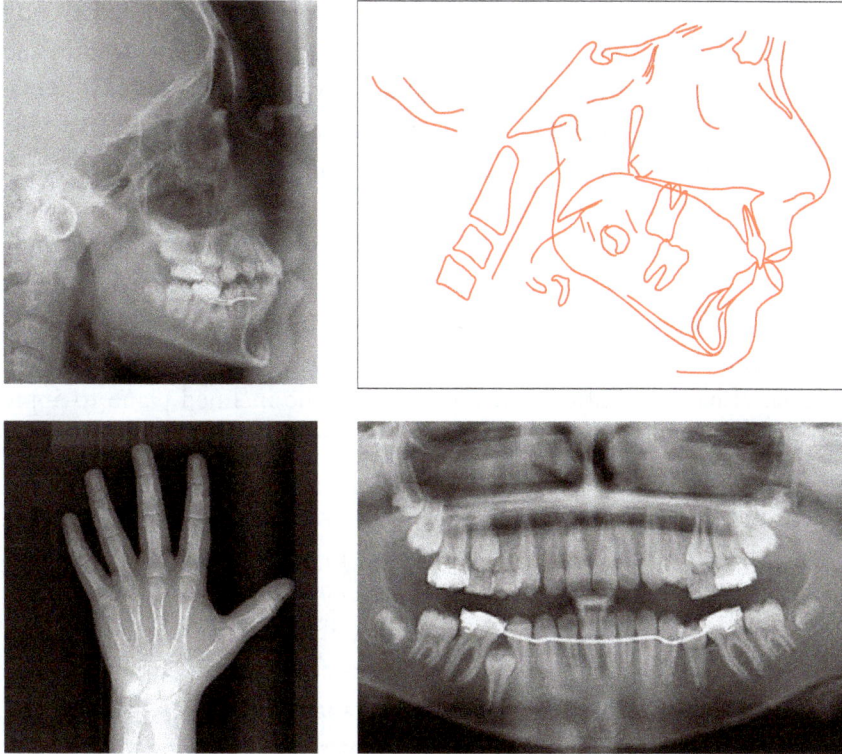

Figure 13 - Radiographs and cephalometric tracing after orthopedic treatment.

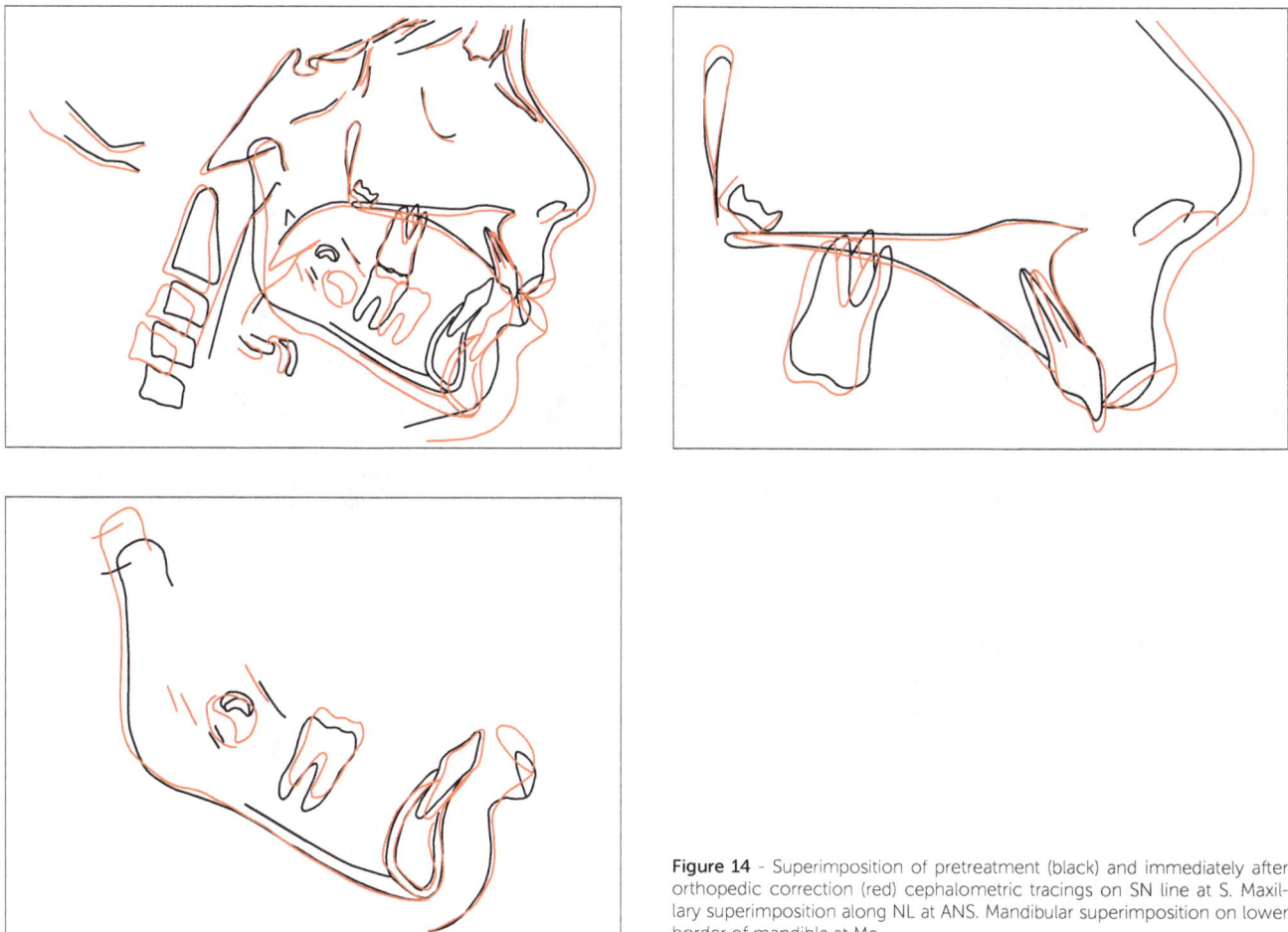

Figure 14 - Superimposition of pretreatment (black) and immediately after orthopedic correction (red) cephalometric tracings on SN line at S. Maxillary superimposition along NL at ANS. Mandibular superimposition on lower border of mandible at Me.

DISCUSSION

In a growing patient, better aesthetic result would ideally be obtained by using orthopedic appliances to accelerate mandible development.[13-17] The FLMGM has effectively been used by the author in skeletal Class II division 1 patients, and a PhD clinical research is now in progress to identify its effectiveness. In the present case, the author attempted to stimulate mandible growth using FLMGM that was well tolerated without complications. Within 8 months of orthopedic treatment, the overjet was considerably enhanced, and the facial harmony was good. The uprighting of incisors was favorable, and this is believed to be resulting from the mechanism of breaking balance between the tongue and lips. While the vertical loops work as a shield relieving the tongue pressure on the incisors, only lingually-directed functional forces generated by the sealed lips affect the incisors and cause lingual crowns tipping.

Conceptually, FLMGM represents an exercise device for the facial and masticatory muscles, in the same way as other functional appliances. It is proven that muscular training is important factor in the normal development of bone.[18] After the appliance is placed,

the patient is asked to keep his mouth closed as long as possible. Once the patient closes his mouth, the inclined plane and the advancement loops will come in contact in the anterior area of the mouth. By continuation of mouth closing, the inclined plane will be forced to slide against the loops, and eventually the mandible will take a predetermined forced anterior position (Fig 15). Functional force, generated by muscles that attempt to return the mandible posteriorly to its original position,[19] causes the upper acrylic button and the lower acrylic inclined plane to apply pressure on the oral mucosa, and this in turn is supposed to cause proprioceptive response that repositions the mandible forward in the same way as the Fränkel II Regulator[20]. In the first period, the patient avoids collision between the loops and the inclined plane by forward-mandibular movement, and with time, the mandible functions without interference in the desired position and the patient will automatically, via neuromuscular reprogramming, close comfortably into the protrusive position. The repetition of the new closure pattern results in orofacial musculature reeducation and induces skeletal adaptation.[19]

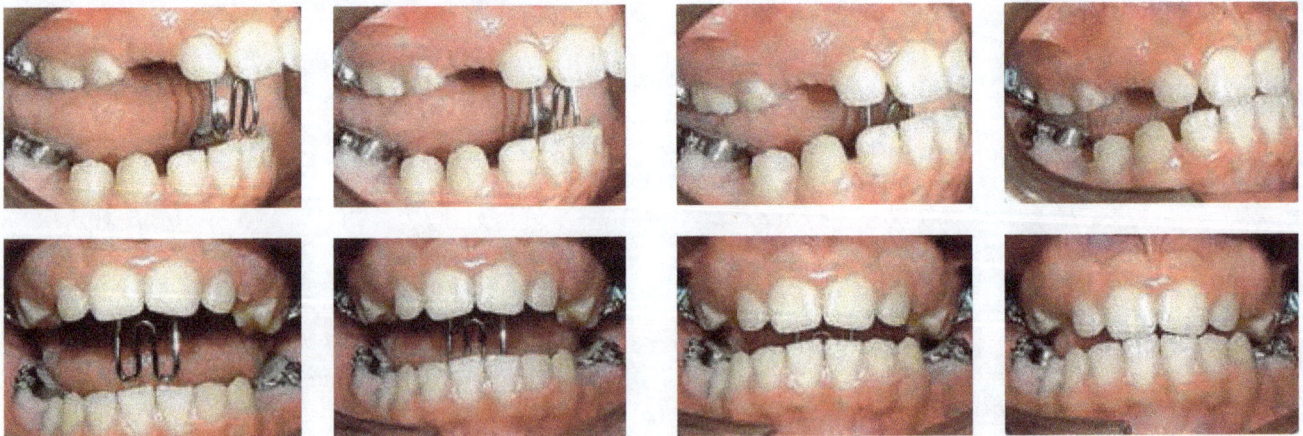

Figure 15 - Mode of action.

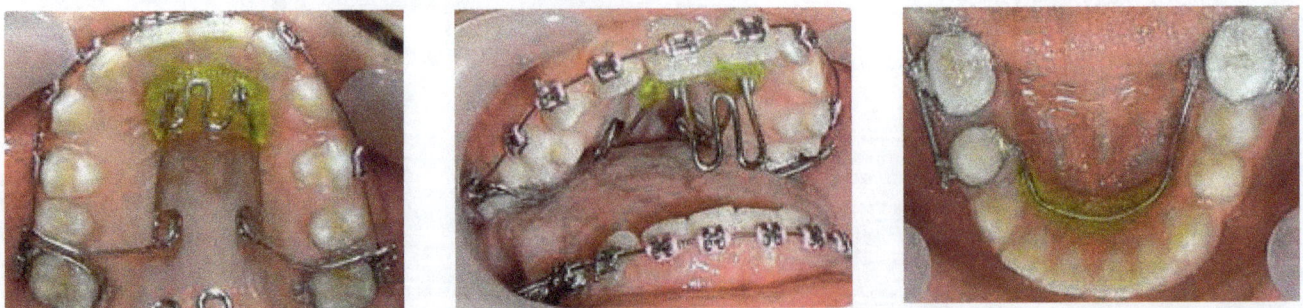

Figure 16 - Coordination of FLMGM with full-bonded appliance.

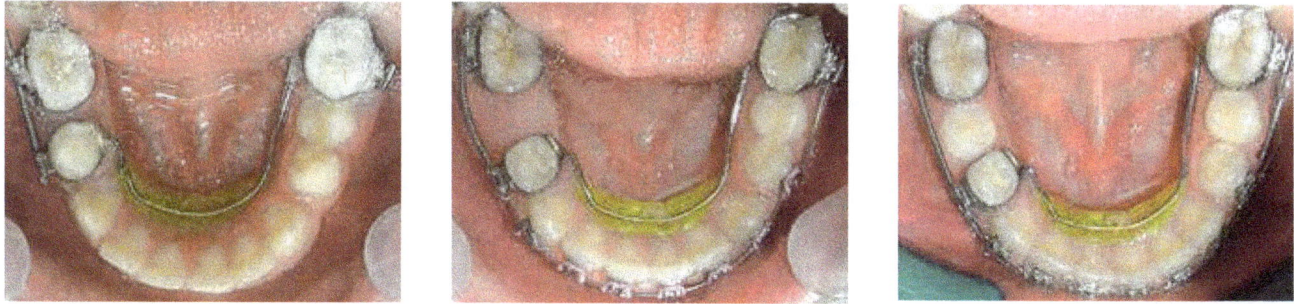

Figure 17 - Mandibular part was modified, and an open coil spring was used to deliver distal force required to distalize the lower right molar. After that, lower right second premolar spontaneously erupted.

Technically, the FLMGM represents a fixed version of the removable double-plate appliance because the two appliances follow an identical mechanism of action, based on incorporating an inclined plane in the mandible and guide bars in the maxilla. The most important two advantages of FLMGM over removable double-plate are: (1) FLMGM is active full-time, regardless of patient cooperation; (2) With FLMGM, the functional appliance phase is not separated from but completely integrated with the bracketed appliance phase (Fig 16). In clinical practices, although not many orthopaedic appliances are suitable for this integration, Dynamax and MARA do approach it.[11,21]

When FLMGM alone in place during orthopaedic or retention phases, fully or partially bracketed appliances can be bonded. Another alternative is to integrate the FLMGM with an existing bracketed appliance. This coordination is a significant feature allowing maximum skeletal Class II correction without extending treatment time and delaying the progress of treatment by eliminating a major drawback of many orthopedic appliances, where there is often a need for an additional interim stabilizing phase, to avoid the relapse which may be seen if the orthopedic phase is abruptly discontinued. Leveling and aligning the dentition and erupting the buccal segment to achieve good interdigitation using fixed appliances, while the FLMGM is maintaining mandibular advancement, is a crucial factor in stability of skeletal correction outcomes.

Extra advantages

• The vertical growth of the alveolus is enhanced during the FLMGM treatment phase, this may be ascribed to two reasons: (1) the upper and lower teeth are free because the FLMGM is supported only by the permanent molars; (2) When the mandible is in a protruded position, there is adequate interocclusal space available for spontaneous eruption.

• The need for permanent extractions may be reduced during mixed dentition FLMGM treatment because the lingual arch maintains the leeway space, and in some cases, it can be modified to help in molar distalization (Fig 17).

• In case of still-active thumb-sucking habit, advancement loops effectively can block the thumb from making contact with the palate.

• In cases associated with lower lip sucking, a lip bumper may be buccally added to the mandibular part of corrector to modify the soft tissue as well.

Disadvantages

• The patient may complain of irritation from the vertically extended advancement loops.

• Swallowing, eating and speaking could be cumbersome, in contrast with buccally positioned appliance, yet the patient accepts it and gets used to it soon.

• Oral hygiene is somewhat difficult in the lower lingual anterior area, but has not been a problem.

CONCLUSIONS

The FLMGM appliance is economic, can be used starting from the mixed dentition and may be effective in stimulating the growth of the mandible and correcting skeletal Class II malocclusions associated with bimaxillary dentoalveolar protrusion. Clinicians can benefit from the unique clinical advantages the FLMGM provides, such as easy handling and full integration with bracketed appliance at any phase.

REFERENCES

1. Bishara S. Functional appliances: a review. Am J Orthod Dentofacial Orthop. 1989;95(3):250-8.
2. McSherry PF, Bradley H. Class II correction-reducing patient compliance: a review of the available techniques. J Orthod. 2000;27(3):219-25.
3. Altuna G, Schumacher HA. Schmuth and Muller Double Plates. J Clin Orthod. 1985;19(6):422-5.
4. Lisson JA, Tränkmann J. Effects of Angle Class II, Division 1 treatment with Jumping-the-Bite appliances: a longitudinal study. J Orofac Orthop. 2002;63(1):14-25.
5. Sander FG. Indikation für die Anwendung der Vorschubdoppelplatte. Prakt Kieferorthop. 1988;2:209-22.
6. Sander FG. Der Nachteffekt bei der Anwendung der Vorschubdoppelplatte. Prakt Kieferorthop. 1989;3:97-106.
7. Sander FG, Lassak C. Die Beeinflussung des Wachstums mit der Vorschubdoppelplatte im Vergleich zu anderen funktionskieferorthopädischen Geräten. Fortschr Kieferorthop. 1990;51:155-64.
8. Cozza P, Baccetti T, Franchi L, De Toffol L, McNamara JA Jr. Mandibular changes produced by functional appliances in Class II malocclusion: a systematic review. Am J Orthod Dentofacial Orthop. 2006;129(5):599.e1-12; discussion e1-6.
9. McNamara JA Jr, Howe RP, Dischinger TG. A comparison of the Herbst and Fränkel appliances in the treatment of Class II malocclusion. Am J Orthod Dentofacial Orthop. 1990;98(2):134-44.
10. Nelson C, Harkness M, Herbison P. Mandibular changes during functional appliance treatment. Am J Orthod Dentofacial Orthop. 1993;104(2):153-61.
11. Pangrazio-Kulbersh V, Berger JL, Chermak DS, Kaczynski R, Simon ES, Haerian A. Treatment effects of the mandibular anterior repositioning appliance on patients with Class II malocclusion. Am J Orthod Dentofacial Orthop. 2003;123(3):286-95.
12. Kinzinger G, Ostheimer J, Förster F, Kwant PB, Reul H, Diedrich P. Development of a new fixed functional appliance for treatment of skeletal Class II malocclusion: first report. J Orofac Orthop. 2002;63(5):384-99.
13. Fränkel R. Decrowding during eruption under the screening influence of vestibular shields. Am J Orthod. 1974;65(4):372-406.
14. Graber TM, Rakosi T, Petrovic A. Dentofacial orthopedics with functional appliances. St. Louis: C.V. Mosby; 1997.
15. Bass NM. Orthopedic coordination of dento-facial development in skeletal class II malocclusion in conjunction with edgewise therapy. Part I. Am J Orthod. 1983;84(6):466-90.
16. Clark WJ. Twin block functional therapy: applications in dentofacial orthopaedics. London: Mosby-Wolf; 1995.
17. Pancherz H. The Herbst appliance: its biological effects and clinical use. Am J Orthod. 1985;87(1):1-20.
18. Fränkel R. Concerning recent articles on Fränkel appliance therapy. Am J Orthod. 1984;85(5):441-7.
19. Graber TM, Neuman B. Removable orthodontic appliances. Philadelphia: WB Saunders; 1984.
20. McNamara JA. On the Fränkel appliance. Part I. Biological basis and appliance design. J Clin Orthod. 1982;16:320-37.
21. Bass NM. The Dynamax System: a new orthopaedic appliance and case report. J Orthod. 2006;33(2):78-89.

13

Surgical-orthodontic treatment of Class III malocclusion with agenesis of lateral incisor and unerupted canine

Bruno Boaventura Vieira[1], Ana Carolina Meng Sanguino[1], Marilia Rodrigues Moreira[1], Elizabeth Norie Morizono[2], Mírian Aiko Nakane Matsumoto[3]

Introduction: Orthodontic-surgical treatment was performed in patient with skeletal Class III malocclusion due to exceeding mandibular growth. Patient also presented upper and lower dental protrusion, overjet of -3.0 mm, overbite of -1.0 mm, congenital absence of tooth #22, teeth #13 and supernumerary impaction, tooth #12 with conoid shape and partly erupted in supraversion, prolonged retention of tooth #53, tendency to vertical growth of the face and facial asymmetry. The discrepancy on the upper arch was -2.0 mm and -5.0 mm on the lower arch. **Methods:** The pre-surgical orthodontic treatment was performed with extractions of the teeth #35 and #45. On the upper arch, teeth #53, #12 and supernumerary were extracted to accomplish the traction of the impacted canine. The spaces of the lower extractions were closed with mesialization of posterior segment. After aligning and leveling the teeth, extractions spaces closure and correct positioning of teeth on the bone bases, the correct intercuspation of the dental arch, with molars and canines in Angle's Class I, coincident midline, normal overjet and overbite and ideal torques, were evaluated through study models. The patient was submitted to orthognathic surgery and then the post-surgical orthodontic treatment was finished. **Results:** The Class III malocclusion was treated establishing occlusal and facial normal standards.
Keywords: Orthodontics. Angle Class III malocclusion. Oral surgery.

» The authors report no commercial, proprietary or financial interest in the products or companies described in this article.

[1] Post-Graduation Student, FORP-USP.
[2] Professor at the Specialization Course in Orthodontics, FORP-USP.
[3] Associated Professor at the Department of Pediatric Clinic, Preventive and Social Dentistry, FORP-USP.

Bruno Boaventura Vieira
Rua Capitão Pereira Lago, 994, apto 07, Ribeirão Preto/SP. CEP: 14.051-130
Email: brn_vieira@hotmail.com

INTRODUCTION

The Class III malocclusions are characterized by more anterior positioning of the mandible in relation to the maxilla, considering that the discrepancy can be caused by the maxilla growth deficit, excessive mandibular prognathism or the combination of both.[5,8,9,16,17] In general, the facial aspect is very compromised, motivating the patient to seek treatment.[4,13,19] Regarding etiology, factors such as heredity and the environmental action are considered relevant. The treatment of the Class III malocclusion in adults is limited, requiring a multidisciplinary planning that provides functional and esthetic benefits for the maxillomandibular complex. The options may be a compensatory treatment or combined treatment, consisted of orthodontic-surgical treatment that may require advancement of the maxilla, retraction of the mandible or a combination of both.[20] The main objectives of the orthognathic surgery are to obtain normal occlusion and improve the facial esthetic, resulting on the balance of the soft tissues of the face, besides the obtainment of functional improvement on mastication, phonation, breathing and occlusion,[15,20] the reported case, also presents dental impaction, prolonged retention of deciduous tooth and presence of supernumerary tooth, that are common characteristics of orthodontic patients.[2,10,12,14] For the success of dental traction, achieving an ideal positioning of the crown and root, previous procedures as the extraction of supernumerary teeth may be necessary.[1,6,11,24,25]

CASE REPORT

Female Caucasian patient, 14 years and 8 months old, presenting Angle Class III malocclusion, skeletal Class III pattern due to mandibular excessive growth, superior and inferior dental protrusion, overjet of -3 mm, overbite of -1 mm, congenital absence of tooth #22, teeth #13 and supernumerary impacted, tooth #12 with conoid shape and partly erupted in supraversion, prolonged retention of tooth #53, tendency to vertical growth of the face and facial asymmetry. Patient main complaint was the malposition of the teeth.

FACIAL AND FUNCTIONAL ANALYSIS

Analysis showed facial asymmetry, with concave profile, normal nasolabial angle, deficiency on the paranasal region, increased lower facial third, normal lip thickness with mentum prominence. On the functional analysis it was found: Nasal breathing, normal phonation, atypical

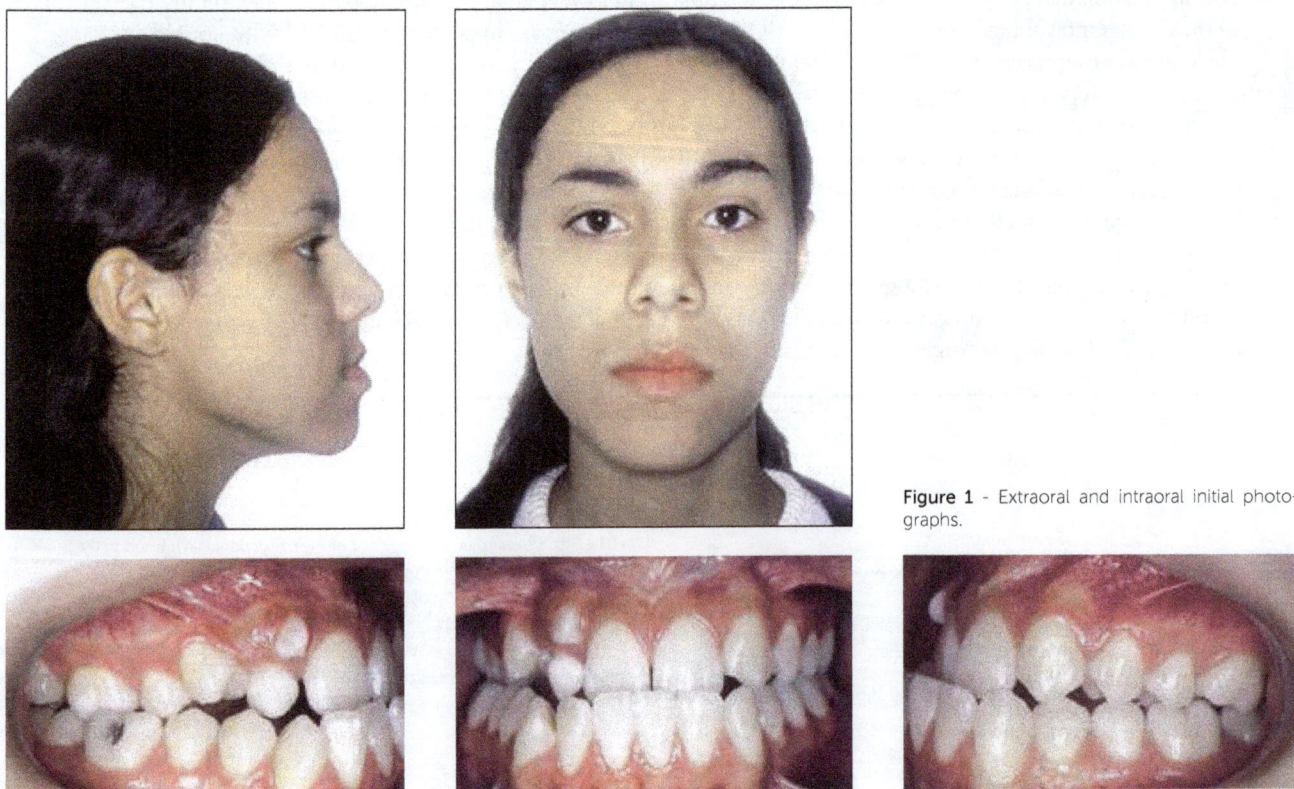

Figure 1 - Extraoral and intraoral initial photographs.

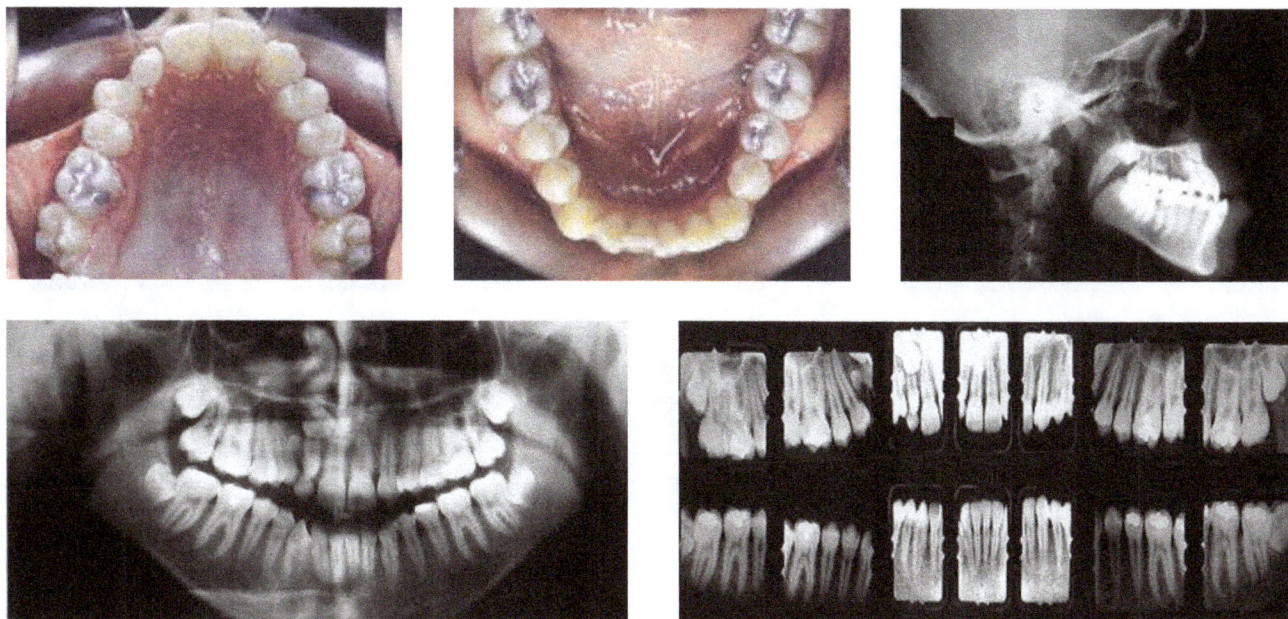

Figure 2 - Occlusal photographs and initial radiographs.

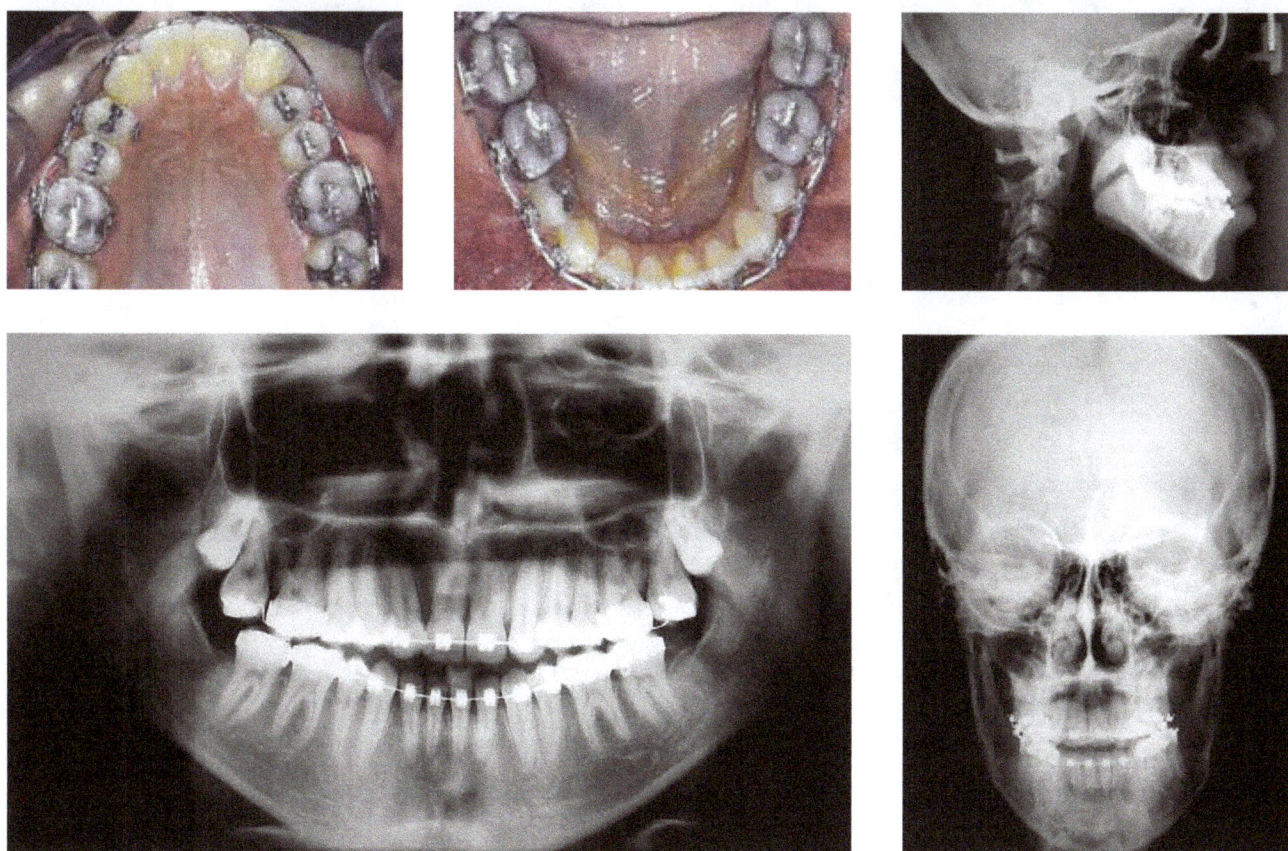

Figure 3 - Occlusal photographs and pre-surgical radiographs.

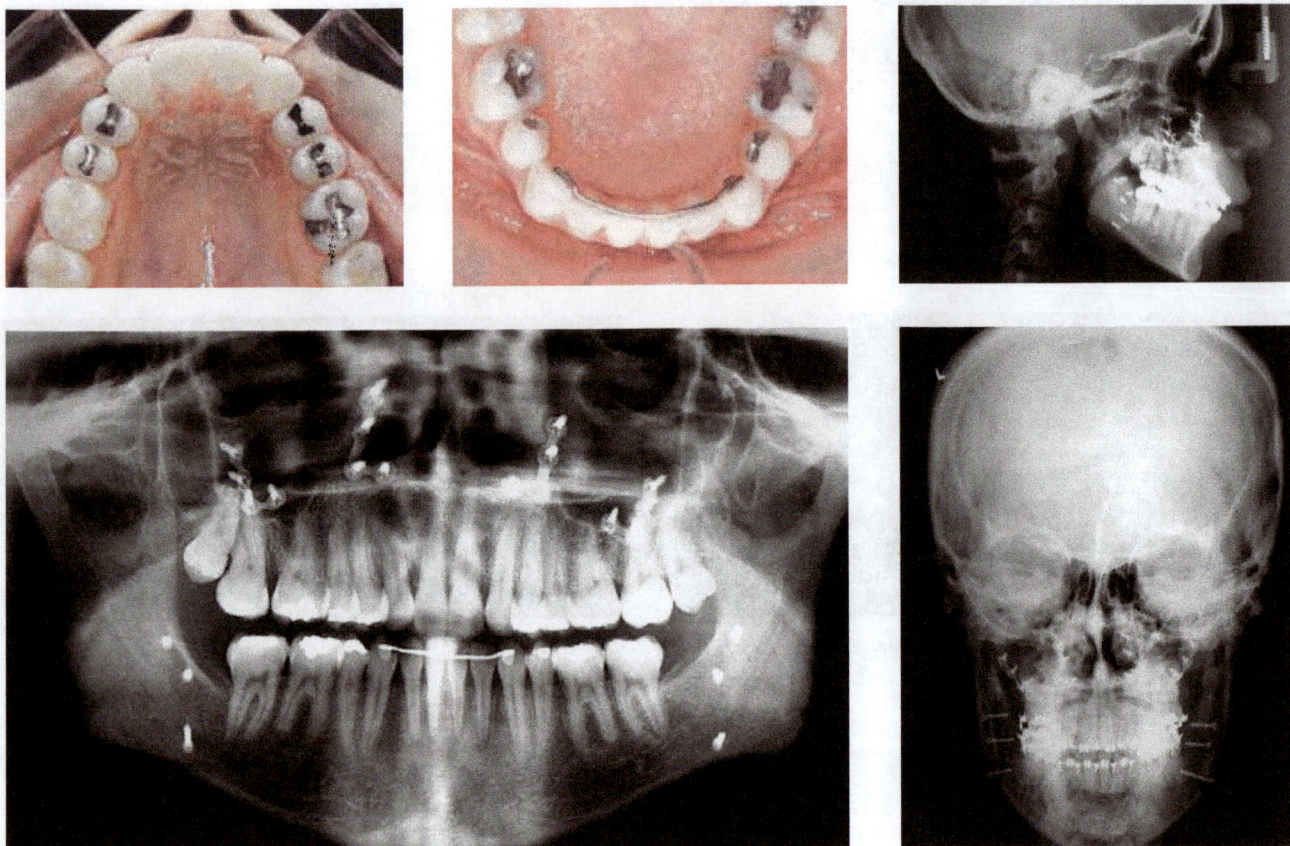

Figure 4 - Occlusal photographs and final radiographs.

swallowing, normal pharyngeal and palatine tonsils, with upper and lower lips in normal function, mandibular closing pattern with deviation to the right and ATM without any anomalies, however, presenting painful symptomatology during intense mastication.

INTRAORAL CLINICAL EXAMINATION

The patient presented good oral hygiene, periodontium with aspect of normality, absence of carious lesions, dental anomaly of number, shape and size, labial and lingual frenum with normal insertions and Class III relation of molars. According to Angle's classification, the patient presented a Class III malocclusion, with superior and inferior midline deviation to the right.

INTERPRETATION OF CEPHALOMETRIC MEASURES AND ANALYSIS OF MODELS

On the analysis of the skeletal pattern it was observed maxillary retrusion, mandibular protrusion, skeletal Class III malocclusion (ANB = -2°), tendency to verti-

cal growth of the face (NSGn = 69°, SN.GoGn = 37°) with dolichofacial morphological pattern, according to Steiner's measures.[23,24] The measures of the dental pattern showed protrusion and increase of axial inclinations of upper incisors (1-NA = 6 mm and 1.NA = 25°) and protruded lower incisors with normal axial inclinations (1-NB = 7 mm and 1.NB = 25°). The occlusal plane was inclined in relation to cranial base. On the model analysis,[5,20] it was verified that the discrepancy on the upper arch was of -2 mm and -5.0 mm for the lower arch, upper arch contracted in relation to the lower and deep ogival palate. The upper midline, evaluated on study models, was 1.5 mm deviated to the right and the lower 3.5 mm to the right side, confirming the facial assessment.

PRE-SURGICAL ORTHODONTIC TREATMENT

The orthodontic treatment was initiated with the installation of the standard edgewise appliance (0.022 x 0.028-in), consisted of bracket bonding on

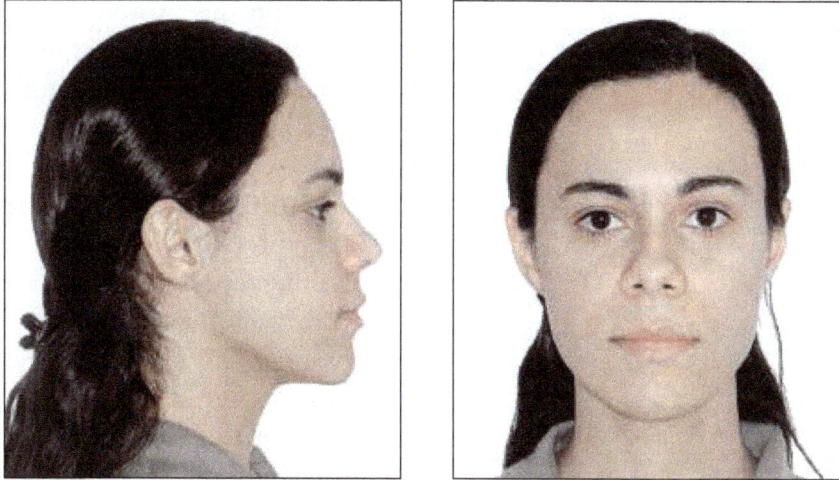

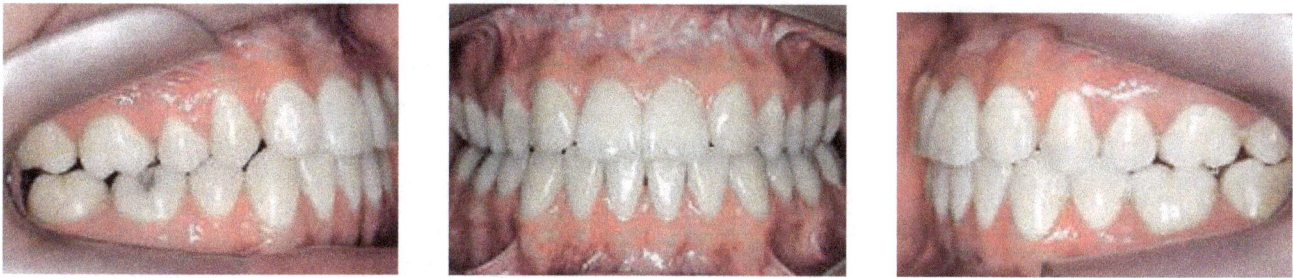

Figure 5 - Final extraoral and intraoral photographs.

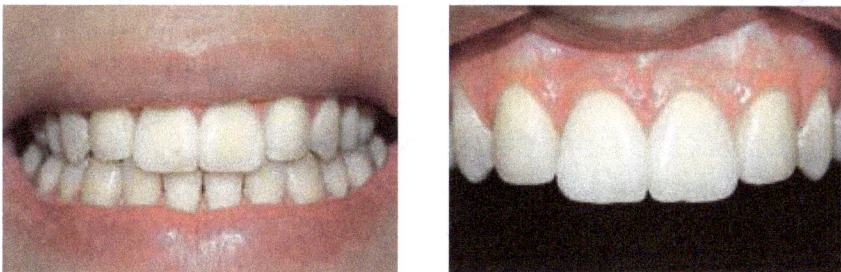

Figure 6 - Observe the canines esthetics.

upper and lower teeth, cemented rings on first molars of both arches and second lower molars.

It was initiated the alignment and levelling of the upper arch with stainless steel 0.014-in, 0.016-in, 0.018-in and 0.020-in archwires.

It was performed extraction of the teeth #53 (deciduous upper right canine), supernumerary and tooth #12 (lateral upper right incisor). On the same surgical act, it was performed button bonding to the tooth #13 in order to perform traction.

It was also indicated extraction of teeth #38 and #48, with a minimum of six months before the orthognathic surgery so that there was enough time for bone formation on the location where it would be performed the mandibular osteotomy.

The traction was done through a chain elastic and rubber type action line (GAC), connected to the tying wire installed during the act of dental extractions.

After traction, the right upper canine, was aligned and leveled through new stainless steel 0.014-in, 0.016 -in, 0.018-in and 0.020-in archwire.

For the lower arch, extraction of the second premolars was required. Alignment and levelling stainless steel 0.014-in, 0.016 -in, 0.018-in and 0.020-in archwires were made and installed, with anchorage type C planned on both sides.

Table 1 - Table with initial and final values of the Steiner analysis.

Measures	Normal values	Age	
		14 years	22 years
SNA	82,0°	80,0°	84,0°
SNB	80,0°	82,0°	82,0°
ANB	2,0°	-2,0°	2,0°
SND	78,0°	78,0°	77,0°
1-NA	4,0 mm	6,0 mm	6,0 mm
1.NA	22,0°	25,0°	25,0°
1-NB	4,0 mm	7,0 mm	6,0 mm
1.NB	25,0°	25,0°	25,0°
Pg-NB		1,0 mm	1,0 mm
Pg-NB / (1-NB)		6,0 mm	5,0 mm
1.1	131,0°	133,0°	127,0°
SN.PIO	14,0°	21,0°	14,0°
SN.GoGn	32,0°	37,0°	32,0°
NSGn	67,0°	69,0°	69,0°
Line S-Ls 0	0 mm	-1 mm	0 mm
Line S-Li 0	0 mm	5 mm	3 mm

On the lower arch 0.020-in, the partial distalization of the first molars and canines, was performed to obtain the alignment of the incisors. After finishing the alignment and leveling, the spaces were closed with loss of anchorage and mesialization of the first and second molars.

With the complete closure of the spaces ideal lower rectangular archwire 0.019 x 0.025-in, coordinated with the opposite and with necessary torques was set.

After alignment and levelling of both arches, closing of spaces from extractions, correct positioning of teeth on the bone base with ideal torques for each tooth, it was obtained study models to evaluate, on the pre-surgical phase, the correct intercuspation (Class I of molars and canines with coincident midlines).

Interdental hooks were welded on the upper and lower arch 0.019 x 0.025-in, for metallic individual tying wire. In this stage the patient was referred to combined orthognathic surgery of maxilla and mandible.

POST-SURGICAL ORTHODONTIC TREATMENT

The post-surgical orthodontic treatment consisted in finishing the intercuspation and the occlusal functions, through the adjustment of torque, characterization of upper canines in lateral incisors and use of intermaxillary elastics.

Functional adjustments of teeth #14 and #24 that substituted the upper canines were performed to obtain guides of disocclusion, Extractions of teeth #18 and #28 were also performed.

The upper and lower fixed appliances were removed and the retainers were installed, being in the upper arch a modified Hawley plate and, in the lower arch, lingual bar bonded to teeth #33 and #43 (Figs 5 and 6).

The patient was orientated to use upper retainer 24 hours a day, during a period of 12 months and after that the period of use should be overnight. The lower retainer should be kept for undetermined period. It was also recommended a speech treatment for adaptation to new muscle functions.

FINAL CONSIDERATIONS

The objectives of the treatment were achieved with the association of the orthodontic-surgical treatment. Molar Class I relation and normal overjet and overbite were obtained. It was performed the traction of tooth #13, which, along with teeth #23, replaced lateral upper incisors. The Class III malocclusion was well corrected, establishing a normal occlusal, facial and functional patterns.

REFERENCES

1. Almeida R, Fuziy A, Almeida MR, Almeida Pedrin RR, Henriques JFC, Insabralde CMB. Abordagem da impactação e/ou irrupção ectópica dos caninos permanentes: considerações gerais, diagnóstico e terapêutica. Rev Dental Press Ortod Ortop Facial. 2001;6(1):93-116.

2. Becker A, Bimstein E, Shteyer A. Interdisciplinary treatment of multiple unerupted supernumerary teeth. Am J Orthod. 1982;81(5):417-22.

3. Bishara SE. Impacted maxillary canines: a review. Am J Orthod Dentofacial Orthop. 1992;101(2):159-71.

4. Bittencourt MAV. Má oclusão Classe III de Angle com discrepância anteroposterior acentuada. Rev Dental Press Ortod Ortop Facial. 2009;14(1):132-42.

5. Cao Y, Zhou Y, Li Z. Surgical-orthodontic treatment of Class III patients with long face problems: a retrospective study. J Oral Maxillofac Surg. 2009;67(5):1032-8.

6. Cappellette M, Cappellette Jr M, Fernandes LCM, Oliveira AP, Yamamoto LH, Shido FT, et al. Caninos permanentes retidos por palatino: diagnóstico e terapêutica: uma sugestão técnica de tratamento. Rev Dental Press Ortod Ortop Facial. 2008;13(1):60-73.

7. Capelozza Filho L, Martins A, Mazzotini R, da Silva Filho OG. Effects of dental decompensation on the surgical treatment of mandibular prognathism. Int J Adult Orthodon Orthognath Surg. 1996;11(2):165-80.

8. Dale HC. Morphologic skeletal asymmetry, with a Class III skeletal discrepancy, treated without surgical intervention. World J Orthod. 2005;6(4):391-7.

9. Ellis E 3rd, McNamara JA Jr. Components of adult Class III malocclusion. J Oral Maxillofac Surg. 1984;42(5):295-305.

10. Fastlicht S. Treatment of impacted canines. Am J Orthod. 1954;40(12):891-905.

11. Frank CA, Long M. Periodontal concerns associated with the orthodontic treatment of impacted teeth. Am J Orthod Dentofacial Orthop. 2002;121(6):639-49.

12. Jacoby H. The etiology of maxillary canine impactions. Am J Orthod. 1983;84(2):125-32.

13. Kerr WJS, O'Donnell JM. Panel perception of facial attractiveness. Br J Orthod. 1990;42(4):299-304.

14. Lewis PD. Preorthodontic surgery in the treatment of impacted canines. Am J Orthod. 1971;60(4):382-97.

15. Medeiros PJD, Quintão CCA, Menezes LM. Avaliação da estabilidade do perfil facial após tratamento orto-cirúrgico. Ortod Gaúch. 1999;3(1):5-23.

16. Miloro M. Combined maxillary and mandibular surgery. In: Fonseca RJ. Oral and maxillofacial surgery: orthognathic surgery. Philadelphia: Saunders; 2000. v. 2, p. 419-32.

17. Iino M, Ohtani N, Niitsu K, Horiuchi T, Nakamura Y, Fukuda M. Two-stage orthognathic treatment of severe Class III malocclusion: report of a case. Br J Oral Maxillofac Surg. 2004;42(2):170-2.

18. Mucha JN, Bolognese AM. Análise de modelos e ortodontia. Rev Bras Ortod. 1985;42(1-3):28-44.

19. Nicodemo D, Pereira MD, Ferreira LM. Effect of orthognatic surgery for class III correction on quality of life as measured by SF-36. Int J Oral Maxillofac Surg. 2008;37(2):131-4.

20. Pangrazio-Kulbersh V, Berger JL, Janisse FN, Bayirli B. Long-term stability of Class III treatment; rapid palatal expansion and protraction facemask vs LeFort I maxillary advancement osteotomy. Am J Orthod Dentofacial Orthop. 2007;131(1):7.e9-19.

21. Steiner CC. Cephalometrics for you and me. Am J Orthod. 1953;39(10):729-55.

22. Steiner CC. Cephalometrics in a clinical pratice. Angle Orthod. 1959;29(1):8-29.

23. Tavares HS, Gonçalves JR, Pinto AS, Rapoport A. Estudo cefalométrico das alterações no perfil facial em pacientes Classe III dolicocefálicos submetidos à cirurgia ortognática bimaxilar. Rev Dental Press Ortod Ortop Facial. 2005;10(5):108-21.

24. Vilas Boas PC, Bernardes LAA, Pithon MM, Engel DP. Tracionamento ortodôntico de incisivos central e lateral superiores impactados: caso clínico. Rev Clin Ortod Dental Press. 2004;3(3):79-86.

25. Wisth PJ, Norderval K, Bøoe OE. Comparison of two surgical methods in combined surgical orthodontic correction of impacted maxillary canines. Acta Odontol Scand. 1976;34(1):53-7.

14

Morphometric evaluation of condylar cartilage of growing rats in response to mandibular retractive forces

Milena Peixoto Nogueira de Sá[1], Jacqueline Nelisis Zanoni[2], Carlos Luiz Fernandes de Salles[3], Fabrício Dias de Souza[4], Uhana Seifert Guimarães Suga[5], Raquel Sano Suga Terada[6]

Introduction: The mandibular condylar surface is made up of four layers, i.e., an external layer composed of dense connective tissue, followed by a layer of undifferentiated cells, hyaline cartilage and bone. Few studies have demonstrated the behavior of the condylar cartilage when the mandible is positioned posteriorly, as in treatments for correcting functional Class III malocclusion. **Objective:** The aim of this study was to assess the morphologic and histological aspects of rat condyles in response to posterior positioning of the mandible. **Methods:** Thirty five-week-old male Wistar rats were selected and randomly divided into two groups: A control group (C) and an experimental group (E) which received devices for inducing mandibular retrusion. The animals were euthanized at time intervals of 7, 21 and 30 days after the experiment had began. For histological analysis, total condylar thickness was measured, including the proliferative, hyaline and hypertrophic layers, as well as each layer separately, totaling 30 measurements for each parameter of each animal. **Results:** The greatest difference in cartilage thickness was observed in 21 days, although different levels were observed in the other periods. Group E showed an increase of 39.46% in the total layer, reflected by increases in the thickness of the hypertrophic (42.24%), hyaline (46.92%) and proliferative (17.70%) layers. **Conclusions:** Posteriorly repositioning the mandible produced a series of histological and morphological responses in the condyle, suggesting condylar and mandibular adaptation in rats.

Keywords: Articular cartilage. Angle Class III malocclusion. Mandibular condyle.

[1] MSc in Integrated Dentistry, State University of Maringá (UEM).
[2] PhD in Cell Biology and Associate professor at the Department of Morphological Sciences, UEM.
[3] PhD in Pediatric Dentistry, University of São Paulo (USP). Adjunct professor at the Department of Dentistry, UEM.
[4] PhD in Endodontics, College of Dentistry — Pernambuco.
[5] Masters student in Integrated Dentistry, UEM.
[6] PhD in Dentistry, USP. Associate professor at the Department of Dentistry, UEM.

» The authors report no commercial, proprietary or financial interest in the products or companies described in this article.

Raquel Sano Suga Terada
Av. Mandacaru, 1550 – Bairro Mandacaru – Maringá/PR — Brazil
CEP: 87080-000 – E-mail: rssterada@uem.br

INTRODUCTION

The surface of the mandibular condyle consists of four layers: an external layer, composed of dense connective tissue, followed by a layer of undifferentiated cells, hyaline cartilage and bone. The condyle features two key functions: joint function and endochondral growth.[16,19] Similarly to other articular cartilages in the body, the mandibular condylar cartilage can withstand biologically-induced stress.

However, it differs in several biological aspects, such as ontogenetic development, postnatal growth and histological structures.[19] One peculiarity of the condylar cartilage is its adaptive capacity due to endochondral ossification.[14,18] This feature may enable orthopedic appliances to modify not only the direction, but also the amount of mandibular growth.[16]

Nevertheless, few studies have shown the behavior of the condylar cartilage when the mandible is positioned posteriorly as in the treatment of functional Class III malocclusion.

The number of studies evaluating the adaptive capacity of rat condylar cartilage under stress significantly increased in the past years. Some authors found an increase in cellular response and growth when the mandible is held in a protrusive position.[8,14,15,21] Other researchers[9,18] have shown modifications in the two condyles when the mandible is deviated laterally. The result obtained in lateral postural deviation indicates that the lateral displacement of the mandible can (a) increase the thickness of the condylar cartilage and proliferation of precondroblasts on the contralateral side, and (b) decrease them on the ipsilateral side.[4,18]

Controversial reports on occlusion and temporomandibular disorder (TMD) can be found in the literature. Some authors believe that there is no scientific evidence that malocclusion is a risk factor for TMD,[7,12] whereas others found a high correlation between TMD and posterior condylar displacement due to malocclusion,[6,11,22] especially deep overbite in patients with Angle Class I or Class II malocclusion. Nevertheless, many changes arising from the posterior positioning of the condyle are still unknown.

In this context, the objective of this study was to assess the characteristics of the condylar cartilage of young rats during mandibular retrusion.

MATERIAL AND METHODS

Thirty 5-week-old male Wistar rats (Fig 1A) were randomly divided into two groups: control (C) and experimental (E). Both groups were fed with a soft diet and water *ad libitum*. Animals were maintained under standard conditions with a 12h light/dark cycle and controlled temperature (23°C).

This study was approved by Maringá State University (UEM) Institutional Review Board, under No. 080/2008.

The 12 animals of group E were fitted with an intraoral device capable of promoting mandibular setback and modifying functional occlusion (Fig 1B). To this end, impressions of the mouths of two animals were taken to enable the devices to be fabricated and adjusted on dental casts. Subsequently, acetate trays were fabricated to allow a standardized technique.

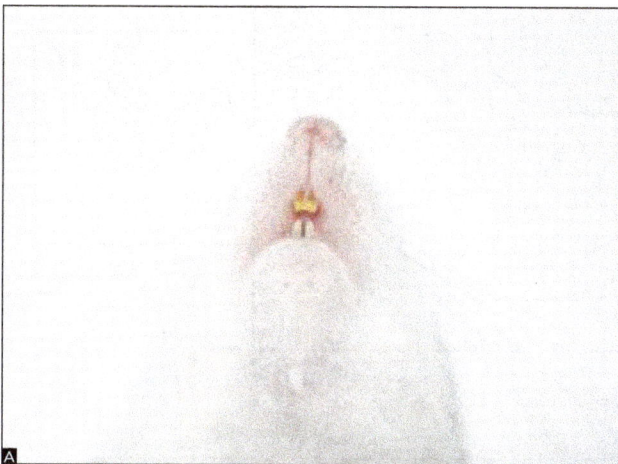

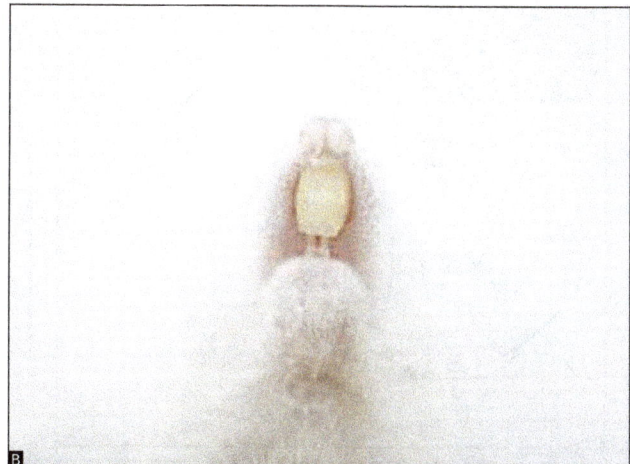

Figure 1 - Occlusal view of Wistar rat. **A)** Control group. **B)** Experimental group.

The devices were fabricated with Z250 composite resin (3M Dental Products, St. Paul, MN / USA) on the upper incisors of group E. The animals were anesthetized with an intramuscular injection of 1:1 combination of Ketamine (10%) and Xylazine (2%) at a dosage of 0.5 mg/100g. Once the animals were under anesthesia, the teeth were etched, self-etching primer was applied, and a thin layer of adhesive was applied and light-activated. The acetate matrix was filled with adhesive and fitted on the teeth of the rats for final light-activation.

Group C received no device and, therefore, corresponded to the characteristics of a normal occlusion (Fig 2). In group E, on the other hand, the presence of the devices and their inclination prevented the mouth from closing in habitual occlusion, which caused mandibular retrusion (Fig 3).

Tissue preparation

The animals were sacrificed with an overdose of anesthetic after a treatment period of 7, 21 and 30 days.

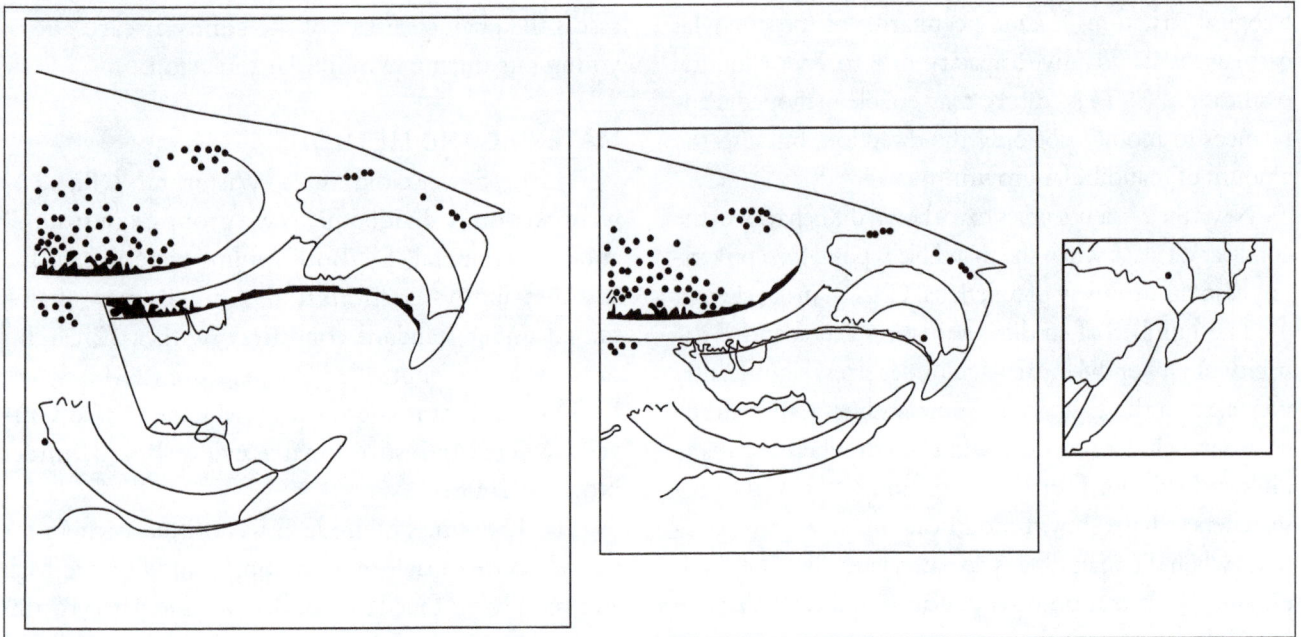

Figure 2 - Schematic sequence of habitual occlusion in a rat (Control Group).

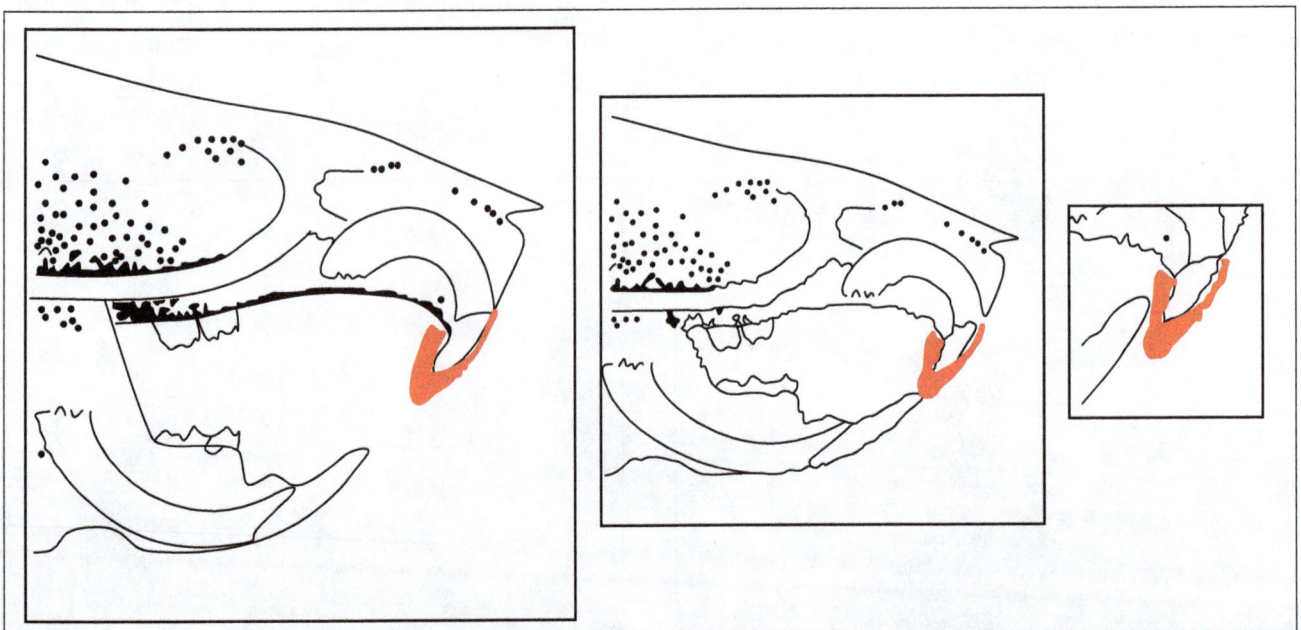

Figure 3 - Schematic sequence showing how the device was fitted onto the upper incisors of the rat, causing mandibular retrusion.

Immediately after death, the animals' heads were dissected and immersed in a fixing solution (Bouin) for 4 days. After consecutive changes of alcohols, the TMJ regions were dissected and decalcified in a solution containing 20% of sodium citrate, formaldehyde and distilled water for 5 days. The pieces were washed in running water for 4 hours in order to have the decalcifier removed. Histological routine was performed and the pieces subsequently embedded in paraffin, using the same plane of orientation with the ramus parallel to the surface of the block. Semi-serial sections were cut into sagittal sections of 7 μm in the region of the condyle using a Leica RM 2145® microtome. Sections were stained with hematoxylin and eosin and mounted under a coverslip using Permount.

Morphometric analysis

The images were captured in high definition by an Optical Microscope (Motic BA400) and exported to a computer. Using ImageProPlus 4 (Media Cybernetics, USA) image analysis software, the various thicknesses of the proliferative, hyaline and hypertrophic layers were measured, totaling 6 sections from each animal.

In each section, 5 measurements were made for each layer, totaling 30 measurements of each animal (Fig 4).

Statistical analysis

Data were obtained through a double-blind study and subsequently processed with Statistica® 7 software for statistical analysis. Data distribution did not show normal characteristics, which prompted the use of non-parametric tests. The groups were broadly assessed with the Kruskal-Wallis test.

RESULTS

Significant differences were found in total cartilage thickness, but only after 21 days (Table 1). In group E, after 7 days, a slight change was observed in the way the hyaline and hypertrophic layers were arranged (Figs 5A and 5B). Total thickness showed no statistically significant difference compared to group C (Table 1), which could be confirmed by superimposing the data distribution curve (Fig 6A). Although the hypertrophic layer of group E seemed to be very similar to that of group C (Figs 5A and 5B), there was a slight decrease (9.60%) in the hyaline layer and a subtle increase of 10.09% (Table 1) in the proliferative layer (Figs 6C and 6D).

After 21 days, histological changes were observed in group E (Figs 5C and 5D), across the entire condylar cartilage. There was an increase of 39.46% in the total layer (Table 1), reflected in an increase in the thickness of the hypertrophic (42.24%), hyaline (46.92%) and proliferative (17.70%) layer, according to the data shown in Table 1 and Figures 6B, 6C and 6D.

Over 30 days of experiment, the condylar cartilage in group E seemed to be histologically similar to that of group C (Figs 5E and 5F). However, total thickness greater than 17.15% was observed due to an increased thickness in the hyaline and proliferative layers of 26.56% and 23.31% respectively, as shown in Table 1.

Both the experimental and the control group showed a significant decrease in the total layer of the condyle at the end of the experiment compared to C7 and E7 times, respectively.

Although the hypertrophic layer of group C showed an increase between C21 and C30 times (see table), such increase was not statistically significant and can be explained by the fact that during natural growth, a decrease in the total thickness of the condylar cartilage occurs (Figs 5A, 5C and 5E). In group E, however, this pattern of development was altered, in particular with regard to thickness of the hyaline and hypertrophic (Figs 5B, 5D and 5F) layers.

DISCUSSION

During growth phase, the chances of achieving a successful treatment which is performed by means of functional orthodontic appliances that promote changes in mandibular posture, is higher, since cellular activity is more dynamic. The ages of the animals used in this study ranged from 5 to 9 weeks, spanning the prepubertal phase

Table 1 - Layer thickness: Total (μm), hypertrophic (μm), hyaline (μm), proliferative (μm) layers of the following groups: control group in 7 (C7), 21 (C21) and 30 (C30) days, and experimental group in 7 (E7), 21 (E21) and 30 (E30) days. N = 5 animals per group.

	Total	Hypertrophic	Hyaline	Proliferative
C7	240.51 ± 39.43	131.06 ± 33.84*	65.92 ± 22.88*	43.54 ± 10.72
E7	245.90 ± 39.46	137.32 ± 33.23	60.15 ± 18.22	48.42 ± 12.70
C21	170.42 ± 23.77**	72.92 ± 17.28**	54.99 ± 13.35**	42.50 ± 10.23**
E21	281.50 ± 52.93	126.26 ± 31.33	103.60 ± 38.99	51.64 ± 28.93
C30	157.29 ± 24.89	73.95 ± 16.69	51.94 ± 13.86#	31.39 ± 12.30#
E30	189.84 ± 28.34	78.18 ± 15.06	70.72 ± 18.27	40.93 ± 13.42

*$p < 0.05$ when compared to E7, **$p < 0.05$ when compared to E21, # $p < 0.05$ when compared to group E30.

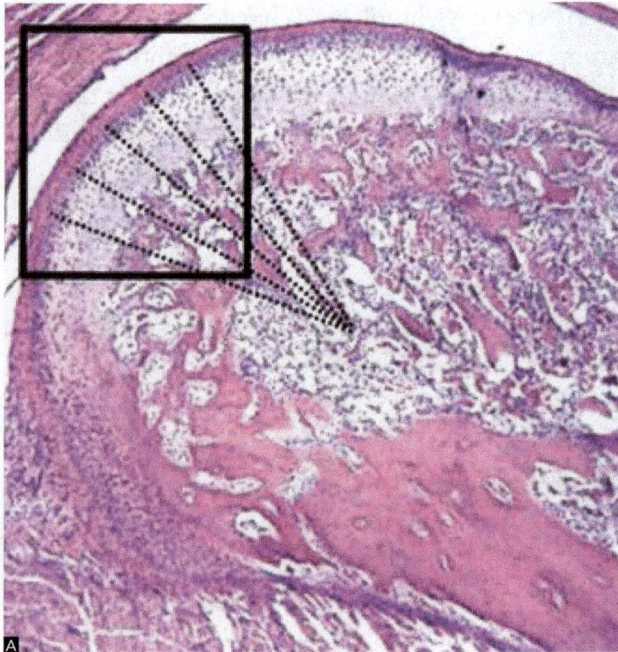

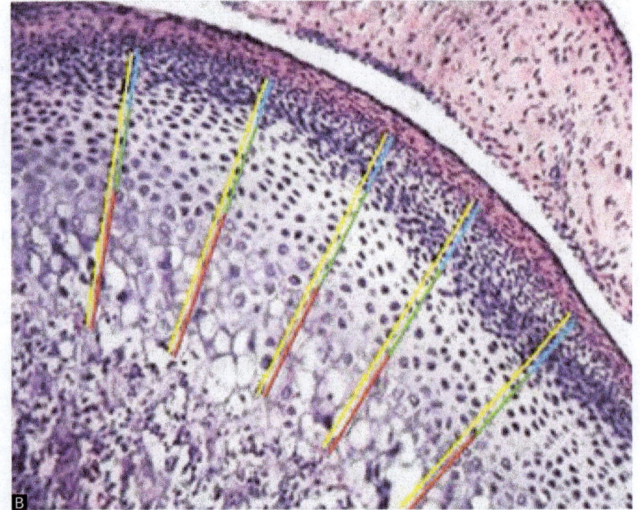

Figure 4 - A) 7-μm histological section of the mandibular condyle of a Wistar rat in the control group, after 7 days. Note the demarcated area where the images were captured for analysis (**B**). Measurements were made following the direction of the dashed line. **B)** Posterior region and part of the median region of the condyle, where total (yellow), proliferative (blue), hyaline (green) and hypertrophic (red) layers were measured.

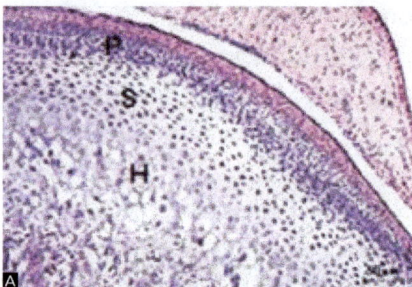

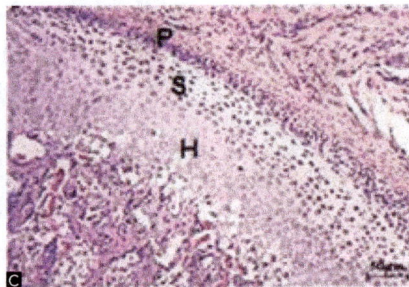

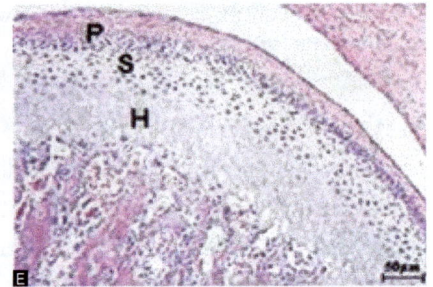

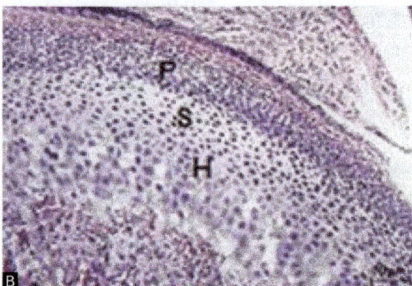

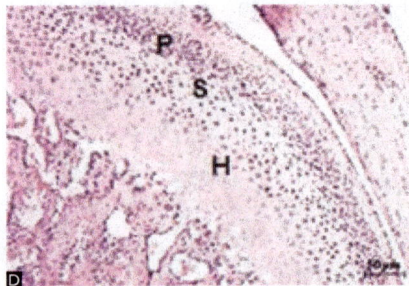

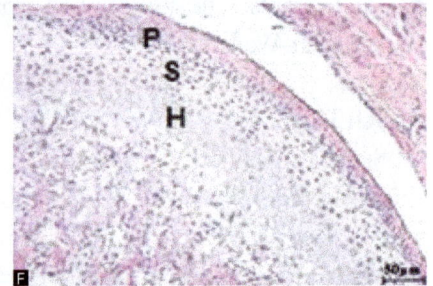

Figure 5 - Photomicrograph of the condylar region of rats showing the proliferative (P), hyaline (S) and hypertrophic (H) regions which belong to the following groups: (**A**) control group after 7 days (**B**) Experimental group after 7 days. (**C**) control group after 21 days (**D**) experimental group after 21 days. (**E**) control group after 30 days (**F**) experimental group after 30 days. Staining: Hematoxylin and eosin. Calibration bar (50 μm).

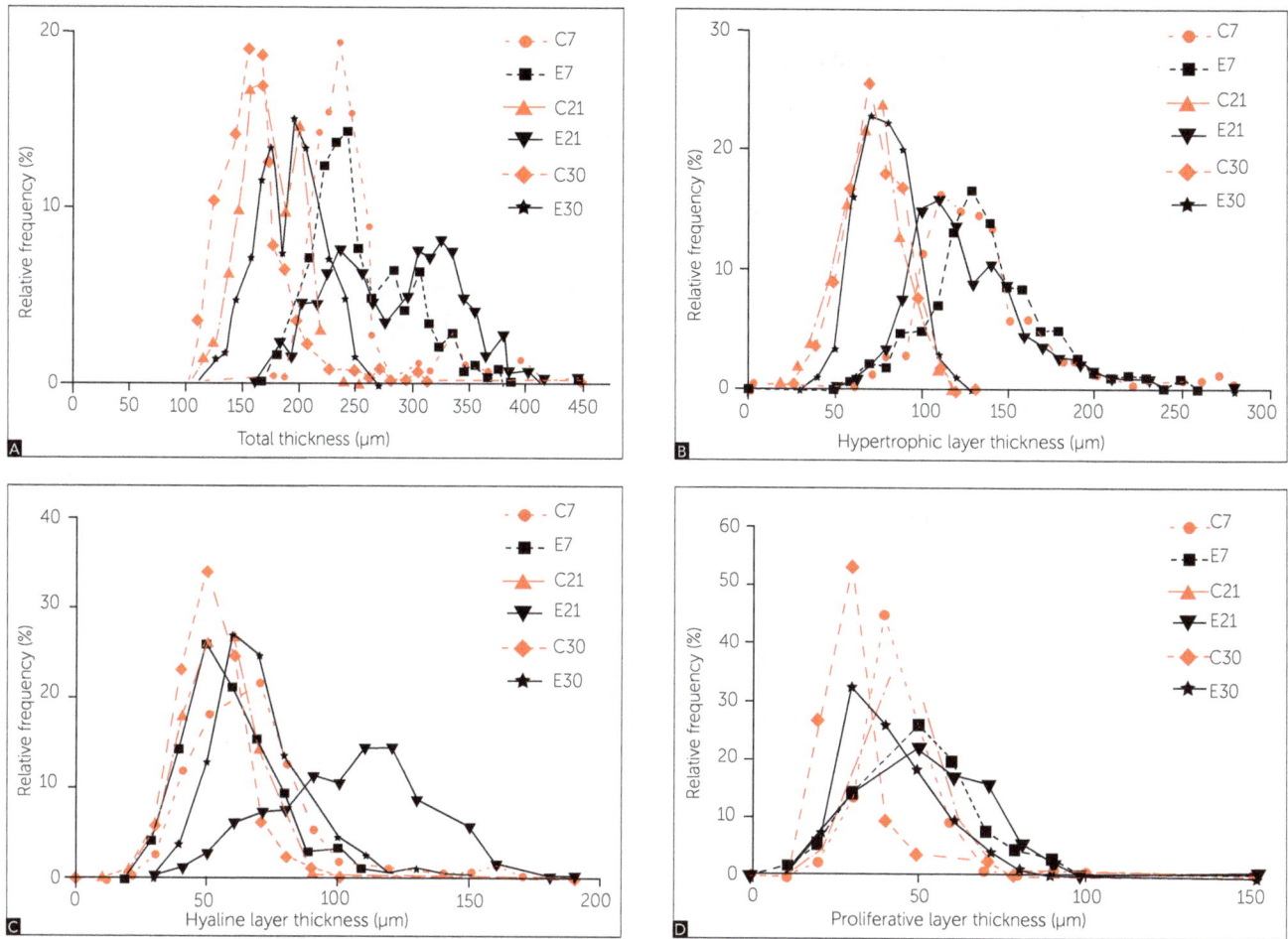

Figure 6 - Distribution of relative frequencies of the different layer thicknesses: (**A**) Total, (**B**) Hypertrophic, (**C**) Hyaline; (**D**) Proliferative, control groups after 7 (C7), 21 (C21) and 30 (C30) days and experimental after 7 (E7), 21 (21) and 30 (E30) days (n = 5).

to the pubertal growth spurt stage.[19] The experimental model that makes use of rat TMJs is widely accepted and studied due to its similarity to the human TMJ.[17]

Few reports in the literature involve changes in posture by mandibular setback.[1,2] Some studies[4,9,18] report cellular changes when the mandible is deviated to one side. The obtained results showed that after 14 days, there was an increase in growth in the condyle in the protruding or contralateral side, and a reduction in the non-protruding or ipsilateral side. Based on these data, the cartilage was expected to yield a total value below that of the control. However, the question is not so simple. The response mechanism of the condylar cartilage was markedly different on the 21st day. There was an increase in total cartilage thickness in group E, with the predominance of the hyaline and hypertrophic layers. It was not possible to determine that this increased cartilage thickness consisted of growth. A greater adaptive capacity of the condylar cartilage can be explored in appositional growth.[19]

It is known that the condylar cartilage has features that are similar to secondary cartilage, and that growth begins with the mesenchymal tissue (undifferentiated cells) covering the prenatal or postnatal condyle.

It should be recalled that during natural growth mesenchymal cells are further divided into smaller cells. Afterwards, these cells will reach their full size, resulting in migration of some of them out of the covering membrane and into the condyle.[5] Differentiation occurs when the mesenchymal cells migrate to the cartilage, becoming immature cartilage cells. The new lineage of cartilage cells will then be added, not by means of mitosis of cartilage progenitor cells (interstitial growth), but by mitosis of undifferentiated mesenchymal cells. This growth mode, in which new external cells are added, consists of appositional increase.[3,10] This study, therefore, did not disclose any increase in the proliferative layer, leading the authors to question any actual growth gains.

According to Liu, Kaneko and Soma,[9] in addition to the amount of growth, direction may also be altered. For example, on the side where the condyle is positioned a decrease occurs in the horizontal direction and an increase in the vertical direction. In this study, thickness of the posterior and middle portion of the cartilage was measured, which revealed an increase within 21 days.

Further studies are warranted to provide greater awareness and understanding of the characteristics of condylar cartilage when the mandible is retropositioned. New data could be observed if bone layer measurement were to be included and if the device were removed after 30 days, thereby promoting mandibular repositioning.

CONCLUSIONS

Application of a device to retrude the mandible modified the characteristics of the condylar cartilage in the experimental period. The most significant difference in cartilage thickness was observed after a period of 21 days, when stimulation promoted the prevalence of growth in the hyaline and hypertrophic layers. Mandibular retrusion produced a number of morphological and histological responses in the condyle and suggests the occurrence of a condylar and mandibular adaptation in rats. Clinically, this indicates that the use of orthopedic/orthodontic treatments can contribute to mandibular adjustments, facilitating mandibular positioning and basal bone interrelation.

REFERENCES

1. Asano T. The effects of mandibular retractive force on the growing rat mandible. Am J Orthod Dentofacial Orthop. 1986;90:464-74.
2. Desai S, Johnson DL, Howes RI, Rohrer MD. Changes in the rabbit temporomandibular joint associated with posterior displacement of the mandible. Int J Prosthodont. 1996;9(1):46-57.
3. Dibbets JM. Mandibular rotation and enlargement. Am J Orthod Dentofacial Orthop. 1990;98(1):29-32.
4. Fuentes MA, Opperman LA, Buschang P, Bellinger LL, Carlson DS, Hinton RJ. Lateral functional shift of the mandible: Part I. Effects on condylar cartilage thickness and proliferation. Am J Orthod Dentofacial Orthop. 2003;123(2):153-9.
5. Garant PR. Oral cells and tissues. Chicago: Quintessence; 2003.
6. Gerber A, Steinhardt G. Disturbed biomechanics of the temporomandibular joint. In: Dental occlusion and the temporomandibular joint. Chicago: Quintessence; 1990. p. 27-47.
7. Goldstein BH. Temporomandibular disorders: a review of current understanding. Oral Surg Oral Med Oral Pathol Oral Radiol Endod. 1999;88:379-85.
8. Hägg U, Rabie AB, Bendeus M, Wong RW, Wey MC, Du X, et al. Condylar growth and mandibular positioning with stepwise vs maximum advancement. Am J Orthod Dentofacial Orthop. 2008;134(4):525-36.
9. Liu C, Kaneko S, Soma K. Effects of a mandibular lateral shift on the condyle and mandibular bone in growing rats. Angle Orthod. 2007;77(5):787-93.
10. Luder HU. Perichondrial and endochondral components of mandibular condylar growth: morphometric and autoradiographic quantitation in rats. J Anat. 1994;185(3):587-98.
11. Owen AH. Orthodontic/orthopedic treatment of craniomandibular pain dysfunction. Part 2: posterior condylar displacement. J Craniomandib Pract. 1984;2(4):333-49.
12. Pullinger AG, Seligman DA, Solberg WK. Temporomandibular disorders. Part II: occlusal factors associated with temporomandibular joint tenderness and dysfunction. J Prosthet Dent. 1988;59(3):363-7.
13. Rabie AB, Hägg U. Factors regulating mandibular condylar growth. Am J Orthod Dentofacial Orthop. 2002;122(4):401-9.
14. Rabie AB, She TT, Hägg U. Functional appliance therapy accelerates and enhances condylar growth. Am J Orthod Dentofacial Orthop. 2003;123(1):40-8.
15. Rabie AB, Xiong H, Hägg U. Forward mandibular positioning enhances condylar adaptation in adult rats. Eur J Orthod. 2004;26(4):353-8.
16. Ramirez-Yañez GO. Cartilagem condilar da mandíbula: uma revisão. Ortop Rev Int Ortop Func. 2004;1(1):85-94.
17. Ren Y, Maltha JC, Kuijpers-Jagtman AM. The rat as a model for orthodontic tooth movement: a critical review and a proposed solution. Eur J Orthod. 2004;26(5):483-90.
18. Sato C, Muramoto T, Soma K. Functional lateral deviation of the mandible and its positional recovery on the rat condylar cartilage during the growth period. Angle Orthod. 2006;76(4):591-7.
19. Shen G, Darendeliler MA. The adaptive remodeling of condylar cartilage: a transition from chondrogenesis to osteogenesis. J Dent Res. 2005;84(8):691-9.
20. Shen G, Hägg U, Rabie AB, Kaluarachchi K. Identification of temporal pattern of mandibular condylar growth: a molecular and biochemical experiment. Orthod Craniofac Res. 2005;8(2):114-22.
21. Shen G, Zhao Z, Kaluarachchi K, Bakr Rabie A. Expression of type X collagen and capillary endothelium in condylar cartilage during osteogenic transition: a comparison between adaptive remodelling and natural growth. Eur J Orthod. 2006;28(3):210-6.
22. Weinberg LA. The role of stress, occlusion, and condyle position in TMJ dysfunction-pain. J Prosthet Dent. 1983;49(4):532-45.

15

Class II malocclusion treatment using Jasper Jumper appliance associated to intermaxillary elastics

Francyle Simões Herrera-Sanches[1], José Fernando Castanha Henriques[2], Guilherme Janson[2], Leniana Santos Neves[3], Karina Jerônimo Rodrigues Santiago de Lima[4], Rafael Pinelli Henriques[5], Lucelma Vilela Pieri[5]

Introduction: Skeletal, dental and profile discrepancies can be amended by using functional orthodontic appliances. **Objective:** This study is a report of the treatment of a patient, 11 years and 4 months old, with Class II, division 1, malocclusion, convex profile, protrusion of upper incisors, pronounced overjet and overbite, and mild crowding. **Methods:** The patient was treated with a Jasper Jumper associated to fixed appliances for 6 months and Class II intermaxillary elastics (3/16-in) during the last 4 months. After debonding, a Hawley retainer was used during daytime and a modified Bionator for night use during one year. In the lower dental arch a bonded lingual retainer was used. This treatment combination improved the profile, as well as the overjet, overbite and molar relation. **Results:** There was clockwise mandibular rotation and increase of lower anterior facial height. The lower incisors were protruded and extruded and the lower molars were extruded. The centric occlusal relation was checked and it was coincident to the maximum usual intercuspation. **Conclusion:** It was demonstrated that the Jasper Jumper is an efficient alternative to Class II malocclusion treatment, providing improvement in the facial profile, although the changes are more dentoalveolar than skeletal.

Keywords: Angle Class II malocclusion. Corrective orthodontics. Functional orthodontic appliances.

[1] MSc in Orthodontics, FOB-USP.
[2] Full Professor, Department of Orthodontics, FOB-USP.
[3] Professor of the Specialization Course in Orthodontics, Federal University of Vale do Jequitinhonha and Mucuri.
[4] Adjunct Professor, Federal University of Paraíba.
[5] PhD in Orthodontics, FOB-USP.

» The authors report no commercial, proprietary or financial interest in the products or companies described in this article.

Francyle Simões Herrera-Sanches
Rua Mário Ranieri, 4-45, lote E-9 – Resid. Jardins do Sul – Bauru/SP, Brazil
CEP: 17.053-902 – E-mail: francyle@gmail.com

INTRODUCTION

The Class II, division 1, malocclusion, is well studied in Orthodontics, being responsible for 12 to 49% of the occlusal problems.[5,7] The most common feature in this type of malocclusion is the mandibular retrusion.[9] Therefore, the redirection of the mandibular growth is the main objective of the Class II treatment. Another treatment goal is the reduction of overjet and overbite and the achievement of molar Class I relationship in a one phase non-extraction treatment.

Besides the skeletal discrepancy, the facial profile can be improved with the use of functional appliances. Several protocols and appliances can be used for this type of treatment, depending on age, sagittal discrepancy and patient cooperation.[11] The beginning of a Class II combined treatment uses mechanics with the purpose of increasing the efficiency of the conventional treatment for this malocclusion, besides it requires less patient cooperation. This technique combines orthodontic and orthopedic mechanics in one phase treatment with fixed appliances.[2]

The Jasper Jumper is a fixed functional appliance considered as an effective option for Class II, division I treatment.[1,10,14] It is made of a flexible intraoral power module, which is comparable to the Herbst appliance, with the advantage of flexibility, and is considered excellent due to great toleration by patients. This appliance was developed to perform light and continuous forces for Class II correction, simulating the effects of the headgear and the activator appliances.[3,6]

On its effects, this appliance corrects the malocclusion by dentoalveolar changes, being useful in cases where growth has ended or is going to end.[12] Another indication is for those patients that refuse orthognathic surgery. This appliance eliminates the need for patient cooperation,[11] but when it faces constant breakage and repair, they can transfer the collaboration to the professional.

Although a number of studies show the clinical efficiency of this appliance on the correction of the Class II, division 1 malocclusion, there are few clinical cases published in the literature.

HISTORY AND DIAGNOSIS

An 11,36 year old boy, with Class II, division 1, malocclusion, in the permanent dentition, with protruded upper incisors, mild crowding of upper and lower incisors, 7 mm overjet, 5,2 mm overbite, convex profile and poor oral hygiene (Figs 1 and 2) sought treatment at the orthodontic clinic of FOB-USP.

TREATMENT OBJECTIVES

1. Correct the molar Class II relationship to a Class I with a mutually protected and maximum intercuspated occlusion.
2. Retraction of upper incisors to correct the overjet and achieve an acceptable interincisal angle.
3. Improve the facial profile by correcting the overjet.
4. Achieve a nice smile providing vertical dimension and reducing the overjet.
5. Ideally align the completely erupted permanent teeth and correct the upper midline discrepancy.

TREATMENT ALTERNATIVES

Three alternatives were offered to the patient and his parents: (1) The use of a headgear, (2) Jasper Jumper appliance associated to fixed appliances, (3) extraction of two upper premolars. They chose the second option, which required less patient cooperation.

TREATMENT PROGRESS

The patient was instructed on oral hygiene before appliance placement. Brackets of the straight arch technique (Roth system, slot 0.022-in. Morelli®) were bonded, as well as bands with triple tubes with a palatal bar cemented to the upper first permanent molars to increase stability and prevent side effects. The leveling and alignment lasted five months (Fig 3) and continuous archwires were used with the following sequence: 0.016-in NiTi; 0.018-in SS, 0.020-in SS and 0.019 x 0.025-in SS. The mandibular arch was tied back to the first or second permanent molars. On the upper arch, the Jumper was inserted in the round tube of the first molars with a ball pin. On the lower arch, the Jumper was inserted in the rectangular archwire with a stop and acrylic spheres over the distal side of the canine bracket. The Jasper Jumpers were selected according the manufacturer's instruction. A rectangular 0.019 x 0.025-in SS archwire was used in both arches during the use of the Jasper Jumper (Fig 3).

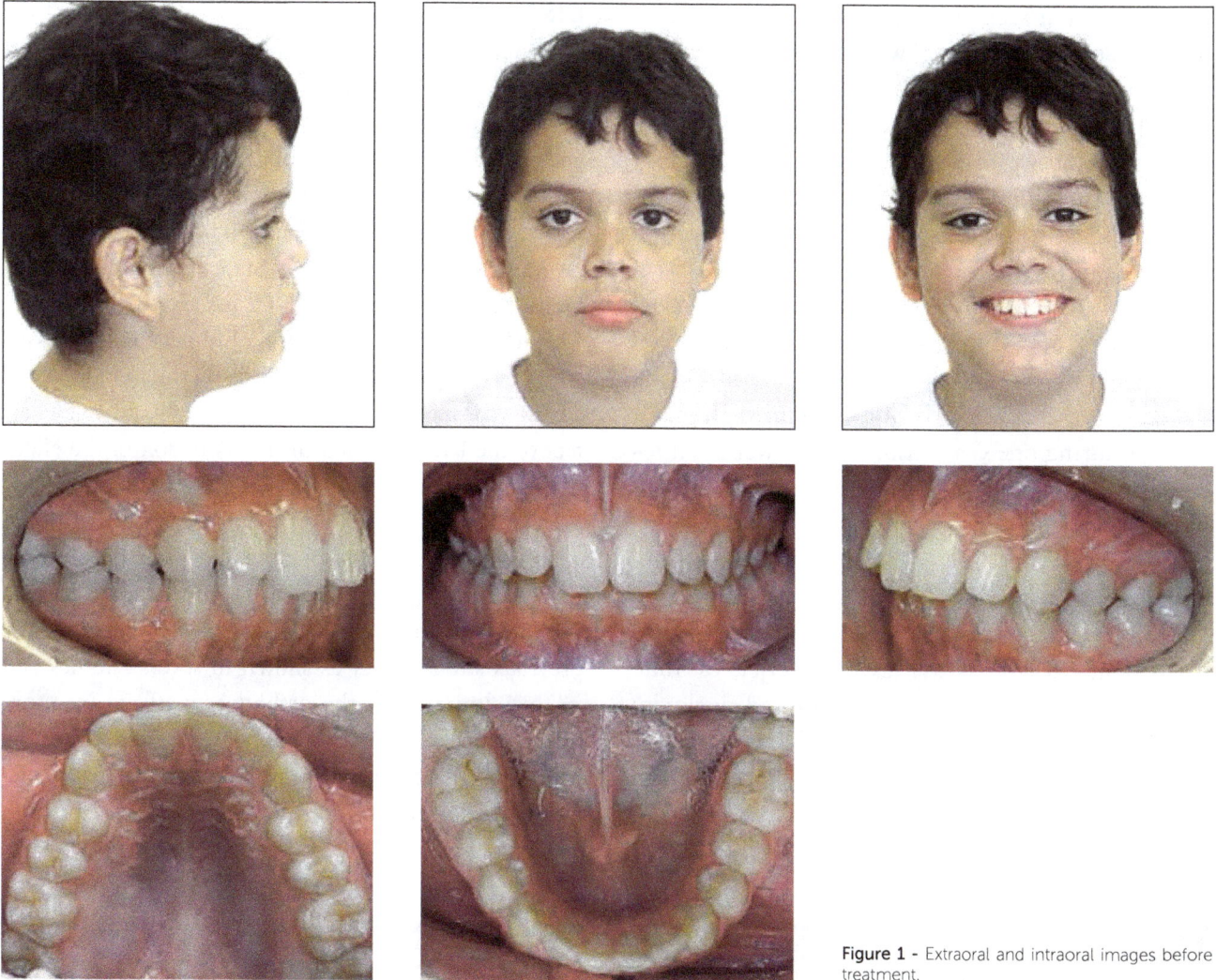

Figure 1 - Extraoral and intraoral images before treatment.

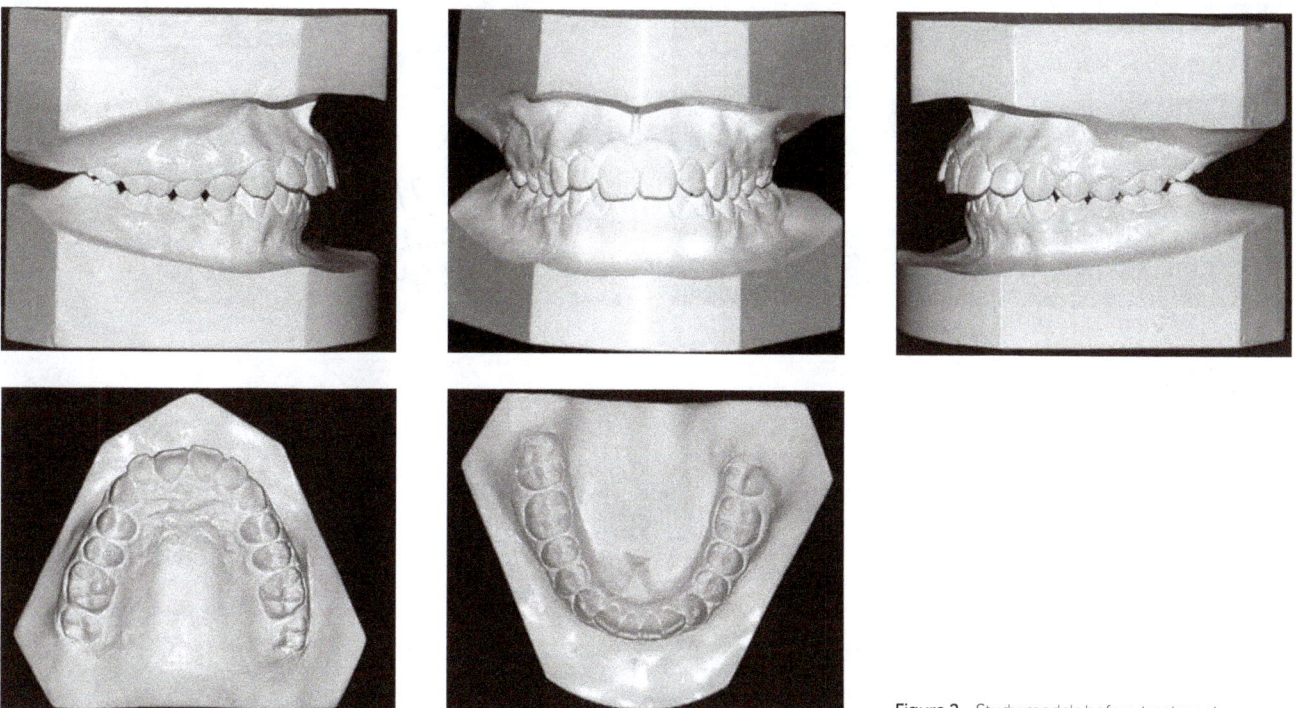

Figure 2 - Study models before treatment.

The patient was seen every four weeks and the Jasper Jumper activated every eight weeks. The Jasper Jumper was removed when the molar and canines reached a Class I relationship or overcorrection (Figs 4 and 5). The treatment period with the Jasper Jumper was six months. After Jumpers removal, the teeth were retained with 3/16-in Class II elastics for a mean period of four months.

The centric occlusal relationship was checked and it was coincident to the centric occlusion. After debonding, a Hawley retainer was used during the day on the upper arch and a modified Bionator at night during one year. Also, a 3x3 lower fixed retainer was used until the end of craniofacial growth (Figs 5, 6 and 7)

RESULTS

The treatment with the Jasper Jumper improved the patient's profile as well as the overjet, overbite and molar relationship. However, it caused clockwise mandibular rotation and increase of lower anterior facial height. The lower incisors were protruded and extruded and the lower molars were extruded.

DISCUSSION

A favorable improvement of the facial profile (Table 1), shows that the Jasper Jumper had a positive effect. As the upper incisors retruded, the upper lip retracted and ceased the interference of the lower lip with the upper incisors. Apart from this, the flaring of the lower incisors gave support to the lower lip. The lip length reduced favorably, due to the retrusion of the upper incisors. Previous studies showed similar soft tissue changes.[8,13]

The mechanism of the Jasper Jumper appliance consists in forward orthodontic force on the mandible and a backward mechanical loading on the maxilla. The effect of the latter resulted in the reduction of the effective length of the maxilla (Co-A). This was the only skeletal change caused by the appliance. This finding agrees with the results of other investigators that reported that the Jasper Jumper had a headgear effect on the maxilla. These effects were expected according to previous studies,[4] but as shown in several studies and in this clinical case, the orthodontic effects are more expressed than the orthopedic. At the same time, the Jumper exerts an intrusive force on the anterior portion of the lower dentition and on the posterior portion

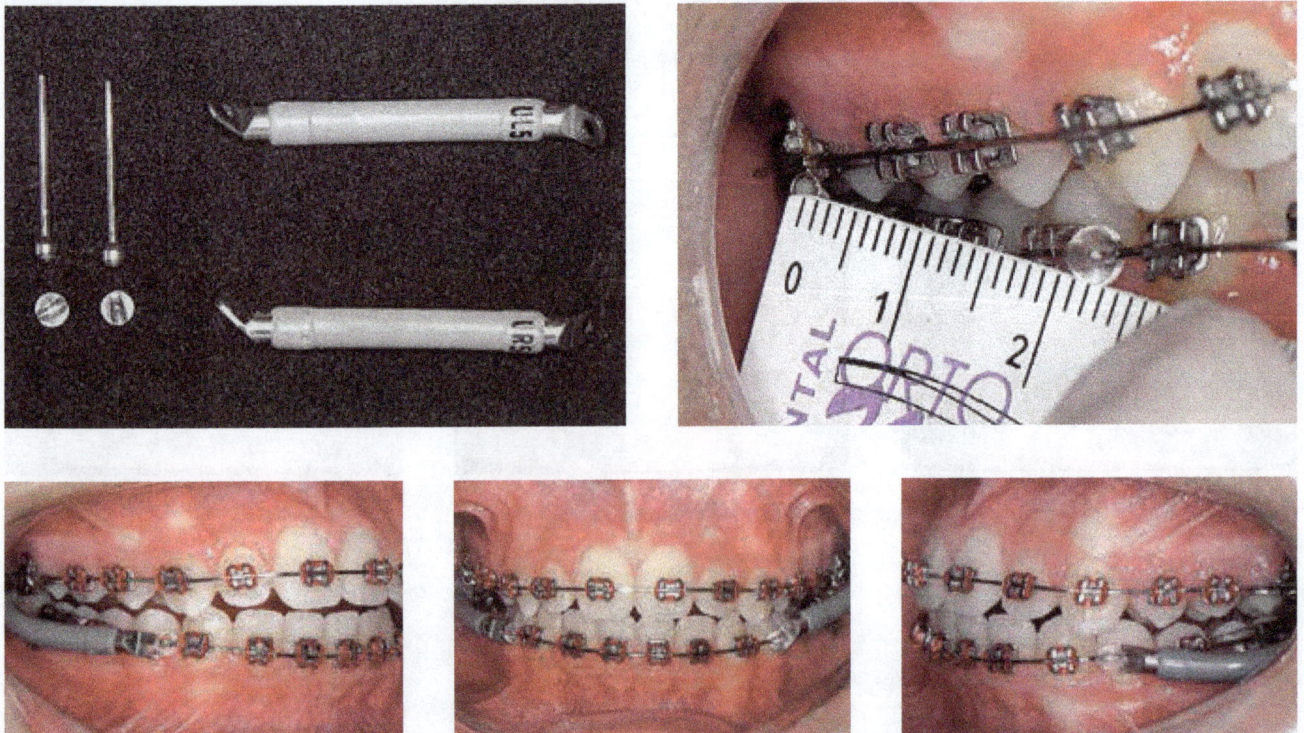

Figure 3 - After alignment and leveling with fixed appliances – Installation of Jasper Jumper and mandibular advancement.

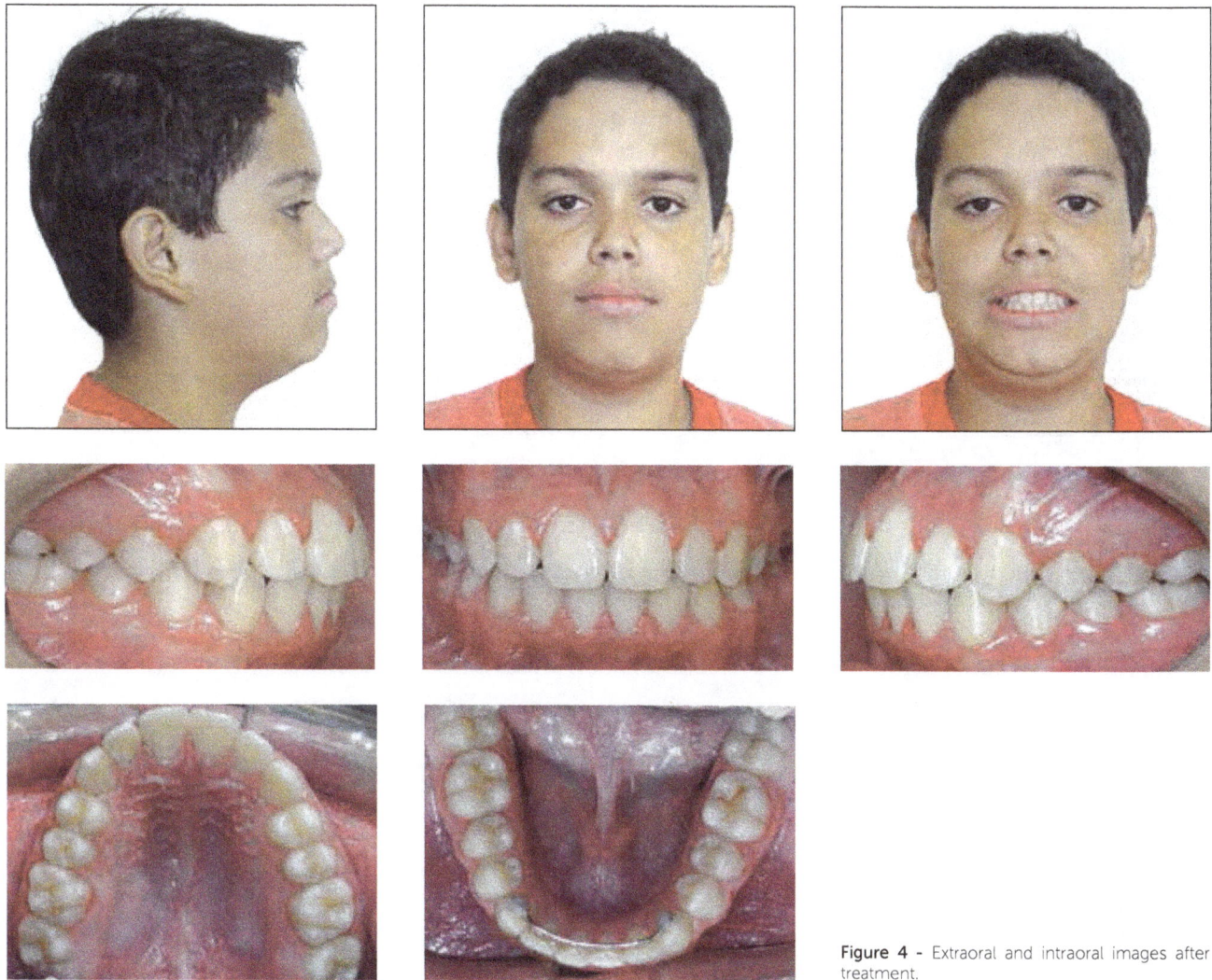

Figure 4 - Extraoral and intraoral images after treatment.

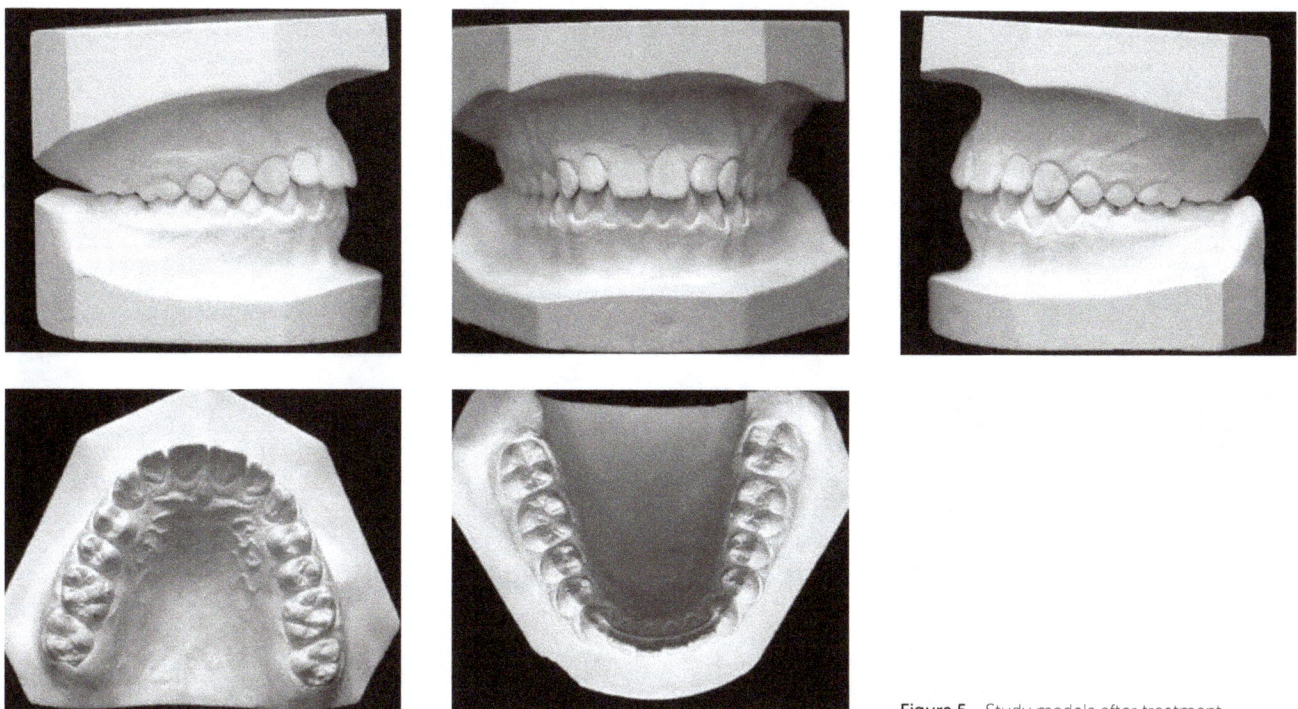

Figure 5 - Study models after treatment.

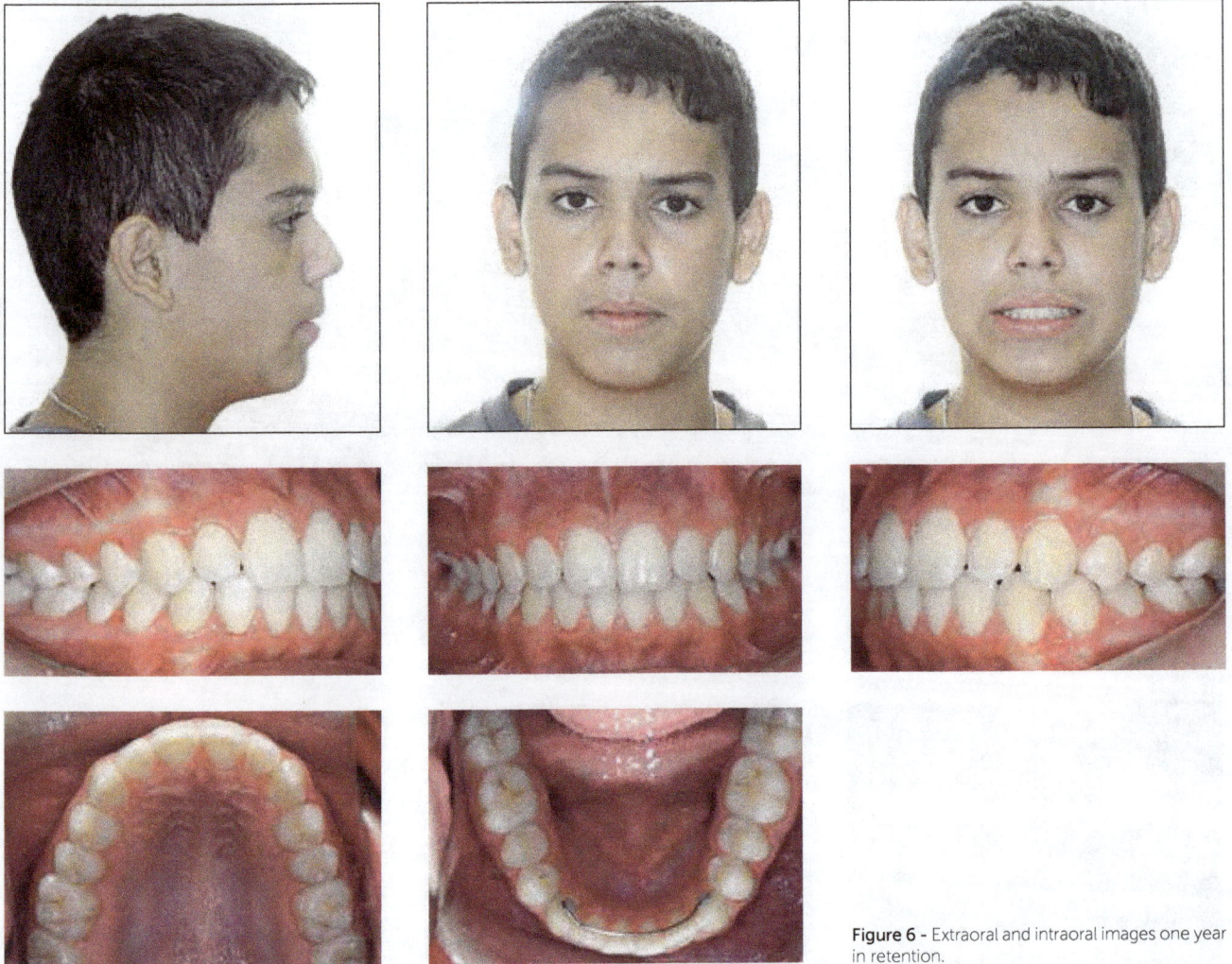

Figure 6 - Extraoral and intraoral images one year in retention.

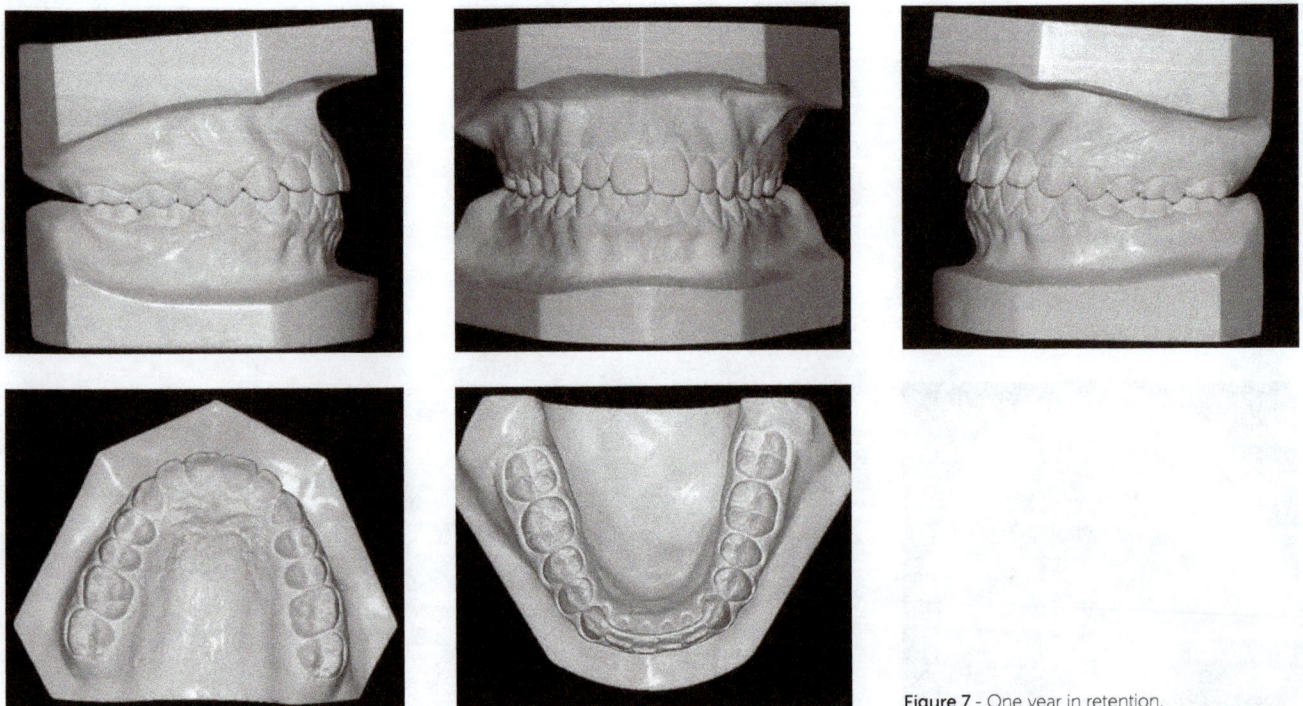

Figure 7 - One year in retention.

Table 1 - Changes in cephalometric variables during and after treatment.

Skeletal variables			
Maxillary			
	Pretreatment	Post-treatment	Retention
SNA	82.2	78.9	78.9
Co-A	81.4	80	80
A-NPerp	3.3	1.5	1.6
Mandibular			
	Pretreatment	Post-treatment	Retention
SNB	77.4	76.6	76.7
Co-Gn	106.9	109.1	109.6
P-NPerp	-0.4	-5.7	-5.8
Maxillomandibular			
	Pretreatment	Post-treatment	Retention
ANB	4.8	2.2	2.2
NAP	8.2	2.9	2.9
Growing			
	Pretreatment	Post-treatment	Retention
SN.GoGn	38.1	39.2	39.1
Sn.PP	7.4	6.1	6.2
LAFH	62.9	67.9	68
Dentoalveolar variables			
Maxillary			
	Pretreatment	Post-treatment	Retention
1.PP	114.6	118.4	118.5
1.NA	25	33.4	33.5
1-NA	5.4	8.9	9.0
1-ENAperp	-2.4	-2.2	-2.2
1-PP	28.6	29.7	29.8
6-PP	20.9	22.3	22.6
6-ENAperp	-28.6	-30.9	-30.8
Mandibular			
	Pretreatment	Post-treatment	Retention
1.NB	28.3	34.7	34.8
1-NB	5.3	8.8	8.8
1-Pogperp	-11.4	-7.4	-7.5
1-GoMe	38.1	39.6	39.8
6-Pogperp	-30.0	-28.9	-28.8
6-GoMe	26.4	29.4	29.5
Dental Relation			
	Pretreatment	Post-treatment	Retention
Molar relation	-1.4	2.5	2.5
Overjet	6.0	2.9	3.0
Overbite	5.2	0.8	1.0
Soft tissues			
	Pretreatment	Post-treatment	Retention
NLA	105.0	108.2	110.0
UL-E	0.7	2.7	2.6
LL-E	-1.6	-1.8	-1.6

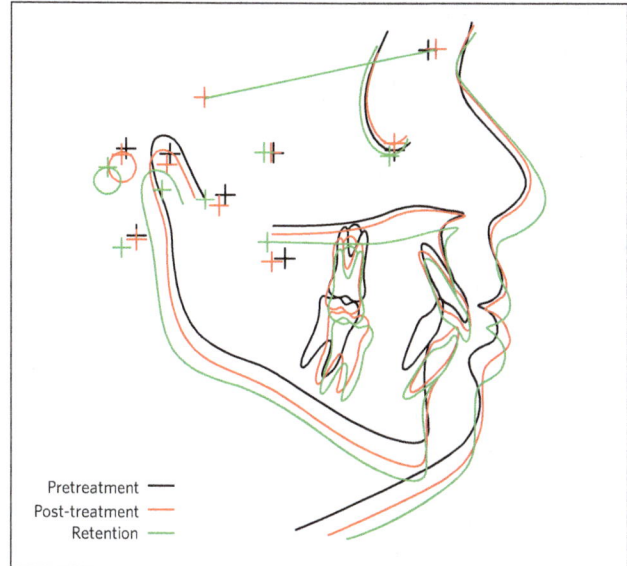

Figure 8 - Cephalometric tracings superimposition: pretreatment (black); post-treatment (red); retention (green).

of the upper dentition. The intrusive force resulted in intrusion of mandibular incisors and upper first molars (1-GoMe and 6-PP) on Table 1. The ANB angle reduced 2.6 degrees. The intrusion of the upper molars and lower incisors caused the functional inclination of the occlusal plane. The lower anterior and total facial height increased from 62.9 to 67.9 mm when the Jasper Jumper was used and remained constant one year later. The smallest reduction on the anteroposterior mandibular position in relation to the cranial base (SNB), –1.2 degrees during the treatment, can be attributed to the clockwise mandibular rotation, as found in previous studies.[4] On the other hand, no skeletal effects were found on mandibular growth. Our results agree with the findings of Cope et al,[4] Küçükkeles and Orgun,[8] but it contradicts Weiland et al.[13] There was a slight mandibular posterior rotation due to extrusion of lower molars (SN.GoGn). In addition to the vertical movement, the lower molars also moved mesially and the upper molars distally, assisting the dentoalveolar Class II correction. The upper incisors uprighted 12.4 degrees in relation to SN, although the lower incisors tended to flare. In this case, the lower incisor angle with line NB increased 6.4 degrees, when added to the upper incisor movement, contributed to most of the reduction of the excessive overjet. The patient was seen one year after treatment and the results were very satisfying (Figs 6, 7 and 8). The overjet and overbite were correct and remained stable one year after the treatment.

CONCLUSION

The Jasper Jumper appliance is an alternative treatment for Class II malocclusion in the permanent dentition in non-cooperative patients correcting this malocclusion through more dentoalveolar than skeletal effects. The only skeletal effect is the restricted growth of the maxilla, but with no significant variations on craniofacial growth standard, although a slight posterior rotation of the mandible occurs. Dental changes, as the protrusion of lower incisors and the uprighting of upper incisors are positive for the correction of Class II malocclusion. The dental relation (overjet, overbite and molar relation) is improved with this individualized treatment.

REFERENCES

1. Bishara SE, Ziaja RR. Functional appliances: a review. Am J Orthod Dentofacial Orthop. 1989;95(3):250-8.
2. Bowman SJ. One-stage versus two-stage treatment: are two really necessary? Am J Orthod Dentofacial Orthop. 1998;113(1):111-6.
3. Champagne M. The Jasper Jumper technique. 1992;9(2):19-21, 24-5.
4. Cope JB, Buschang PH, Cope DD, Parker J, Blackwood HO. Quantitative evaluation of craniofacial changes with Jasper Jumper therapy. Angle Orthod. 1994;64(2):113-22.
5. Ingervall B. Prevalence of dental and occlusal anomalies in Swedish conscripts. Acta Odontol Scand. 1974;32(2):83-92.
6. Jasper JJ. The Jasper Jumper: a fixed functional appliance. Sheboygan, Wisconsin: American Orthodontics; 1987.
7. Kim YH. A comparative cephalometric study of Class II, Division 1 nonextraction and extraction cases. Angle Orthod. 1979;49(2):77-84.
8. Kuçükkles N, Orgun A. Correction of Class II malocclusions with a Jasper Jumper in growing patients. Eur J Orthod. 1995;17(5):445.
9. McNamara JA Jr. Components of Class II malocclusion in children 8-10 years of age. Angle Orthod. 1981;51(3):177-202.
10. Quintão C, Helena I, Brunharo VP, Menezes RC, Almeida MA. Soft tissue facial profile changes following functional appliance therapy. Eur J Orthod. 2006;28(1):35-41.
11. Salzmann JA, editor. Practice of Orthodontics. Philadelphia: J. B. Lippincott; 1966.
12. Stucki N, Ingerval B. The use of the Jasper Jumper for the correction of Class II malocclusion in the young permanent dentition. Eur J Orthod. 1998;20(3):271-81.
13. Weiland FJ, Ingerval B, Bantleon HP, Droacht H. Initial effects of treatment of Class II malocclusion with the Herren activator, activator-headgear combination, and Jasper Jumper. Am J Orthod Dentofacial Orthop. 1997;12(1):19-27.
14. Woodside DG. Do functional appliances have an orthopedic effect? Am J Orthod Dentofacial Orthop. 1998;113(1):11-4.

16

Influence of initial occlusal severity on time and efficiency of Class I malocclusion treatment carried out with and without premolar extractions

Ruben Leon-Salazar[1], Guilherme Janson[2], José Fernando Castanha Henriques[2], Vladimir Leon-Salazar[3]

Introduction: The aim of this retrospective study was to compare the occlusal outcomes, duration and efficiency of Class I malocclusion treatment carried out with and without premolar extractions in patients with different degrees of initial malocclusion severity. **Methods:** Complete records of 111 patients were obtained and divided into two groups: Group 1 consisted of 65 patients at an initial mean age of 13.82 years old treated with four premolar extractions; whereas Group 2 consisted of 46 patients at an initial mean age of 14.01 years old treated without extractions. Two subgroups were obtained from each group (1A, 1B, 2A and 2B) with different degrees of malocclusion severity according to the initial values of PAR index. Compatibility was assessed using chi-square and t-tests. The subgroups were compared by means of Analysis of Variance (ANOVA). The variables that might be related to treatment duration and efficiency were assessed using the multiple linear regression analysis. **Results:** Initial malocclusion severity was positively related to the amount of occlusal correction and consequently to a higher efficiency index. Moreover, extraction protocol showed a positive relationship with treatment duration and a negative relationship with treatment efficiency. **Conclusion:** Extraction and non-extraction protocols for correction of Class I malocclusion provide similar satisfactory results; however, the extraction protocol increases the overall treatment duration. Orthodontic treatment is more efficient in cases with high initial malocclusion severity treated with a non-extraction protocol.

Keywords: Class I malocclusion. Efficiency. Time. Tooth extraction.

[1] Masters student in Orthodontics, School of Dentistry — USP/ Bauru.
[2] Full professor, School of Dentistry — USP/ Bauru.
[3] PhD resident in TMD and Orofacial Pain, School of Dentistry — University of Minnesota.

» The authors report no commercial, proprietary or financial interest in the products or companies described in this article.

Ruben Leon-Salazar
Al. Dr. Octávio Pinheiro Brizola, 9-75 — CEP: 17043-101 — Bauru/SP — Brazil

INTRODUCTION

Assessing treatment outcomes by means of occlusal indexes allows us to understand the effects different types of appliances, techniques and treatment protocols produce on dental occlusion,[1,4,8,13,20,28,33] treatment time[2,3,10,21,34] and efficiency. In this context, efficiency is described as the achievement of the best results within a shorter period of time.[19,31]

Some authors have observed the influence of dental extractions on correction of initial malocclusion severity, showing better occlusal results when a non-extraction protocol was used.[6] However, they observed that in Class II malocclusion cases, the protocol that included the extraction of two maxillary premolars yielded better occlusal outcomes than the non-extraction and the four-premolar extraction protocols.[19,20]

Regarding treatment time, the literature generally highlights dental extractions as one of the main factors for increased treatment time.[6,10,34] Contrary to those findings, Beckwith et al[3] stated that the difference in treatment time between extraction and non-extraction protocols is not significant. Other authors also assessed the influence of malocclusion severity on treatment time and found no relation between treatment duration and initial malocclusion severity.[16]. Nevertheless, other studies have shown that there is a direct correlation between initial malocclusion severity and the treatment duration.[6,10]

Unfortunately, these previous studies used mixed samples that included different types of malocclusions and treatment protocols. Therefore, the applicability of their findings is limited and cannot be extrapolated to Class I malocclusion.

The objective of this study was to compare the occlusal outcomes, treatment duration and efficiency of two different protocols for Class I malocclusion: non-extraction and four-premolar extractions, in order to elucidate the effects of dental extractions on orthodontic treatment performed for this specific malocclusion.

MATERIAL AND METHODS
Material

The sample of this retrospective study comprised patients with Class I malocclusion and similar pretreatment characteristics who were treated with four premolars extractions or without extractions. Patients were selected from the Master's and Postgraduate Orthodontic programs at the School of Dentistry of University of São Paulo, Bauru, Brazil. In selecting the sample, the following inclusion criteria were applied:

- » Class I malocclusion treated without extractions or with extraction of four premolars, two maxillary and two mandibular.
- » Presence of all permanent teeth up to the first molar.
- » Presence of crowding not greater than 8 mm.
- » Absence of supernumerary teeth.
- » Absence of impacted teeth.
- » Absence of abnormalities in tooth size and / or shape.
- » Treatment with full fixed Edgewise appliances.
- » No history of orthognathic surgery.
- » Full orthodontic records available for review.

The sample comprised the initial and final orthodontic records of 111 patients who were divided into two groups according to the extraction protocol used as part of the orthodontic treatment.

Group 1 consisted of 65 patients, 24 males (36.92%) and 41 females (63.08%), with initial mean age of 13.82 years old (ranging from 10.69 to 22.04 years), who had Class I malocclusion and were treated with extraction of four premolars, two maxillary and two mandibular (Tables 4 and 5).

Group 2 consisted of 46 patients treated without extractions, 16 males (34.78%) and 30 females (65.22%) with initial mean age of 14.01 years old (ranging from 11.04 to 21.54 years) (Tables 4 and 5). Both groups were treated with full fixed appliances using the simplified Edgewise technique.

Since previous studies have shown that severity of malocclusion could influence the treatment duration,[6,10] we further divided each group, based on their initial occlusal index, into two subgroups with different malocclusion severity (high and low). Thus, the four subgroups, two in each group, with high and low initial malocclusion severity had the following characteristics (Table 6).

Subgroup 1A (High severity; n = 22) comprised 8 males and 14 females with initial mean age of 13.54 ± 2.18 years (minimum 10.69, maximum 21.25). Subgroup 1B (Low severity; n = 22) comprised 6 males and 16 females with a initial mean age of 13.34 ± 1.25 years (minimum 11.15, maximum 15.53). Subgroup 2A (High severity; n = 15) comprised 5 males and 10

Table 1 - Criteria applied to score each component of PAR index[9].

	Occlusal relationships	Discrepancy	Score	Weight
POSTERIOR OCCLUSION	Anteroposterior	Good interdigitation – Class I, II or III	0	2
		Less than half of premolar width	1	
		Half of premolar width	2	
	Vertical	No discrepancy in intercuspation	0	2
		Posterior open bite on at least two teeth greater than 2 mm	1	
	Transverse	No cross-bite	0	2
		Cross-bite tendency	1	
		Single tooth in cross-bite	2	
		More than one tooth in cross-bite	3	
		More than one tooth in scissor bite	4	
OVERJET	Positive	0 - 3 mm	0	5
		3.1 - 5 mm	1	
		5.1 - 7 mm	2	
		7.1 - 9 mm	3	
		Greater than 9 mm	4	
	Negative	No discrepancy	0	5
		One or more teeth edge-to-edge	1	
		One single tooth in cross-bite	2	
		Two teeth in cross-bite	3	
		More than two teeth in cross-bite	4	
OVERBITE	Negative	No open bite	0	3
		Open bite less than and equal to 1 mm	1	
		Open bite 1.1 - 2 mm	2	
		Open bite 2.1 - 3 mm	3	
		Open bite greater than or equal to 4 mm	4	
	Positive	Less than or equal to 1/3 coverage of lower incisor	0	3
		Greater than 1/3. but less than 2/3 coverage of lower incisor	1	
		Greater than 2/3 coverage of lower incisor	2	
		Greater than or equal to full coverage of lower incisor	3	
DISPLACEMENT	Crowding Spacing Impaction	0 - 1 mm displacement	0	1
		1.1 - 2 mm displacement	1	
		2.1 - 4 mm displacement	2	
		4.1 - 8 mm displacement	3	
		Greater than 8 mm	4	
		Impacted teeth	5	
	Midline	Coincident and up to 1/4 lower incisor width	0	3
		Deviated 1/4 to 1/2 lower incisor width	1	
		Deviated more than 1/2 lower incisor width	2	

Table 2 - Description of variables used.

ABBREVIATIONS	DESCRIPTION
PARi	Initial PAR index
APINH	Initial amount of mandibular crowding
AGE	Age at the beginning of treatment
PARf	Final PAR index
PARi-PARf	Improvement of occlusal discrepancy
PC-PAR	Improvement of occlusal discrepancy (percentage)
Time	Treatment duration in months
IET-PAR	Treatment Efficiency Index

Table 3 - Results of systematic and random errors assessed using depended t-test and Dahlberg's formula.

Variables	1st Measurement (n = 20) Mean ± SD	2nd Measurement (n = 20) Mean ± SD	gl	p	Dahlberg
PARi	19.25 ± 6.07	19.40 ± 6.28	19	0.527	0.72
PARf	5.00 ± 3.15	5.25 ± 3.31	19	0.234	0.65

Table 4 - Compatibility of groups.

Sex	GROUP 1 (Extraction) n = 65	GROUP 2 (Non-extraction) n = 46	Total
Females	41	30	71
Males	24	16	40
Total	65	46	111
X^2 = 0.535	GL = 1	p = 0.817	

Table 5 - Comparison of the initial characteristics using t-test.

VARIABLES	GROUP 1 (Extraction) n = 65 Mean ± SD	GROUP 2 (Non-extraction) n = 46 Mean ± SD	DF	p
PARi	19.92 ± 8.08	17.89 ± 6.96	109	0.170
CROWDING	4.94 ± 1.59	4.32 ± 1.87	109	0.065
AGE	13.82 ± 2.11	14.01 ± 1.78	109	0.620

Table 6 - Results of ANOVA and Tukey's test regarding the initial characteristics of subgroups 1A, 1B, 2A e 2B. Subgroups were classified according to their initial malocclusion severity.

Variables	GROUP 1 (Extraction)		GROUP 2 (Non-extraction)		ANOVA	
	Subgroup 1A High Severity n = 22 Mean ± SD	Subgroup 1B Low Severity n =22 Mean ± SD	Subgroup 2A High Severity n =15 Mean ± SD	Subgroup 2B Low Severity n = 15 Mean ± SD	F	p
PARi	29.09[a] ± 5.32	11.68[b] ± 2.40	25.60[a] ± 5.15	10.87[b] ± 2.97	97.28	0.000*
CROWDING	5.17 ± 1.67	4.64 ± 1.62	4.08 ± 2.39	4.19 ± 1.72	1.35	0.265
AGE	13.54 ± 2.18	13.34 ± 1.25	13.88 ± 1.06	14.09 ± 1.45	0.79	0.504

* Statistically significant: P < 0.05.

females with a initial mean age of 13.88 ± 1.06 years (minimum 11.90, maximum 15.82). Subgroup 2B (Low severity; n =15) comprised 4 males and 11 females with a initial mean age of 14.09 ± 1.45 years (minimum 11.40, maximum 15.99).

Methods
Clinical records

Patients' orthodontic records were used to obtain the demographic and clinical information included in the analysis: sex, date of birth, age at treatment onset, proposed treatment protocol, including extraction and non-extraction of premolars, and length of active orthodontic treatment.

To estimate total treatment time, the starting date was defined as the date when placement of first molar bands or first direct bonding occurred, whereas final date was defined as the date when orthodontic retainers were delivered.

Dental cast analysis
Assessment of mandibular crowding

The amount of mandibular crowding was calculated based on the difference between the arch perimeter (circumference measured from the mesial of one permanent first molar to its antimere) and the sum of the mesio-distal width of all mandibular permanent teeth except molars.[26]

Calculation of occlusal index

The occlusal index was calculated according to the weighted Peer Assessment Rating (PAR index) advocated by DeGuzman et al[9] which includes the assessment of five occlusal features (posterior occlusion, overjet, overbite, midline and maxillary tooth displacements) with well-defined measurement criteria (Table 1).

The scores for PAR index calculation[30] are recorded according to the following:

1. Posterior occlusion.

Posterior occlusion, also described as "buccal segment relationship" in the original PAR index, comprises the zone from the distal anatomical contact point of canine to the mesial anatomical contact point of first permanent molar. Posterior dental relationship is assessed in three planes of space and scores are given to anteroposterior, vertical and transverse discrepancies according to Table 1. These scores are added and the final value is multiplied by two. Each posterior segment, right and left, is recorded separately.

2. Overjet.

Positive or negative overjet is recorded using the most prominent surface of any central or lateral incisors as reference. During this measurement, the ruler is held parallel to the occlusal plane and radial to the line of the arch. The magnitude of the overjet is transformed into a score according to Table 1 and then multiplied by 5.

3. Overbite.

Overbite is recorded as the proportion of the lower incisor crown that is covered by upper incisors or the amount of open bite, in millimeters, taking as reference the tooth with greater overlap. The score obtained according to Table 1 is then multiplied by 3.

4. Midline.

Discrepancy of maxillary midline is assessed in relation to lower central incisors using the score in Table 1 which is then multiplied by 3.

5. Maxillary tooth displacement.

Displacements such as crowding, spacing and impacted teeth are recorded in the maxillary anterior region, only. These occlusal features are recorded considering the shortest distance between contact points of adjacent teeth parallel to the occlusal plane. These measurements are transformed into scores and added according to the criteria defined in Table 1. A tooth is considered impacted when the space available for this tooth is less than 4 mm.

We calculated the PAR index for each of the pretreatment and post treatment dental casts (n = 222) using the criteria described above and using the scores specified in Table 1. PAR index was termed initial PAR (PARi) when obtained from the pretreatment models, and final PAR (PARf) when calculated in post-treatment casts. The higher the numerical value obtained in these indexes, the more severe the malocclusion, because PAR index is obtained by applying scores to the intra-arch (e.g. crowding) and inter-arch (e.g. overbite, overjet, crossbite, midline) dental relationships as well as by using an ordinal scale starting at 0 for a normal value. All measurements in the initial and final casts were obtained using a digital caliper (Mitutoyo, Kawasaki, Japan) with accuracy closed to 0.1 mm.

Assessing changes in occlusal discrepancy

Changes in occlusal discrepancy produced by each treatment protocol were calculated by subtracting PARf from PARi values (PARi - PARF). The numerical reduction in the index accounted for occlusal changes directly related to treatment protocol.[29,30] In addition, the percentage of PAR reduction (PcPAR) during treatment was calculated to verify the amount of improvement produced in relation to the initial severity of malocclusion.[29,30]

For this calculation, we applied the following mathematical formula:

$$PcPAR = \frac{PARi - PARf}{PARi} \times 100$$

Treatment efficiency index (TE)

Treatment efficiency was defined as the greatest occlusal index change produced within the shortest treatment time. It was calculated using the following formula, in which the denominator is the total treatment time expressed in months:[19,31]

$$T_E = \frac{PcPAR}{TIME}$$

Statistical analysis

Errors of the method were assessed by repeating the measurements on 20 initial and 20 final dental casts randomly selected from the sample. Repeated measurements were taken approximately one month after the first occlusal index calculation (Table 3). The formula proposed by Dahlberg[7] ($S^2 = \Sigma d^2/2n$) was applied to estimate random errors, while paired t-test was used to analyze systematic errors.[18]

Initial compatibility regarding gender distribution between the two study groups was assessed using the non-parametric chi-square test (Table 4). T-test was also used to assess other baseline characteristics, such as age, malocclusion severity, and amount of mandibular crowding (Table 5). Subgroups 1A, 1B, 2A and 2B were compared using Analysis of Variance (ANOVA). Tukey's test was used to investigate the hypothesis that severity of PARi influences the treatment duration (Tables 6 and 7). Multiple linear regression was used to assess the influence of initial malocclusion severity, mandibular crowding and the extraction/non-extraction protocols over treatment efficiency (Tables 8 and 9). All statistical analyses were performed using Statistica software. P value ≤ 0.05 was considered significant.

RESULTS

No systematic errors[18] were found for repeated measurements one month after the initial assessment. Random errors[7] were considered negligible (Table 3).

Groups were compatible regarding age, sex, mandibular crowding and PARi (Tables 4 and 5). As shown in Table 6, malocclusion severity was significantly different between subgroups with high PARi (1A, 2A) and low PARi (1B, 2B) severity. The difference between PARi was of approximately 16 points. Subgroups were compatible in all other variables.

Final occlusal outcome, assessed by means of PARf, was similar in all subgroups (Table 7). However, numerical and proportional reduction in the occlusal index was significantly greater in subgroups with high PARi (1A, 2A) than in subgroups with low PARi (2A, 2B). The treatment duration for the non-extraction subgroups was about four (2A) to six (2B) months less than the extraction subgroups; however, treatment time was only significantly reduced in subgroup 2B that started with a low PARi. Treatment was also more efficient in the group with high malocclusion severity treated without extractions (Table 7).

Multiple linear regression analysis showed that of the three variables evaluated (PARi, CROWDING and PROTOCOL), only the treatment protocol with extractions showed significant positive correlation with treatment duration (Table 8). Regarding treatment efficiency, initial malocclusion severity showed a positive influence on the efficiency index, while treatment protocol influenced it negatively (Table 9).

DISCUSSION

Sample and compatibility

The overall objective of this study was to compare two different treatment protocols for Class I malocclusion. For this reason, the sample only included patients with Class I malocclusion who were treated with or without extraction of four premolars. We focused on this specific type of malocclusion because the compatibility of groups regarding initial malocclusion severity decreased the risk of bias. As showed in previous studies, treatment length and efficiency varies according to the amount of initial anteroposterior discrepancy.[6,19,31,34] Distribution of sex, age, PARi, and mandibular crowding were also compatible between groups, which reduced the risk of confounding and selection bias.

During preliminary data collection, we realized that most patients treated without extractions had mandibular crowding of 8 mm or less, while cases treated with extractions showed greater amount of crowding. Therefore, we only included patients with initial mandibular crowding not greater than 8 mm in order to eliminate the influence of this variable on the results of our study.[32]

Cases that had their initial treatment plan changed during the course of treatment (e.g. non-extraction cases that ended up with extractions) were excluded from the study to avoid the influence of this factor on treatment duration.[21]

The aforementioned inclusion and exclusion criteria were applied to 4000 clinical charts belonging to the Department of Orthodontics' archives of the School of Dentistry — University of São Paulo/Bauru. A sample of 111 subjects was obtained. Considering that the incidence of Angle Class I malocclusion is of approximately 55 %,[15] we expected to come up with a larger study sample. However, the meticulous application of these criteria resulted in

Table 7 - Comparison of occlusal changes, treatment duration and treatment efficiency between subgroups 1A, 1B, 2A e 2B.

| Variables | GROUP 1 (Extraction) | | GROUP 2 (Non-extraction) | | ANOVA | |
	Subgroup 1A High Severity N = 22 Mean ± SD	Subgroup 1B Low Severity N =22 Mean ± SD	Subgroup 2A High Severity N =15 Mean ± SD	Subgroup 2B Low Severity N = 1 Mean ± SD	F	p
PARf	5.95 ± 3.93	5.36 ± 3.92	4.33 ± 3.90	5.53 ± 3.44	0.55	0.652
PARi-PARf	23.14^a ± 5.05	6.32^b ± 3.82	21.27^a ± 7.70	5.33^b ± 4.34	60.90	0.000*
PC-PAR	80.00^a ± 12.54	54.81^b ± 32.26	81.36^a ± 17.91	45.74^b ± 40.70	7.40	0.000*
TIME	24.84^a ± 4.18	24.57^a ± 7.33	20.39^{ab} ± 8.15	18.24^b ± 7.24	4.09	0.010*
IET-PAR	3.32^{ab} ± 0.83	2.42^a ± 1.67	4.37^b ± 1.38	3.31^{ab} ± 3.22	3.24	0.027*

* * Statistically significant: P < 0.05.

Table 8 - Multiple regression analysis using treatment duration as a dependent variable.

Variables	Coefficient	SE	t	p
(Constant)	22.748	2.657	8.562	0.0000
PARi	0.031	0.087	0.344	0.7316
CROWDING	0.080	0.389	0.870	0.3864
PROTOCOL	0.332	1.369	-3.593	0.0005*

SE: standard error
R^2= 0.1297. Length of treatment=22.75 + 0.33(Protocol) + 0.080(Crowding) + 0.031 (PARi). *Protocol: 0 – Non-extraction; 1 – Extraction.

Table 9 - Multiple regression analysis using treatment efficiency as a dependent variable.

Variables	Coefficient	SE	t	p
(Constant)	2.075	0.639	3.247	0.0016
PARi	0.238	0.021	2.589	0.0110*
CROWDING	-0.057	0.094	-0.615	0.5397
PROTOCOL	-0.261	0.329	2.808	0.0059*

R^2=0,1149. Treatment efficiency = 2.075 - 0.261(Protocol) - 0.057(Crowding) + 0.238 (PARi). *Protocol: 0 – Non-extraction; 1 – Extraction.

the elimination of a large number of potential participants with Class I malocclusion. The study sample reduced even further because some of the clinical charts did not have the orthodontic documentation that met the specific needs of this study.

METHODS

We used the PAR occlusal index to quantify both, pre-treatment discrepancy and post-treatment occlusal outcomes, since its accuracy and reliability has been previously validated. Moreover, the PAR index is an objective and user friendly analysis method that has been extensively used in similar studies.[1,4,8,9,13,19,30] Besides allowing us to compare our findings with previous studies, the use of PAR index allowed us to investigate the compatibility of both groups regarding the severity of initial malocclusion,[4,9,19,29,30] as well as the numerical and the percentage of improvement obtained in each group at the end of treatment. We associated the percentage of occlusal improvement with treatment duration in order to obtain an index capable of objectively expressing the degree of treatment efficiency (T_E), as previously described by other studies.[19,31]

Lack of significant systematic errors and reduced value of random errors found in this study reflect standardization and accuracy of measurements (Table 3) and are related to the calibration of the examiner prior to data collection. The simple and objective assessment of dental casts by means of PAR index also allowed us to obtain a high degree of precision and reproducibility.

COMPARISON BETWEEN GROUPS AND VARIABLES

Post-treatment occlusal outcomes

The comparison of PARf values between subgroups showed that final occlusal relationships in all subgroups were similarly satisfactory (Table 7). PARf index of non-extraction and extraction groups ranged from 4.33 to 5.95, thus showing a good occlusal outcome in all patients regardless of severity of their initial occlusal discrepancy. These values were similar to those found in prior studies conducted with Class I patients. For instance, Birkeland et al[4] found PARf values of 5.9 and 6.2 for cases treated with and without extractions, respectively. Likewise, other authors, such as Willems et al,[38] Freitas et al,[8,13] found pooled PARf

values of 5.1, 6.32, and 5.65, respectively. However, these studies used different criteria for sample selection. Birkeland et al[4] included cases treated with fixed appliances in both maxillary and mandibular arches and cases treated with fixed appliances in a single arch. Willems et al[38] included patients treated with removable orthodontic or functional orthopedic appliances and cases treated with fixed appliances in one or two dental arches. Freitas et al[8,13] only included patients treated with extraction of four premolars and fixed appliances in both dental arches.

Several other studies have assessed the amount of correction of initial occlusal discrepancy using PAR index. Nevertheless, these studies included different types of malocclusion in their samples because their main objectives were to audit the quality of orthodontic treatment provided and the factors that may influence treatment duration and efficiency provided in private practice, university-based and hospital-based clinics. Some of these studies reported similar PARf values,[6,12,17,24] while others showed higher PARf[11,12,24,33] and lower PARf values than our study.[25,28,31,39] The difference in samples and methodology prevented us to make further comparison with these studies.

The high PARf values found in some previous studies were related to cases treated with removable functional orthopedic appliances,[11,12,24,33] or cases receiving treatment for only one of the dental arches, or the use of historical samples that do not show results as good as recently treated cases.[11] Additionally, the experience of the treatment provider was also found to be directly associated with the quality of occlusal outcomes.[11,12,28,31,33] Moreover, the common characteristic among studies that showed low PARf values was that orthodontic treatment was provided by a certified specialist, regardless of being a private or public setting.

Treatment-related occlusal improvement

The amount of occlusal improvement, measured as the numerical and percentage reduction in PAR index, was significantly greater in subgroups with high initial malocclusion severity (1A and 2A) than in subgroups with low initial malocclusion severity (1B and 2B) (Table 6). The direct correlation between the amount of initial occlusal discrepancy and the amount of occlusal improvement has been previously reported.[4,6,12,13,24,27,33] The higher the initial occlusal discrepancy, the greater reduction in PARf and the greater percentage of occlusal improvement.

For instance, Robb et al[31] observed percentages of PAR index reduction of 84.5% in adults and 88.1% in adolescents while Woods, Lee and Crawford,[39] found 82.2% and 87.2% of occlusal improvement in patients treated with and without extractions, respectively. These high levels of occlusal improvement could be attributed to the inclusion of patients with high PARi (24.9 to 26.6) treated by specialist in private practices.[11,12,28,33]

Treatment duration

To analyze treatment duration, we took into account initial malocclusion severity (high and low) and differences between subgroups regarding age, sex, mandibular crowding, and dentition. Our results showed that patients treated without extractions had overall shorter treatment than those treated with extraction of four premolars. However, difference was significant only in the non-extraction subgroup with low severity (Table 7). As shown in the multiple regression analysis and in agreement with previous studies,[6,10,34] extractions had a direct incremental effect on the length of treatment (Table 8). Our results corroborate the conclusions by Turbill, Richmond and Wrigh,[34] indicating that treatment with extractions in Class I malocclusion has an additional phase (closure of extraction spaces) as compared to treatment without extractions, thus resulting in increased total treatment time.

Previous studies have shown that there is a direct influence of initial malocclusion severity over treatment duration, meaning that severe malocclusions require longer treatment time.[6,10] Our findings, however, are similar to Grewe and Hermanson's[16] results:

we did not find a significant correlation between initial malocclusion severity and treatment duration.

Total treatment time found in our study was similar to several other studies investigating Class I malocclusion. For instance, Wes Fleming et al[37] reported a treatment time of 20.6 ± 6 months for non-extraction cases, whereas Freitas et al[8,13] and Nakamura[23] reported treatment times of 24.96, 25.08 and 28.95 months, respectively, for patients treated with extractions. Kocadereli[22] found greater treatment time for non-extraction and extraction cases, 26.35 ±13.25 months and 31.53 ± 14.10 months, respectively. Interestingly, Germec and Taner[14] found that borderline Class I cases treated with extraction lasted 24.8 ±6.9 months while those treated with stripping lasted 17 ± 4 6 months. On the other hand, Skidmore et al[32] reported that treatment duration of their Class I sample was 21.9 months, despite the fact that they used different treatment protocols. Minor variations in treatment time between studies are probably related to differences in methodology and sample.

Treatment efficiency

Treatment efficiency is defined as the satisfactory occlusal relationship obtained within the shortest treatment time, assuming that the outcomes meet clinician's and patient's expectations. Treatment efficiency index allowed us to objectively assess and compare the degree of efficiency of the two protocols used in this study.

Results showed a higher efficiency ratio (4.37) for the subgroup with high malocclusion severity treated without extractions and a lower efficiency ratio (2.42) for the subgroup with low severity treated with extractions (Table 7), while the two other subgroups showed an intermediate value (3.3). These findings were mainly due to the following factors:

Initial malocclusion severity

Similarly to previous studies,[4,6,12,13,24,27,33] our results revealed a direct relationship between initial malocclusion severity and its correction, as analyzed numerically and in percentage (Table 7). Thus, knowing that the percentage of correction (PcPAR) has a direct relationship with efficiency, it would be expected that initial severity also influence it, as shown by multiple regression analysis (Table 9). Therefore, treatment efficiency was positively influenced by high initial occlusal discrepancy (subgroups 1A and 2A) and negatively influenced by low initial severity (subgroups 1B and 2B).

Treatment duration

While the occlusal changes resulting from treatment have a proportional relationship with efficiency ratio, treatment duration showed an inversely proportional relationship.[19,31] Thus, the lower values in the length of treatment in subgroups treated without extractions resulted in higher values for the efficiency ratio.

Treatment protocol

The multiple regression analysis showed a direct relationship between the extraction protocol and longer treatment time (Table 8), and an inverse relationship with the efficiency ratio (Table 9). This result was expected, as several studies have also shown a direct relationship between the number of extractions and a longer treatment time,[6,10,20,34] which suggests that extractions negatively influence treatment efficiency.

Therefore, the significant greater efficiency found in the subgroup with high PARi values treated without extractions (subgroup 2A) was mainly due to the positive influence of a high value of initial severity

and treatment protocol. An opposite effect was observed in the subgroup with low PARi treated with extractions (subgroup 1B), which showed a low efficiency index.

Clinical considerations

Extraction of permanent teeth for orthodontic purposes has been used for a long time.[5,36] However, the controversy surrounding its use is far from being resolved. The popularity of extraction and non-extraction protocols have alternated in orthodontic history,[5,36] showing a "pendulum" effect, i.e., favoring one protocol for a period of time and then the other in the next period. New appliances and techniques have also influenced the use of tooth extraction as part of the orthodontic treatment (e.g. cephalometry, expanders, distalization, brackets, archwire alloys).[36] Currently, the search for better esthetic, functional and stable results has decreased this discussion, and extractions are more accepted as means and not as objectives of orthodontic treatment. Its use has also decreased and it is only considered after careful evaluation of all factors involved in each particular case.[19,20,22,35]

In this study, we found that initial malocclusion severity did not significantly influence the duration of orthodontic treatment. However, initial severity was directly related to the amount of its correction and, as a consequence, to a higher degree of efficiency, which corroborates the results reported in previous studies.[4,6,12,13,24,27,33]

Extraction of premolars as part of Class I treatment showed a direct relationship with treatment duration and an inverse relationship with treatment efficiency. This positive relationship between the extraction of premolars and treatment duration had already been observed in other studies;[6,10,34] however, the high heterogeneity of the methodology, sample, types of malocclusion, and appliances used limited the application of their results to specific situations, such as treatment of Class I malocclusion. Moreover, Beckwith et al[3] showed that there was no relationship between extractions and an increased treatment time, making it difficult to generalize these conflicting results.

The treatment objectives regarding the occlusal outcomes in all subgroups were the same (tooth alignment, ideal overjet and overbite, and maintenance of Class I molar relationship). Therefore, the main difference between groups was whether or not their treatment included extraction of four premolars. The greater treatment time in the extraction group could be explained by the need for an additional phase that involved closure of the extraction space by retraction of maxillary and mandibular anterior teeth. The size of the remaining extraction space depended on the amount of initial crowding.[34]

This study confirms the positive influence of initial malocclusion severity on treatment efficiency and the negative influence of dental extractions on orthodontic treatment duration. Clinicians can expect satisfactory occlusal outcomes with a greater amount of correction in cases with severe occlusal discrepancy and a longer treatment time when it involves dental extractions. Our findings can be used to inform patients and parents about the expected treatment time for correction of Class I malocclusion. Additionally, it can be used to calculate professional fees.

CONCLUSIONS

The methodology and results of this study led us to the following conclusions:

1. Occlusal outcomes were satisfactory and similar in the four subgroups evaluated, regardless of the protocol (extraction or non-extraction) used.

2. Initial malocclusion severity showed a significant direct relationship with the amount of occlusal improvement and with the efficiency ratio; but no influence on orthodontic treatment duration.

3. Extraction of premolars for treatment of Class I showed a direct relationship with treatment duration and an inverse relationship with treatment efficiency.

REFERENCES

1. Andrews LF. The six keys to normal occlusion. Am J Orthod. 1972;62(3):296-309.
2. Angle EH. Classification of malocclusion. Dent Cosmos. 1899;41:248-64; 350-7.
3. Capelozza Filho L, Silva Filho O, Ozawa T, Cavassan A. Individualização de braquetes na técnica de straight-wire: revisão de conceitos e sugestão de indicações para uso. Rev Dental Press Ortod Ortop Facial. 1999;4(4):87-106.
4. Ceylan I, Baydas B, Bolukbasi B. Longitudinal cephalometric changes in incisor position, overjet, and overbite between 10 and 14 years of age. Angle Orthod. 2002;72(3):246-50.
5. Cotton WN, Takano WS, Wong WM. The Downs analysis applied to three other ethnic groups. Angle Orthod. 1951;21(4):213-20.
6. Downs WB. Variations in facial relationship: their significance in treatment and prognosis. Am J Orthod. 1948;34:812-40.
7. Engel G, Spolter BM. Cephalometric and visual norms for a Japanese population. Am J Orthod. 1981;90(1):48-60.
8. Fêo OS, Interlandi S, Martins DR, Almeida RR. Avaliação cefalométrica da inclinação dos lábios e relações com a estrutura dento-esquelética. Estomat Cult. 1971;5(2):166-77.
9. Fernandes TMF. Estudo comparativo do padrão cefalométrico de jovens mestiços nipo-brasileiros - Grandezas tegumentares e esqueléticas [dissertação]. Bauru (SP): Universidade de São Paulo; 2009.
10. Hayasaki SM, Henriques JFC, Janson G, Freitas MR. Influence of extraction and nonextraction orthodontic treatment in Japanese-Brazilians with class I and class II division 1 malocclusions. Am J Orthod Dentofacial Orthop. 2005;127(1):30-6.
11. Houston WJ. The analysis of errors in orthodontic measurements. Am J Orthod. 1983;83(5):382-90.
12. Interlandi S. O cefalograma padrão do curso de pós-graduação de Ortodontia da Faculdade de Odontologia da USP. Rev Fac Odontol S Paulo. 1968;6(1):63-74.
13. Ioi H, Nakata S, Nakasima A, Counts AL. Anteroposterior lip positions of the most-favored Japanese facial profiles. Am J Orthod Dentofacial Orthop. 2005;128(2):206-11.
14. Iwasawa T, Moro T, Nakamura K. Tweed triangle and soft-tissue consideration of Japanese with normal occlusion and good facial profile. Am J Orthod. 1977;72(2):119-27.
15. Ludwig M. A cephalometric analysis of the relationship between facial pattern, interincisal angulation and anterior overbite changes. Angle Orthod. 1967;37(3):194-204.
16. Margolis HI. The axial inclination of the mandibular teeth. Am J Orthod Oral Surg. 1943;29(10):571-94.
17. Merrifield LL. The profile line as an aid in critically evaluating facial esthetics. Am J Orthod. 1966;52(11):804-22.
18. Miura F, Inoue N, Suzuki K. Cephalometric standards for japanese according to the steiner analysis. Am J Orthod. 1965;51(4):288-95.
19. Miyajima K, McNamara Jr JA, Kimura T, Murata S, Iizuka T. Craniofacial structure of Japanese and European-American adults with normal occlusions and well-balanced faces. Am J Orthod Dentofacial Orthop. 1996;110(4):431-8.
20. Parker CD, Nanda RS, Currier GF. Skeletal and dental changes associated with the treatment of deep bite malocclusion. Am J Orthod Dentofacial Orthop. 1995;107(4):382-93.
21. Pepicelli A, Woods M, Briggs C. The mandibular muscles and their importance in orthodontics: a contemporary review. Am J Orthod Dentofacial Orthop. 2005;128(6):774-80.
22. Pinzan A. Estudo cefalométrico longitudinal das medidas SNA, Nperp-A, SNB, SND, Nperp-P, ANB, SN.GoGn, SN.Gn, PoOr.GoMe e BaN.PtGn, em jovens leucodermas brasileiros de ambos os sexos, com oclusão normal dos 5 aos 11 anos [tese]. Bauru (SP): Universidade de São Paulo; 1994.

23. Raddi I. Determinação da linha "I" em xantodemas nipo-brasileiros, dos 12 aos 18 anos e 6 meses, com "oclusão normal" [dissertação]. Bauru (SP): Universidade de São Paulo; 1988.

24. Steiner CC. Cephalometrics for you and me. Am J Orthod. 1953;39(10):729-55.

25. Takahashi R. Padrão cefalométrico FOB-USP para jovens nipo-brasileiros com oclusão normal [dissertação]. Bauru (SP): Universidade de São Paulo; 1998.

26. Taylor WH, Hitchcock HP. The Alabama analysis. Am J Orthod. 1966;52(4):245-65.

27. Tweed CH. Frankfort Mandibular Incisor Angle (FMIA) in diagnosis treatment planning and prognosis. Angle Orthod. 1954;24(3):121-69.

28. Uesato G, Kinoshita Z, Kawamoto T, Koyama I, Nakanishi Y. Steiner cephalometric norms for Japanese and Japanese-Americans. Am J Orthod. 1978;73(3):321-7.

29. Williams R. The diagnostic line. Am J Orthod. 1969;55(5):458-76.

30. Williamson EH, Caves SA, Edenfield RJ, Morse PK. Cephalometric analysis: comparisons between maximum intercuspation and centric relation. Am J Orthod. 1978;74(6):672-7.

17

Transverse maxillary and mandibular growth during and after Bionator therapy: Study with metallic implants

André da Costa Monini[1], Luiz Gonzaga Gandini Júnior[2], Luiz Guilherme Martins Maia[3], Ary dos Santos-Pinto[4]

Introduction: This study evaluated posteroanterior cephalograms before and after treatment and long term follow-up of Class II division 1 patients treated with bionator. **Objective:** The objective was to demonstrate the transverse growth of maxilla and mandible during and after bionator therapy. **Methods:** Measurement of transverse dimensions between posterior maxillary and mandibular implants, as well as the distances between the buccal, gonial and antegonial points were recorded. Measurements were analyzed at three periods: T_1 = before bionator therapy, T_2 = after bionator therapy and T_3 = 5.74 years after T_2. **Results:** There was statistically significant transverse increase due to growth and/or treatment for all variables, except for the distance between the anterior maxillary implants. **Conclusions:** During the study period only the anterior maxillary area did not show transverse growth.

Keywords: Activator appliances. Angle Class II malocclusion. Maxillofacial development.

[1] Specialist and Master in Orthodontics UNESP-Araraquara.
[2] Professor, School of Dentistry of Araraquara, UNESP. Assistant Professor, Baylor College of Dentistry, Dallas, Texas, USA.
[3] Master and Doctorate student in Orthodontics UNESP- Araraquara.
[4] Professor, School of Dentistry of Araraquara, UNESP.

» The authors report no commercial, proprietary or financial interest in the products or companies described in this article.

Luiz Gonzaga Gandini Júnior
Av. Casemiro Perez, 560 – Vila Harmonia – Araraquara/SP – Brazil
CEP: 14.802-600 – E-mail: luizgandini@uol.com.br

INTRODUCTION

Few studies evaluating the transverse growth of the face were carried out so far, especially regarding sagittal growth. This is due to problems such as difficulty on identification and consequent reproducibility of cephalometric points,[18,21] standardization of the head positioning,[20,11] radiographic magnification[9,11,15,27] and standardization of the sample.[19] In the last years, some studies assessed the facial skeletal growth without interference of functional orthopedic appliances.[9,10,13,16,17,25] Several studies showed the potential of increase on transverse growth of the jaws by the use of functional appliances[1,8,12,14,23,26] and three of them[12,14,26] followed longitudinally the patients after treatment, but without radiographic evaluation. The longitudinal examination using metallic implants carried out so far refers to Class I patients with or without treatment[4,5,10,17] or to mixed samples.[16]

The cephalometric studies in teleradiographs with metallic implants proved to be the most efficient method to longitudinally assess the craniofacial growth[3,5] due to the difficulty of identification of cephalometric points and remodeling that occurs on the surface of the jaws. The objective of the present study is to evaluate the maxillary transverse growth and its relation to the treatment, through posteroanterior radiographs, during 6 years after the use of Balters' bionator in patients with metallic implants.

MATERIAL AND METHODS

The sample consisted of 25 patients that used bionator (15 boys and 10 girls), participants on a prior study[1] and treated in the Department of Orthodontics at the School of Dentistry of Araraquara – Unesp. Each one of them presented skeletal Class II with mandibular retrusion, upper and lower incisors erupted or in eruption, overbite, no dental loss, absence of crowding and/or posterior cross bite. The subjects of the sample had metallic implants inserted in the maxilla (four implants) and mandible (three implants), according to proposed by Björk.[6,7] From the original sample of 25 patients (mean age of 9.2 years), it was possible to obtain long term radiographs of 13 patients (9 boys and 4 girls) with mean age of 16.95 years. The other patients could not be contacted. On the final sample, one patient did not present the posterior implants on the maxilla in T_3

and on the mandible in T_1, other patient did not present one anterior implant in T_3 and another patient did not present one of the posterior implants on the mandible. Table 1 shows age and gender of the sample and Table 2 characterizes the sample.

Lateral and posteroanterior teleradiographs were obtained in three time periods: T_1 at the beginning of treatment with bionator, T_2 at the end of the bionator therapy and (T_3) 5.74 years, on average, after T_2. The teleradiographs were manually traced and the cephalometric points were digitized twice on Dentofacial Planner Plus (DFP Plus, version 2.0, Toronto, Ontario, Ca) by a single examiner and the digitalization mean was used for cephalometric measurements. The cephalometric points used on the posteroanterior teleradiographs are described on Table 3 and Figure 1.

The transverse growth was calculated by the transverse linear distance between the cephalometric points on the right and on the left. Corrections for magnification on transverse linear measurements were necessary before classifying the growth data, because although the posteroanterior teleradiographs had been taken with cephalostat, the radiographic magnification of the region of the metallic implants is different from the region of the acoustic meatus center plane because it is closer to the radiographic film, especially compared to the anterior implants on the maxilla. Another reason for correction is that, with the facial growth, maxilla move forward carrying together the metallic implants making them closer to the radiographic film. These variations on radiographic magnification were mathematically corrected by a combination of information of lateral and posteroanterior teleradiograph using correction method recommended by Hsiao et al.[15] A reference system, comprised by Frankfurt's horizontal plane and a vertical line perpendicular from the Porion, built in each lateral teleradiograph allowed the calculation of distance from the position of the implants mean to the acoustic meatus center plane (Fig 2).

With these measures it was possible to calculate the radiographic magnification on the region of metallic implants for each patient based on the formula described by Hsiao et al:[15] Inter-implants real distance = inter-implants radiographic distance x focus-ear rods distance + ear rods-implant distance / distance focus-film (Fig 3).

Table 1 - Characteristics of the studied sample.

Individuals	n	T₁ Mean (years) ± SD	T₂ Mean (years) ± SD	T₃ Mean (years) ± SD
Male	9	9.25 ± 1.39	11.08 ± 1.28	16.99 ± 1.62
Female	4	9.55 ± 1.01	11.52 ± 1.7	16.86 ± 2.17
Total	13	9.34 ± 1.25	11.21 ± 1.36	16.95 ± 1.71

T_1 - (beginning of treatment).
T_2 - (end of treatment with bionator).
T_3 - (final evaluation).

Table 2 - Sagittal and vertical angular cephalometric measures.

MEASURES	T₁ Mean (years) ± SD	T₂ Mean (years) ± SD	T₃ Mean (years) ± SD
SNA	82.92 ± 4.0°	81.53 ± 3.9°	81.26 ± 4.4°
SNB	76.75 ± 3.5°	77.56 ± 3.9°	78.20 ± 4.3°
ANB	6.17 ± 1.9°	3.96 ± 2.3°	3.05 ± 2.6°
SN.GoMe	32.91 ± 5.3°	33.57 ± 5.9°	31.73 ± 6.4°
FMA	23.49 ± 3.8°	23.86 ± 4.4°	22.33 ± 5.4°
SN-ANS-PNS	5.98 ± 2.7°	6.78 ± 4.2°	6.43 ± 3.5°

Table 3 - Cephalometric points digitized on the posteroanterior teleradiograph.

CEPHALOMETRIC POINTS	DESCRIPTION
1) R PIMX	Right posterior implant of the maxilla
2) L PIMX	Left posterior implant of the maxilla
3) R AIMX	Right anterior implant of the maxilla
4) L AIMX	Left anterior implant of the maxilla
5) RJ	Intersection of the right maxillary tuber with the zygomatic wall
6) LJ	Intersection of the left maxillary tuber with the zygomatic wall
7) R PIMD	Right posterior implant of the mandible
8) L PIMD	Left posterior implant of the mandible
9) R Go (Right Gonion)	Most posterior and inferior point of the right gonial angle
10) L Go (Left Gonion)	Most posterior and inferior point of the left gonial angle
11) R Ag (Right Antegonion)	Deeper point of the right antegonial notch
12) L Ag (Left Antegonion)	Deeper point of the left antegonial notch

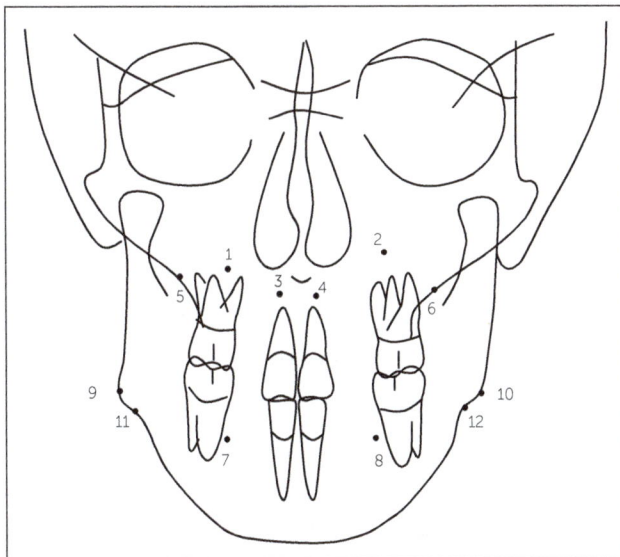

Figure 1 - Cephalometric points digitized on the posteroanterior teleradiograph. Table 3 identifies each cephalometric point.

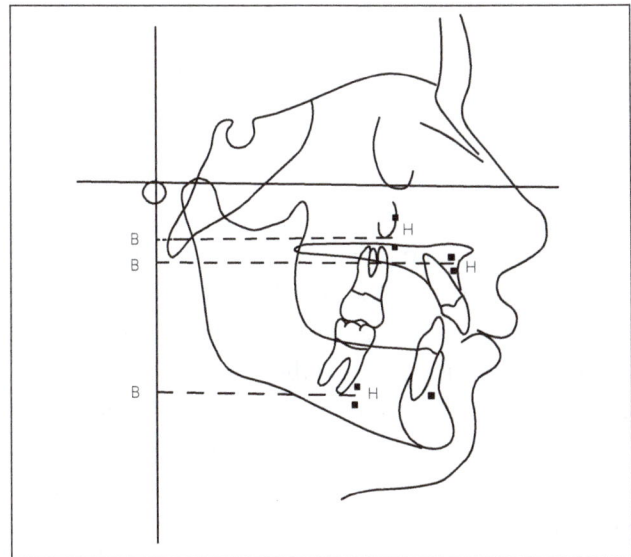

Figure 2 - Traced line shows the calculation of distance from the position of implants (mean point between implants) to the acoustic meatus center plane.

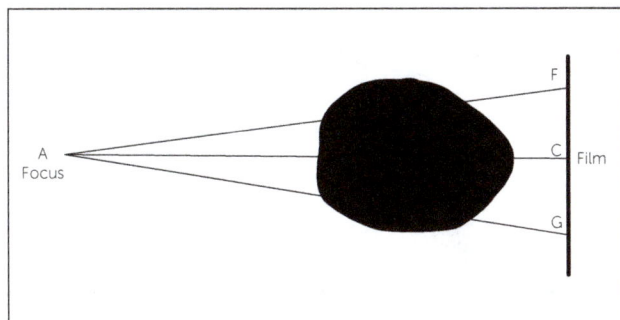

Figure 3 - AB: Distance focus-olive; BH: ear rods-implant distance; AC: focus-film distance; DE: inter-implants real distance (posterior inter-implants of the maxilla, anterior inter-implants of the maxilla and posterior inter-implants of the mandible); FG: inter-implants. radiographic distance (Source: Hsiao et al.[15]).

The following transverse measurements were performed:

» R PIMX - L PIMX: Distance inter-posterior implants of the maxilla.

» R AIMX - L AIMX: Distance inter-anterior implants of the maxilla.

» RJ - LJ: Distance inter-jugal, in relation to the maxilla width.

» R PIMD - L PIMD: Distance inter-posterior implants of the mandible.

» R Go - L Go: Distance inter-gonial, in relation to mandibular width on point Go.

» R Ag - L Ag: Distance inter-antegonial, in relation to mandibular width on point Ag.

Statistical analysis

The mean and standard deviation were calculated for each variable. The different variables presented normal distribution and the Student's t test was used to evaluate the significance of the changes during evaluation periods (T_2–T_1, T_3–T_2, and T_3–T_1). The level of significance used was $p \leq 0.05$. All calculations were performed with SPSS for Windows (version 10.0, SPSS Inc., Chicago, Ill).

Method error

To evaluate the error on the localization of cephalometric points and digitalization procedures all tracings were digitalized again after two weeks by the same examiner. The random error was evaluated using Dahlberg's formula and the systematic errors were evaluated using paired t test. The method random error (Dahlberg's formula) did not exceed 0,33 mm. The paired t test did not show statistically significant systematic error.

RESULTS

Table 4 shows the transverse dimension of the maxilla and mandible on the three periods of evaluation. Table 5 shows that there was statistically significant increase of the maxillary transverse distances on the region of anatomic cephalometric points (Go, Ag and J) and of implants in all evaluated periods, except for the region of anterior implants of the maxilla that did not show statistically significant growth at no time. The lowest gains obtained were on the distance between mandibular implants and the highest were found on the inter-gonial distance.

DISCUSSION

The size of the sample cannot be considered representative of the population in a statistical sense, on the other side, due to the use of metallic implants, a detailed analysis can provide information on the facial growth.[16] Studies with posteroanterior radiographs present some limitations such as variability on the magnification of the projected transverse dimension,[9,16,22] problem of standardization of the head positioning on the cephalostat[16,22,25] due to slight up and down movements of the head and difficulty on identification of points.[16,18,22]

Table 4 - Means and standard deviation of the maxillary and mandibular dimension by period of evaluation.

Variable	T_1 Mean ± SD	T_2 Mean ± SD	T_3 Mean ± SD
R Go – L Go	82.37 ± 4.8	84.71 ± 5.1	91.04 ± 5.5
R Ag – L Ag	75.56 ± 5.5	77.63 ± 5.8	81.05 ± 5.6
R J – L J	57.46 ± 2.0	59.32 ± 2.4	63.01 ± 2.8

Table 5 - Transverse alterations of the distances between implants and of the maxilla and mandible widths.

Variable	T_2 – T_1 Mean ± SD	p	T_3 – T_2 Mean ± SD	p	T_3 – T_1 Mean ± SD	p
R PIMX – L PIMX	1.27 ± 0.5	0.000 *	2.52 ± 1.5	0.000*	3.77 ± 1.6	0.000*
R AIMX – L AIMX	0.12 ± 0.4	0.356	-0.53 ± 1.3	0.209	-0.35 ± 1.4	0.414
R PIMD – L PIMD	0.66 ± 0.8	0.027*	0.83 ± 1.2	0.049*	1.49 ± 1.6	0.015 *
R Go – L Go	2.33 ± 1.1	0.000 *	6.33 ± 2.6	0.000*	8.66 ± 2.2	0.000*
R Ag – L Ag	2.06 ± 1.6	0.001 *	3.42 ± 2.1	0.000*	5.48 ± 2.0	0.000*
R J – L J	1.85 ± 1.3	0.000 *	2.68 ± 2.2	0.000*	5.54 ± 1.8	0.000*

* = statistically significant values p ≤ 0.05.

The problem on identification of points is corrected when metallic implants are used, the variability of magnification was individually corrected for the distances between implants in each period of evaluation, but the problems of standardization of the head positioning are impossible to solve because slight movements of the head are inevitable,[14] however, some studies[11,20] did not find statistically significant differences among measures taken with up to 10° of difference.

The study confirmed the increase of bone bases and evidenced that the maxillary growth was greater than the mandibular.[1,10,17] The distance between posterior implants of the maxilla increased more than the distance between the anterior implants confirming the findings of other studies[4,5,10,17] and showing that the maxillary growth on the posterior region was greater than the anterior besides confirming the existence of transverse growth until the studied age. The mean increase of the distance between posterior implants of the maxilla during all evaluated period, T_1-T_3, was of 3.77 mm. Björk and Skieller[5] found 3 mm increase from 10-11 years to 21 years and in a previous study[4] they found 2.8 mm from 11 to 19 years of age. The result in this work was a little higher, but considering the standard deviation the values are similar because they also observed great variability.[5] The amount of maxillary transverse growth between the implants when compared to the increase related to Jugal point agrees with the present literature[4,5] confirming the median palatine suture as the main site for the maxillary transverse growth and, less expressive, the bone apposition in other areas completing the transverse growth (Table 5).

The differential maxillary transverse increase regarding the anterior and posterior region implies in a transverse rotation between the sides.[4,5,10,17] Our findings agree with other study[10] about the posterior move of the maxillary transverse rotation center with aging in function of the immutability of the anterior maxillary transverse distance.

Table 6 shows that the annual growth of the posterior region of the maxilla was the greatest among the studies that used metallic implants. This result may be associated to the influence of the facial pattern since the patients with horizontal growth pattern present larger transverse facial dimensions when compared to other patterns,[27] may be due to the fact that the sample is composed mostly by male that presents facial widths larger than female[9,17,24,25,28] and/or stimulation of transverse growth by the use of bionator.[1,8] During the treatment with bionator there was an increase of 1.85 mm on the distance RJ - LJ. A previous study[19] showed 1.72 mm increase during the same period in Class II division 1 patients and 2.03 mm in Class I patients. This difference may be related to the therapy used because when comparing Class II our results were higher and when compared Class I they were lower, but it must be emphasized that Class II patients present the maxillary transverse dimension smaller than Class I patients.[19] Besides, the remodeling of the Jugal point during this period was also greater than the presented by other works.[2,9,13] The annual transverse increase between the maxillary implants calculated on the same period was 0.73 mm. In one year of treatment with Frankel's appliance, a study[8] showed 0.57 mm of increase in patients with age and gender distribution similar to the present study. It was concluded that the treatment was capable to increase the basal transverse distances of the maxilla. As the values of annual growth in the present study, were higher it is believed that the bionator also has the capacity to increase the maxillary bone base,[1] although it is not clinically significant.

Table 6 - Annual changes (mm/year) and standard deviation in transverse growth with metallic implants according to the location.

Authors	Anterior of the maxilla	Posterior of the maxilla	Posterior of the mandible	n	Age (years)
Björk, Skieller[4,5]	0.12 ± 0.06	0.42 ± 0.12	Did not report	9	10 to 20
Korn, Baumrind[17]	0.15 ± 0.11	0.43 ± 0.18	0.28 ± 0.15	31	8.5 to 15.5
Gandini, Buschang[10]	-0.10 ± 0.18	0.27 ± 0.13	0.19 ± 0.20	13	13.9 to 16.7
Iseri, Solow[16]	Did not report	Did not report	0.13 ± 0.06	10	6 a 18
Marotta Araujo et al.[1]	-0.14 ± 0.53	0.40 ± 0.17	0.03 ± 0.25	14	8.9 to 9.9
Present study	-0.04 ± 0.18	0.49 ± 0.22	0.18 ± 0.18	13	9.34 to 16.95

During the bionator therapy, the presented mandibular basal transverse growth was 0.66 mm. Another study,[16] on the same period of evaluation, found 0,46 mm and despite not presenting similar sample to the present study, it could be assumed that the bionator has the ability of increasing the mandibular bone base, when used appropriately. This information was already reported by another study[1] that did not find statistically significant mandibular transverse increase during one year of treatment with bionator, but observed higher value on the treated group. Evaluating the annual changes of growth on the two periods it is observed that on the stage of treatment with bionator the maxillary and mandibular basal transverse growth was 0.73 mm/year and 0.37 mm/year, respectively. After therapy, the normal growth showed 0.43 mm/year and 0.14 mm/year for maxilla and mandible showing the stimulation of growth with bionator (Figs 4 to 8). The mandibular basal transverse increase is a supposition, but at a dental and dentoalveolar matter it was already identified in studies with functional appliances.[12,14,23,26] The width of the mandibular implants increased 0.18 mm/year, value similar to the one found previously[10] in older Class I patients. This result may represent that Class II patients have lower potential of mandibular basal transverse growth even if treated at a young age, however some authors[19] did not identify difference on the mandible between Class I and II patients.

After therapy with bionator, the remodeling on the Jugal point found by the present study was greater than the ones shown by several articles with similar period of observation.[2,9,13,19,27] Differently from the maxilla,

the contribution of the basal growth on the mandibular transverse increase is lower than the remodeling[10] (Table 5). Regarding the mandibular remodeling, after therapy with bionator, our results were lower than the ones presented by other works,[2,9,19,27] and observing the increase of the distance R Ag-L Ag during therapy with bionator, the amount of remodeling was identical to one found in the same period (2 mm),[9] but inferior to other works.[2,19,27] However the values of annual growth obtained during the treatment were systematically higher (Fig 4).

The mandibular transverse distance, both on the region of Gonion and Antegonion, evaluated in T_3, is lower than the presented by Lux et al[19] evaluating 15 years old

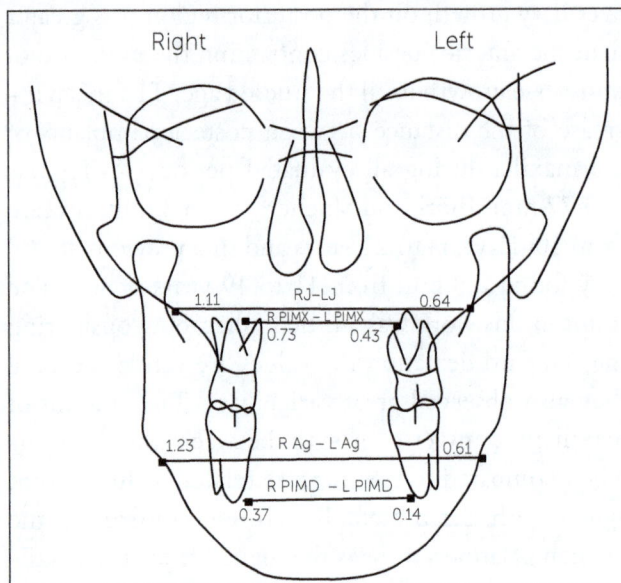

Figure 4 - Annual changes in transverse growth during bionator therapy (values on the right) and after bionator therapy (values on the left).

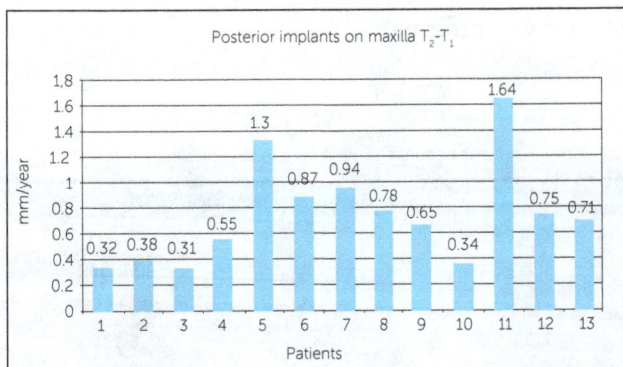

Figure 5 - Individual annual changes in transverse growth on the region of posterior implants of the maxilla during bionator therapy.

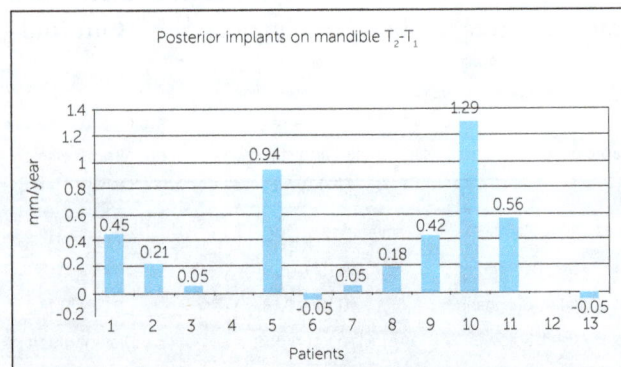

Figure 6 - Individual annual changes in transverse growth on the region of posterior implants of the mandible during bionator therapy.

Class I or II patients. It was also lower than presented in other studies.[2,13,27] Thus, our results suggest that the Class II patients, present mandibular transverse growth and dimensions lower that Class I patients, not confirming the result by Lux et al,[19] although the found differences of size probably have little clinical meaning once they were not greater than 4 mm. Besides, the gonial region showed wide remodeling during growth and it is the transverse dimension of the lower third of the face that presents greater growth and possibility of morphological variation. On Table 7 it can be noticed the influence of gender and malocclusion on the mandibular transverse growth since

the lowest annual growths are related to studies evaluating female patients and/or with Class II malocclusion. Another aspect is that the comparison of normative values between the studies is not appropriated due to radiographic magnification. Some articles do not mention the correction and other do not describe appropriately the used methodology. Due to these problems some studies[9,27] suggest the use of proportion (JJ/AgAg) instead of normative values to minimize the problem although not solving it because some centers take posteroanterior radiographs with Frankfurt's plane parallel to the ground and others with Frankfurt plane inclined 35° down.

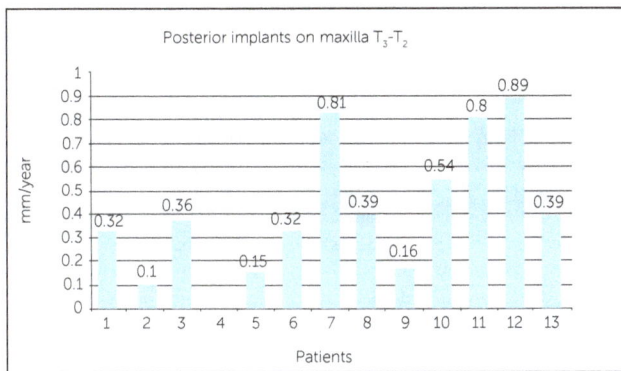

Figure 7 - Individual annual changes in transverse growth on the region of posterior implants of the maxilla after bionator therapy.

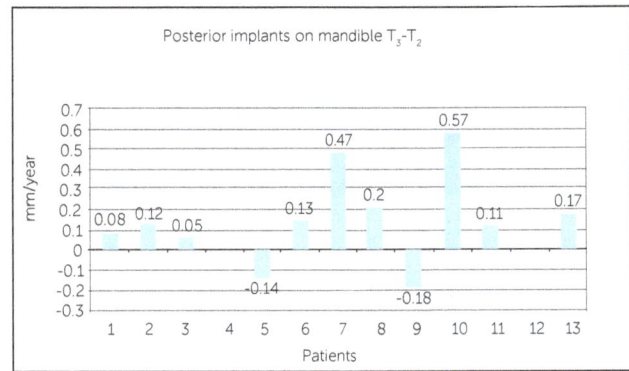

Figure 8 - Individual annual changes in transverse growth on the region of posterior implants of the mandible after bionator therapy.

Table 7 - Annual changes (mm/year) in transverse growth of anatomic points according to the location.

Author	R J – L J	R Go – L Go	R Ag – L Ag	Age (years)	Corrected magnification	Type of malocclusion
Cortella et al[9]	0.58	Not informed	1.03	5 to 18	Yes	I
Snodell et al[25]	0.73	1.53	Not informed	6 to 18	Not informed	I
Hesby et al[13]	0.76	1.42	1.24	7.6 to 16.5	Yes	I
Yavuz et al[28]	1.05	Not informed	1.98	10 to 14	Not informed	I
Lux et al[19] (boys)	0.98	1.68	1.40	7.64 to 15.61	Yes	I
Lux et al[19] (girls)	0.66	1.37	1.21	7.6 to 15.66	Yes	I
Lux et al[19] (boys)	0.65	1.54	1.15	7.49 to 15.6	Yes	II
Lux et al[19] (girls)	0.61	1.36	1.13	7.52 to 15.59	Yes	II
Athanasiou et al[2]	0.70	Not informed	1.41	6 to 15	No	Several
Wagner and Chung[27] (girls)	0.56	Not informed	1.16	6 to 18	Yes	I and II
Present study	0.73	1.14	0.72	9.34 to 16.95	Yes	II

The findings in this study are limited by the size of the sample, bias of the treatment potential and lack of control group. Although the size of the sample is small, the highly significant probabilities obtained (p < 0.001) suggest that the changes observed in growth are real. Besides, additional studies with larger samples are necessary to provide better estimates of variation on transverse increase by growth. There is also the possibility of influence of the treatment subsequent to the bionator on the transverse increase although it is hardly likely that conventional fixed appliances have some potential of orthopedic effect.

CONCLUSIONS

1) The maxillary and mandibular bone bases seem to be affected by bionator therapy, during treatment, returning to a normal pattern on the posttreatment.

2) The maxillary and mandible remodeling pattern followed the same tendency of transverse growth of metallic implants.

3) With aging, the center of transverse rotation of the maxilla is displaced posteriorly.

REFERENCES

1. Marotta Araujo A, Buschang PH, Melo AC. Transverse skeletal base adaptations with Bionator therapy: a pilot implant study. Am J Orthod Dentofacial Orthop. 2004;126(6):666-71.
2. Athanasiou AE, Droschl H, Bosch C. Data and patterns of transverse dentofacial structure of 6- to 15-year-old children: a posteroanterior cephalometric study. Am J Orthod Dentofacial Orthop. 1992;101(5):465-71.
3. Baumrind S, Ben-Bassat Y, Korn EL, Bravo LA, Curry S. Mandibular remodeling measured on cephalograms: 2. A comparison of information from implant and anatomic best-fit superimpositions. Am J Orthod Dentofacial Orthop. 1992;102(3):227-38.
4. Björk A, Skieller V. Growth in width of the maxilla studied by the implant method. Scand J Plast Reconstr Surg. 1974;8(1-2):26-33.
5. Björk A, Skieller V. Growth of the maxilla in three dimensions as revealed radiographically by the implant method. Br J Orthod. 1977;4(2):53-64.
6. Björk A. Facial growth in man, studied with the aid of metallic implants. Acta Odontol Scand. 1955;13(1):9-34.
7. Björk A. Variations in growth pattern of the human mandible: Longitudinal radiographic study by the implant method. J Dent Res. 1963;42(1):400-11.
8. Brieden CM, Pangrazio-Kulbersh V, Kulbersh R. Maxillary skeletal and dental change with Frankel appliances: an implant study. Angle Orthod. 1984;54(3):226-32.
9. Cortella S, Shofer FS, Ghafari J. Transverse development of the jaws: Norms for the posteroanterior cephalometric analysis. Am J Orthod Dentofacial Orthop. 1997;112(5):519-22.
10. Gandini LG Jr, Buschang PH. Maxillary and mandibular width changes studied using metallic implants. Am J Orthod Dentofacial Orthop. 2000;117(1):75-80.
11. Ghafari J, Cater PE, Shofer FS. Effect of film-object distance on posteroanterior cephalometric measurements: suggestions for standardized cephalometric methods. Am J Orthod Dentofacial Orthop. 1995;108(1):30-7.
12. Gibbs SL, Hunt NP. Functional appliances and arch width. Br J Orthod. 1992;19(2):117-25.
13. Hesby RM, Marshall SD, Dawson DV, Southard KA, Casko JS, Franciscus RG, et al. Transverse skeletal and dentoalveolar changes during growth. Am J Orthod Dentofacial Orthop. 2006;130(6):721-31.
14. Hime DL, Owen AH 3rd. The stability of the arch-expansion effects of Fränkel appliance therapy. Am J Orthod Dentofacial Orthop. 1990;98(5):437-45.
15. Hsiao TH, Chang HP, Liu KM. A method of magnification correction for posteroanterior radiographic cephalometry. Angle Orthod. 1997;67(2):137-42.
16. Işeri H, Solow B. Change in the width of the mandibular body from 6 to 23 years of age: an implant study. Eur J Orthod. 2000;22(3):229-38.
17. Korn EL, Baumrind S. Transverse development of the human jaws between the ages of 8.5 and 15.5 years, studied longitudinally with use of implants. J Dent Res. 1990;69(6):1298-306.
18. Leonardi R, Annunziata A, Caltabiano M. Landmark identification error in posteroanterior cephalometric radiography. A systematic review. Angle Orthod. 2008;78(4):761-5.
19. Lux CJ, Conradt C, Burden D, Komposch G. Dental arch widths and mandibular-maxillary base widths in Class II malocclusions between early mixed and permanent dentitions. Angle Orthod. 2003;73(6):674-85.
20. Major PW, Johnson DE, Hesse KL, Glover KE. Effect of head orientation on posterior anterior cephalometric landmark identification. Angle Orthod. 1996;66(1):51-60.
21. Major PW, Johnson DE, Hesse KL, Glover KE. Landmark identification error in posterior anterior cephalometrics. Angle Orthod. 1994;64(6):447-54.
22. Malkoc S, Sari Z, Usumez S, Koyuturk AE. The effect of head rotation on cephalometric radiographs. Eur J Orthod. 2005;27(3):315-21.
23. Owen AH. Morphologic changes in the transverse dimension using the Fränkel appliance. Am J Orthod. 1983;83(3):200-17.
24. Savara BS, Singh IJ. Norms of size and annual increments of seven anatomical measures of maxillae in boys from three to sixteen years of age. Angle Orthod. 1968;38(2):104-20.
25. Snodell SF, Nanda RS, Currier GF. A longitudinal cephalometric study of transverse and vertical craniofacial growth. Am J Orthod Dentofacial Orthop. 1993;104(5):471-83.
26. Vargevik K. Morphologic evidence of muscle influence on dental arch width. Am J Orthod. 1979;76(1):21-8.
27. Wagner DM, Chung CH. Transverse growth of the maxilla and mandible in untreated girls with low, average, and high MP-SN angles: a longitudinal study. Am J Orthod Dentofacial Orthop. 2005;128(6):716-23.
28. Yavuz I, Ikbal A, Baydaş B, Ceylan I. Longitudinal posteroanterior changes in transverse and vertical craniofacial structures between 10 and 14 years of age. Angle Orthod. 2004;74(5):624-9.

18

Mini-implants: Mechanical resource for molars uprighting

Susiane Allgayer[1], Deborah Platcheck[2], Ivana Ardenghi Vargas[3], Raphael Carlos Drumond Loro[4]

Introduction: The early orthodontic treatment allows correction of skeletal discrepancies by growth control, and the elimination of deleterious habits, which are risk factors for the development of malocclusions, favoring for the correction of tooth positioning later in a second treatment stage. During development of teeth and occlusion, the mandibular second molars commonly erupt in the oral cavity after all other teeth of the anterior region. In their eruptive process there may be a condition known as tooth impaction, which precludes its complete eruption and requires proper uprighting treatment. The temporary anchorage devices allow disimpaction and movement of these teeth directly to their final position, without the need of patient compliance or reaction movements in other parts of the arch. **Objective:** This paper aims at describing a case report of the treatment of a patient with Angle Class II malocclusion, performed in two phases, in which mini-implants were used for uprighting the impacted mandibular second molars.

Keywords: Corrective orthodontics. Orthodontic anchorage procedures. Impacted tooth.

[1] PhD student of Orthodontics and Facial Orthopedics, PUC-RS.
[2] PhD and Professor of Orthodontics, ABO/RS.
[3] PhD in Dentistry, ULBRA.
[4] PhD in Oral and Maxillofacial Surgery and Professor at Graduation and Post-graduation courses, PUCRS.

Susiane Allgayer
PUCRS – Pontifícia Universidade Católica do Rio Grande do Sul
Av. Ipiranga, 6681 – Prédio 06 – Sala 209
CEP: 90619-900 – Porto Alegre / RS, Brazil
E-mail: susianeallgayer@gmail.com

INTRODUCTION

Tooth impaction is a condition in which the eruption of a tooth is interrupted as a consequence of its contact with other tooth or teeth.[1] A tooth is considered impacted when, after completion of root formation, the tooth does not erupt in up to six months compared to the contralateral tooth.[2]

The prevalence of impaction of mandibular second molars is relatively low, nearly 1 to 3 teeth in 1,000.[3,4,5,6] The most probable causes of impaction of second molars seem to be related to the excessive size of these teeth, deficient mandibular growth, inadequate length of the mandibular arch or only due to an abnormal eruption pathway.[7,8]

The treatment options may involve or not surgery for exposure of the molar crown and utilization of fixed and/or removable appliances.[7-10]

The utilization of temporary implants for orthodontic anchorage allowed a new perspective in the orthodontic treatment, especially in the permanent dentition. Mini-implants, palatal implants and mini-plates are currently used in several clinical situations, as the treatment of open bites and uprighting of molars without adverse effects on the adjacent teeth.[11-18]

Class II is the severe malocclusion most frequently found and is characterized by "distal positioning" of the mandibular teeth compared to the maxillary teeth, which may be caused by bone dysplasia or forward positioning of the alveolar process or maxillary dental arch, or even by the combination of skeletal and dental factors.[9]

This case report describes the orthodontic treatment of a patient with Angle Class II malocclusion with impaction of the mandibular second molars, in which two mini-implants were used as an anchorage aid for uprighting of the teeth, which were impacted on the distal aspect of mandibular first molars.

CASE REPORT

Caucasian patient of female gender sought for initial orthodontic treatment at the age of 9 years and 5 months. The general health status was good and there was no history of severe diseases or traumas. On the clinical examination, it was observed that the patient was in the intermediate mixed dentition and presented tongue thrusting and speech disorder.

The patient exhibited symmetric face with a slightly convex profile and competent lips. The facial thirds were proportional and the smile line was normal (Fig 1). The cephalometric evaluation revealed skeletal Class II pattern with ANB of 5° due to maxillary protrusion (SNA 84°) (Fig 2 and Tab 1). Considering the values of the occlusal plane angle (SN-Occlusal Plane 15°), mandibular plane (GoGn-SN 28°) and Y axis (Frankfurt plane-SGn 65°), the patient presented a favorable mandibular growth pattern in both horizontal and vertical directions. Concerning the dental relationships, the maxillary and mandibular incisors were slightly buccally tipped and protruded (1-NA 6 mm, 1-NA 25°, 1-NB 6 mm, 1-NB 25°, and IMPA 95°). The patient presented overjet of 3.5 mm, anterior open bite, negative tooth size discrepancy of 4 mm in the maxillary arch and

Table 1 - Cephalometric measurements.

Measure	Initial	Follow-up	Final
SNA	84	82	81
SNB	79	77	77
ANB	5	5	4
1-NA	6	5	7
1.NA	25	22	25
1-NB	6	7	9
1.NB	26	31	35
1.1	125	122	106
SN.Occlusal plane	15	17	15
GoGn.SN	28	31	32
S-UI	2	1	-1
S-LI	3	3	1
Y-axis	65	58	60
Facial angle	80	87	87
Convexity angle	8	9	5
Witts	-2	1	2
FMA	30	26	28
FMIA	55	54	50
IMPA	95	100	102
Nasolabial angle	95	109	105
A-NPerp	- 4	- 2	- 1
Co-A	88	91	87
Co-Gn	106	110	114
Mx-Mn difference	18	19	27
AFAI	65	66	73
Facial axis	0	- 4	- 5
Pog-NPerp	-14	-12	-7

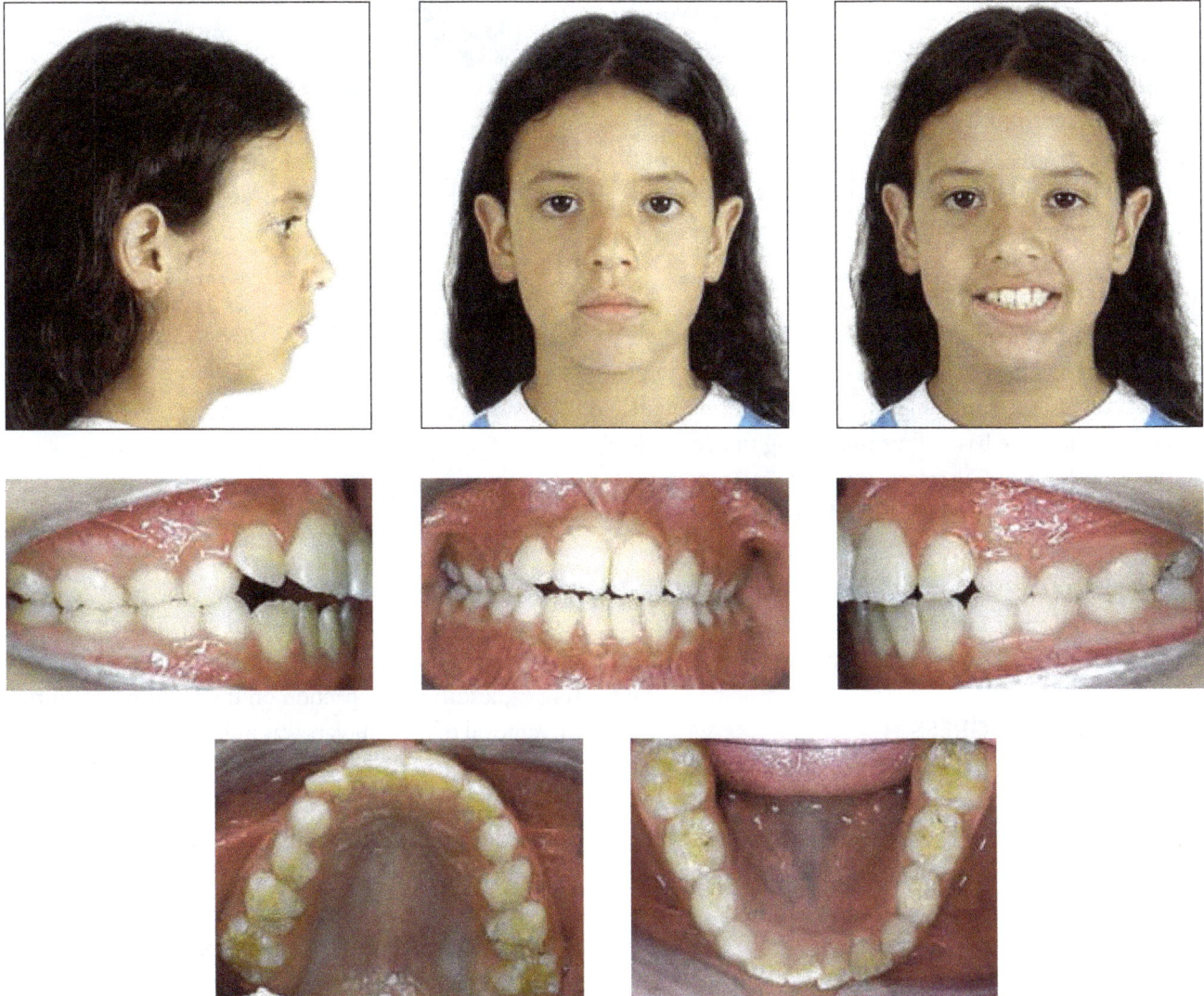

Figure 1 - Pretreatment facial and intraoral photographs.

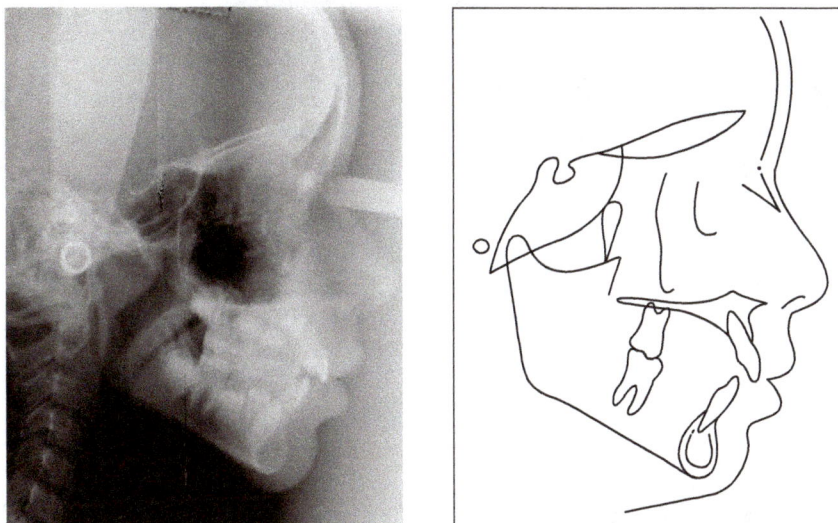

Figure 2 - Initial lateral cephalometric radiograph and tracing.

2 mm in the mandibular arch, with mild crowding in both arches. Analysis of panoramic (Fig 3) and periapical radiographs revealed the presence of all permanent teeth, including the third molars, besides deciduous canines and molars still present in the oral cavity. The hand-wrist radiograph revealed that the patient was not in the pubertal growth spurt yet.

TREATMENT OBJECTIVES

The treatment objectives were to correct the skeletal and dental Class II malocclusion and intercept the malocclusion, providing conditions for adequate growth of the bone bases, thus improving the dentoalveolar morphology. Therefore, it was necessary to control the maxillary protrusion by redirecting growth, to eliminate oral habits, to re-establish normal lip and tongue functions to correct the overbite, and to control the eruption of mandibular second molars, which presented a mesial eruption pathway.

TREATMENT PROGRESS

Initially, a maxillary appliance with tongue crib was used for six months, for tongue reeducation. After achievement of adequate overbite (Fig 3), correction of the skeletal discrepancy was initiated by redirecting maxillary growth with an extraoral traction appliance, during 10 months (Fig 5).

The fixed orthodontic appliance was placed using standard edgewise brackets, and the alignment and leveling stage was initiated.

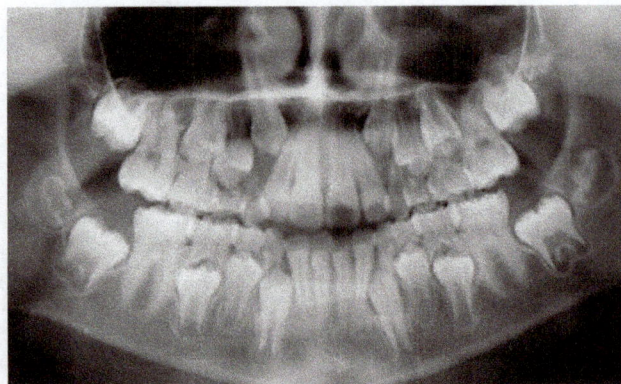

Figure 3 - Initial panoramic radiograph.

During the eruption process, the mandibular second molars presented a marked mesial eruption pathway (Fig 6), leading to impaction on the first molars. Surgical removal of third molars was indicated to enhance the uprighting of second molars. The same procedure comprised surgical exposure and bonding of a bracket on the cusp of these teeth and placement of mini-implants (Ortoimplante Conexão, 2.0 x 9.0, medium transmucous profile) for anchorage on the retromolar region, distal and occlusal to the second molars, using a mucoperiosteal flap[11]. This site was selected to allow support for orthodontic eruption of the impacted second molars in distal and occlusal direction (Fig 7A).

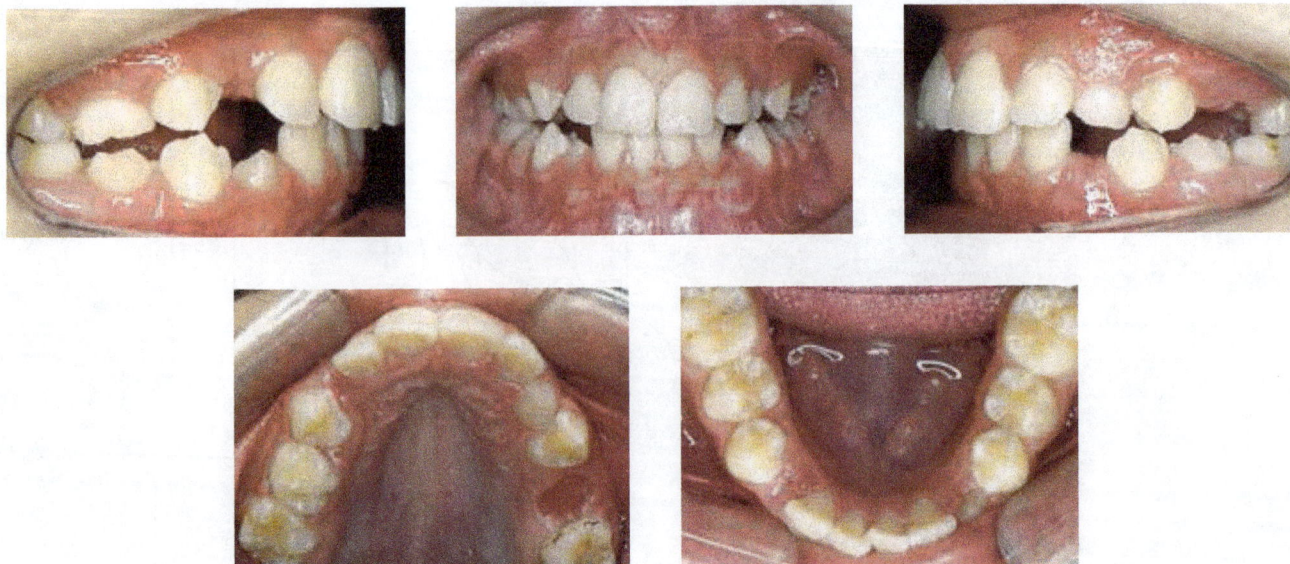

Figure 4 - Intermediate intraoral photographs.

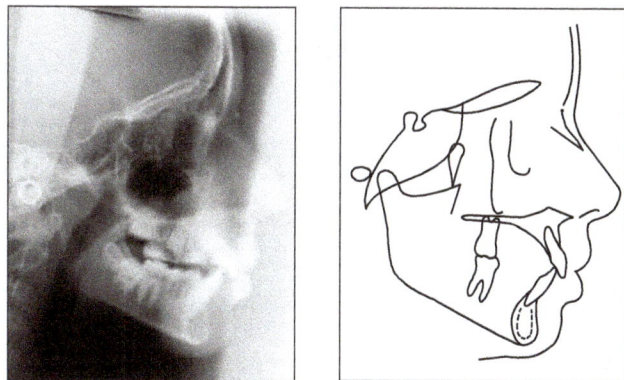

Figure 5 - Intermediate lateral cephalometric radiograph and tracing.

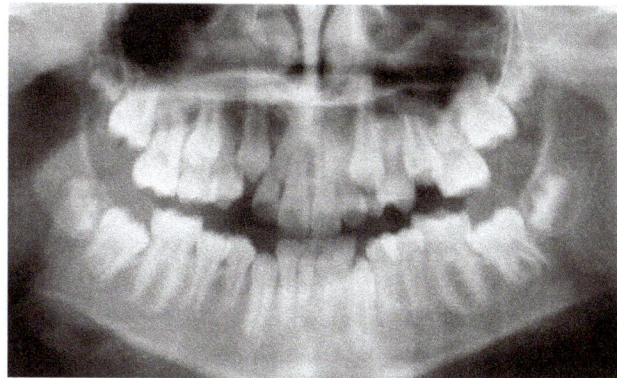

Figure 6 - Intermediate panoramic radiograph.

The affected teeth were gradually moved using chain elastics, improving their positioning (Fig 7B). The period required for uprighting was 18 months. The mini-implants did not present mobility and the patient hygiene was excellent.

The maxillary second molars did not erupt (Fig 7B). After surgical removal of fibrosis, they erupted with palatal tipping and the mandibular second molars were in buccoversion, which caused a crossbite that was treated by placement of a contracted lingual archwire, besides expansion of the maxillary arch. Simple cross vertical elastics were also used on brackets bonded on the palatal aspects of maxillary right and left second molars and buccal aspect of the mandibular right and left second molars. After 18 months, they presented good inclination in the bone base (Fig 7C), were included in the archwire, the lingual arch and mini-implants were removed and corrective fixed appliances were placed for treatment finalization. There was resorption of the distal root of the mandibular right first molar, which was followed up radiographically (Figs 7C and D).

The total treatment time with the fixed appliances was eight years, due to the period elapsed to wait for eruption of the maxillary and mandibular second molars. After orthodontic finishing and improvement of occlusion, the appliance was removed and a wraparound removable orthodontic retainer was placed in the maxillary arch, as well as a mandibular 3x3 bonded lingual retainer.

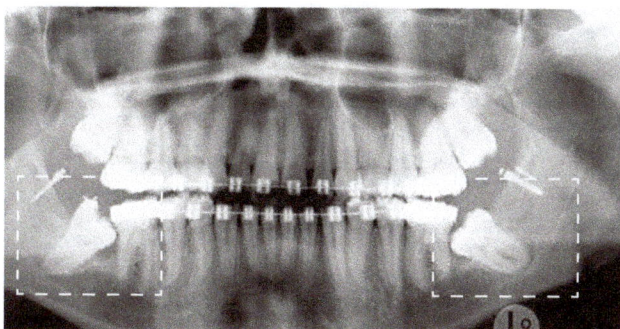

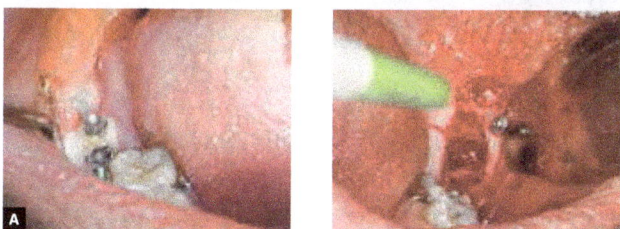

Figure 7A - Intermediate radiograph and photographs.

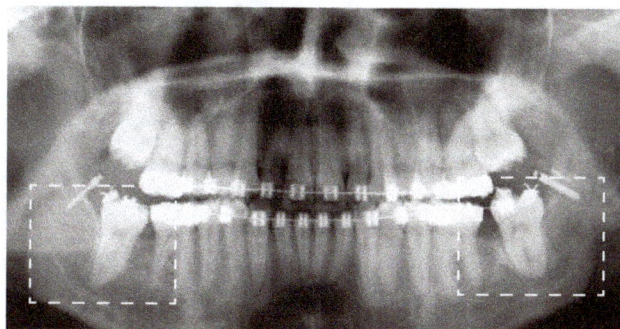

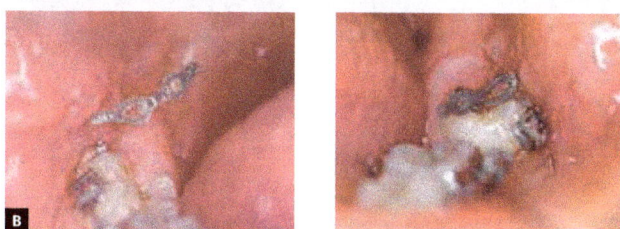

Figure 7B - Intermediate radiograph and photographs.

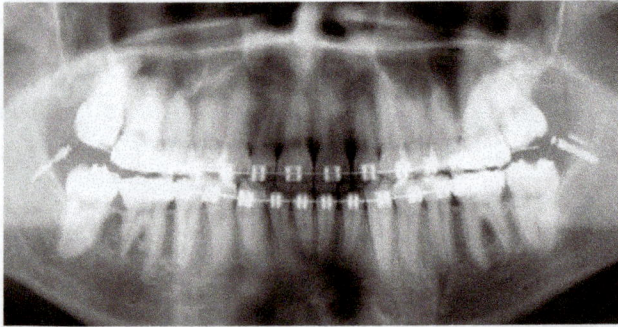

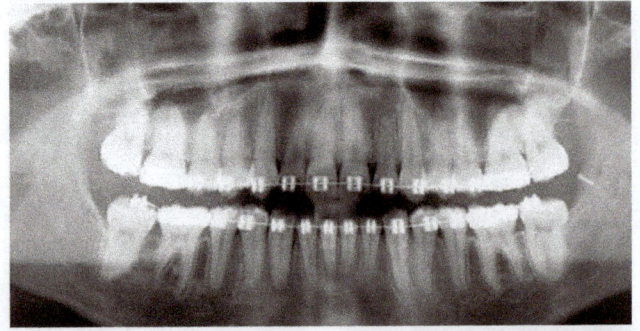

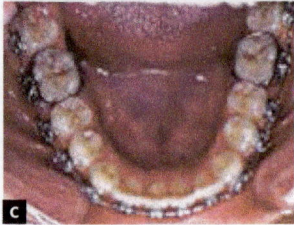

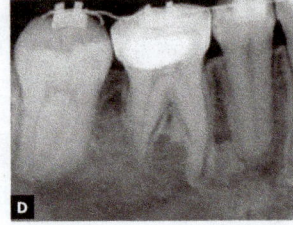

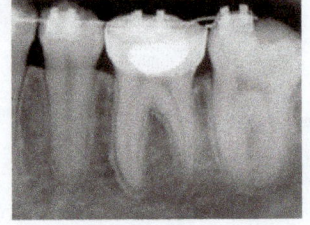

Figure 7C - Intermediate radiograph and photograph.

Figure 7D - Intermediate radiographs.

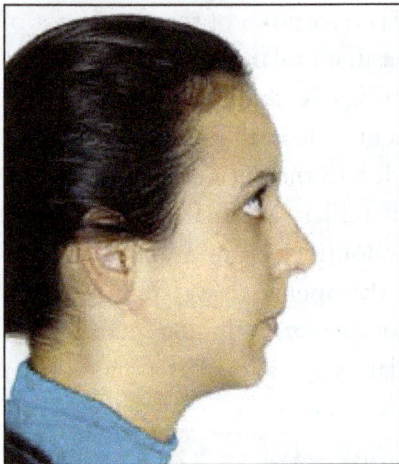

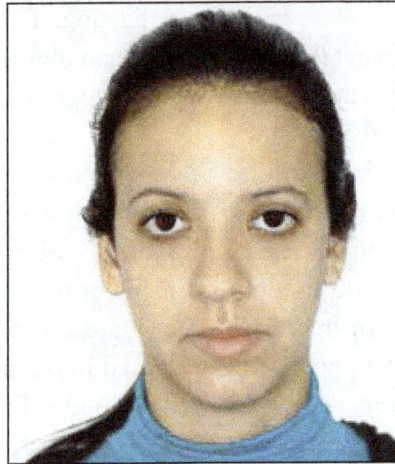

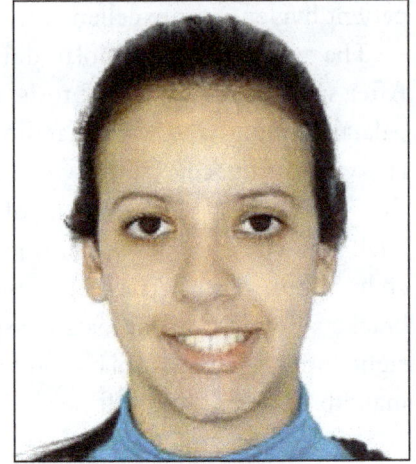

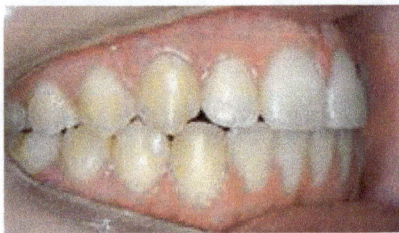

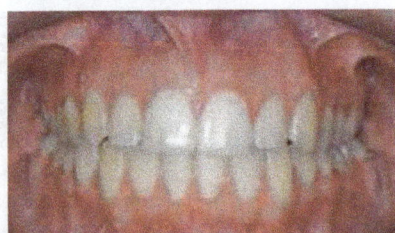

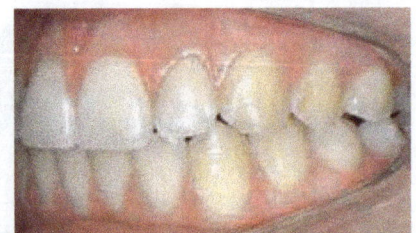

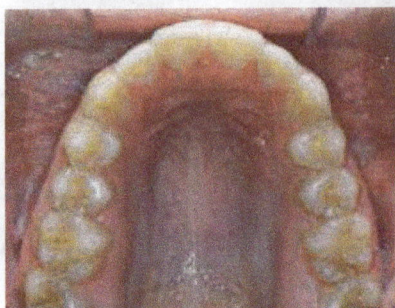

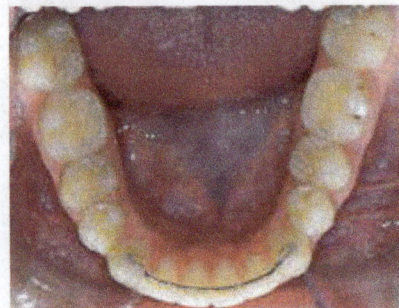

Figure 8 - Final facial and intraoral photographs.

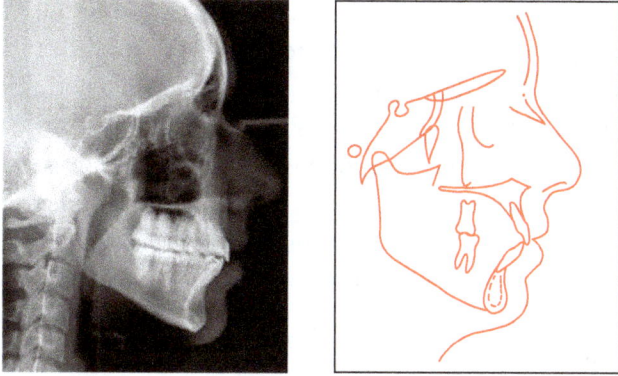

Figure 9 - Final lateral cephalometric radiograph and tracing.

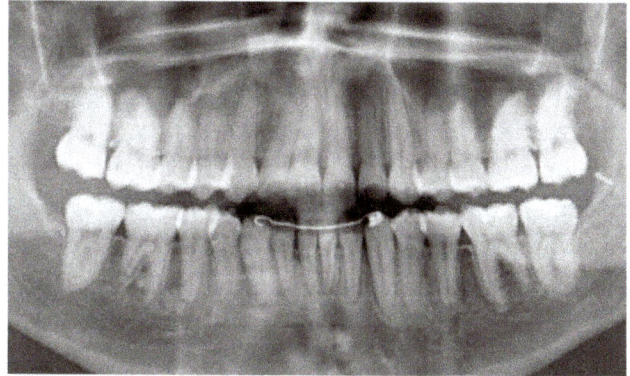

Figure 10 - Final panoramic radiograph.

TREATMENT RESULTS

At treatment completion, the facial outcome was excellent. The intraoral analysis revealed Class I molar and canine relationship, adequate overjet and overbite, coincident midlines and adequate intercuspation between the dental arches, including the second molars. The panoramic radiograph evidenced correct parallelism between the roots, and the cephalometric tracing and superimposition on the cephalogram revealed the dental and skeletal changes achieved at treatment completion (Figs 8 - 11, Tab 1).

DISCUSSION

Tooth impaction may be caused by factors as heredity, malposition of the tooth germ, overretention of deciduous teeth, localized pathological lesions, reduced arch length and deficient growth of the mandibular ramus.[9] The mandibular second molars may be impacted or severely malpositioned and are often blocked under the distal convexity of permanent first molars. Their early repositioning is usually advantageous during active root development.[9,10,19]

The utilization of mini-plates was initially suggested as orthodontic anchorage for distal movement of mandibular molars, which was necessary in cases like this. The placement and removal require invasive surgery, which may lead to infection.[13,18] The utilization of endosseous implants as anchorage in retromolar,[21,22] palatal and edentulous areas has been successfully described in the literature,[11,16,23,24] however they require osseointegration before the orthodontic force is applied, thus increasing the treatment time, besides the limited sites for placement.

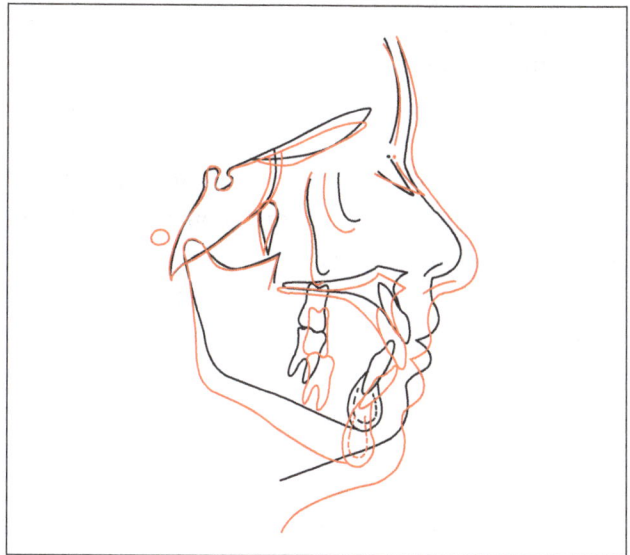

Figure 11 - Superimposition of cephalometric tracings at pretreatment (black) and posttreatment (red), with parallel Sella-Nasion lines and register at Sella for growth analysis. The redirection of maxillary growth combined to the favorable mandibular horizontal growth corrected the malocclusion.

Both mini-plates and endosseous implants are costly and difficult to be removed.[13,18,25]

However, skeletal anchorage has surely been an important tool in Orthodontics. These treatments require minimum patient compliance and a good oral hygiene can be more easily maintained. Even in patients who do not need prosthetic rehabilitation, recent studies have used the retromolar, palatal and alveolar regions for the placement of implants only for orthodontic purposes, for induced movement of teeth or segments.[16]

Different from the aforementioned resources, the mini-implants are easy to insert and remove, may be used immediately, are less costly and may be placed in several sites, increasing their versatility.[12,15,25] The anchorage using mini-implants is as effective as the aforementioned mechanisms and has the advantages of being minimally invasive, the insertion technique is simple and facilitates the surgical procedure, providing reduced surgical time.[16] For these reasons, in several clinical situations, they are preferred as a skeletal anchorage method[25].

The site for fixation of the orthodontic mini-implant should present sufficient quantity of cortical bone tissue to assure immediate mechanical stability, minimum discomfort to the patient, safety to anatomical structures, as well as to allow the application of adequate biomechanics. The retromolar region[21,22] is indicated to promote the uprighting of molars because it increases the distal force component. When mini-implants are placed at this region, it is also possible to achieve extrusion forces with a distal component, another reason for selecting this treatment.[26]

One of the goals of orthodontic treatment is to achieve a harmonious arch shape. Transverse problems should be corrected soon after diagnosis to prevent bone deficiencies.[27] When a tooth presents crossbite, it rarely presents alterations only in its axial inclination. The opposing tooth in the other arch is often also malpositioned. Thus, the mandibular tooth may be in buccoversion and the maxillary tooth in palatoversion. In these cases, both should be corrected and simple cross elastics are indicated. In the present case, brackets bonded on the surfaces of molars were used to position the elastics to correct the crossbite. The technique is relatively easy, but requires patient compliance.[28] Combined to elastics, a contracted lingual archwire soldered to the bands on the mandibular right and left second molars was placed, because they presented with marked buccoversion.

Similar to the aforementioned problem, deleterious habits should be interrupted as early as possible, to reestablish the normal lip and tongue functions in order to allow a correct overbite. In the present case, a maxillary removable appliance fabricated with clear acrylic and a tongue crib fabricated with 0.7mm stainless steel wire was used for tongue reeducation. This appliance — which is easy to be made and is fixed in the oral cavity using Adams clasps in the molars and Kennedy clasps in the canines — intercepted the local factors that precluded tooth eruption in their normal position and allowed stable outcomes during treatment.

External root resorption is a common complication of orthodontic treatment. The esthetic and function improvement often compensate the treatment risks.[29] Reduction of the root length does not reduce the longevity or functional capacity of the affected teeth; after the force is removed, there is the repair process and reestablishment of the periodontal ligament.[30] In the present case, resorption of the mandibular right first molar observed during treatment was controlled by radiographic follow-up and force control. Considering the large movement of the second molar, repair of the periodontal ligament of the mandibular right first molar and reestablishment of the normal functions of the two teeth, resorption of the first molar was clinically acceptable (Figs 7C and D).

Ultimately, the mini-implants provide biomechanical advantages that allow an easier and more effective treatment, without the need of patient compliance.[17,26] The preference of clinicians for a certain treatment modality must not be necessarily followed. After deciding that the utilization of mini-implants is safe and necessary for the treatment, the area of insertion should be selected considering the accessibility, conditions of soft and hard tissues, biomechanical utility in orthodontics, comfort to the patient and possibility of irritation of the adjacent oral tissues.[26]

CONCLUSION

Disimpaction of the mandibular second molar, comprising extraction of the third molar, exposure of the crown of the impacted tooth for bonding of orthodontic bracket followed by orthodontic mechanics demonstrated to be a safe and effective approach with minimum discomfort to the patient. The mechanics required only two mini-implants placed at the retromolar region, which allowed correct positioning of the second molars impacted in the dental arch. Good results were obtained and the orthodontic treatment objectives were achieved; also, the Class II molar relationship and open bite were corrected, thus yielding an occlusion with excellent function and esthetics.

REFERENCES

1. Hitchin AD, Durh MDS, Edin RCS. The impacted maxillary canine. Br Dent J. 1956;100(1):1-14.

2. Lindauer SJ, Rubenstein LK. Canine impaction identified early with panoramic radiographs. J Am Dent Assoc. 1992;123(3):91-7.

3. Grover PS, Lorton L. The incidence of unerupted permanent teeth and related clinical cases.Oral Surg Oral Med Oral Pathol. 1985;59(4):420-5.

4. Varpio M, Wellfelt B. Disturbed eruption of the lower second molar: clinical appearance, prevalence, and etiology. ASDC J Dent Child. 1988;55(2):114-8.

5. Montelius GA. Impacted teeth: a comparative study of chinese and canadian dentitions. J Dent Res. 1932;12(6):931-8.

6. Johnsen DC. Prevalence of delayed eruption of permanent teeth as a result of local factors. J Am Dent Assoc. 1977;94(1):100-6.

7. Lima CEO, Henriques JFC, Janson GRP, Freitas MR. Segundo molar inferior impactado: revisão e apresentação de um caso clínico. Rev Clín Orthod Dental Press. 2004;2(6):68-75.

8. Teixeira RG, Vidal BC, Bastos EPS. Reposicionamento cirúrgico de um segundo molar inferior direito impactado com cárie: relato de caso. J Bras Ortodon Ortop Facial. 2000;5(30):76-81.

9. Moyers RE. Ortodontia. 4ª ed. Rio de Janeiro: Guanabara Koogan; 1991.

10. Pogrel MA. The surgical uprighting of mandibular second molars. Am J Orthod Dentofacial Orthop. 1995;108(2):180-3.

11. Faber J, Velasque F. Titanium miniplate as anchorage to close a premolar space by means of mesial movement of the maxillary molars. Am J Orthod Dentofacial Orthop. 2009;136(4):587-95.

12. Cope JB. Temporary anchorage devices in orthodontics: a paradigm shift. Semin Orthod. 2005;11(1):3-9.

13. Faber J, Morum TFA, Leal S, Berto PM, Carvalho CKS. Miniplacas permitem tratamento eficiente e eficaz da mordida aberta anterior. Rev Dental Press Ortod Ortop Facial. 2008;13(5):144-57.

14. Faber J. Ancoragem esquelética com miniplacas. In: Lima Filho RMA, Bolognese AM. Ortodontia: arte e ciência. Maringá: Dental Press; 2007. p. 449-73.

15. Kuroda S, Katayama A, Takano-Yamamoto T. Severe anterior open-bite case treated using titanium screw anchorage. Angle Orthod. 2004;74(4):558-67.

16. Erverdi N, Keles A, Nanda R. The use of skeletal anchorage in open bite treatment: a cephalometric evaluation. Angle Orthod. 2004;74(3):381-90.

17. Sugawara J, Kanzaki R, Takahashi I, Nagasaka H, Nanda R. Distal movement of maxillary molars in nongrowing patients with the skeletal anchorage system. Am J Orthod Dentofacial Orthop. 2006;129(6):723-33.

18. Sugawara J, Daimaruya T, Umemori M, Nagasaka H, Takahashi I, Kawamura H, et al. Distal movement of mandibular molars in adult patients with skeletal anchorage system. Am J Orthod Dentofacial Orthop. 2004;125(2):130-8.

19. Vedtofte H, Andreasen JO, Kjaer I. Arrested eruption of the permanent lower second molar. Eur J Orthod. 1999;21(1):31-40.

20. Rindler A. Effects on lower third molars after extraction of second molars. Angle Orthod. 1977;47(1):55-8.

21. Higuchi KW, Slack JM. The use of titanium fixtures for intraoral anchorage to facilitate orthodontic tooth movement. Int J Oral Maxillofac Implants. 1991;6(3):338-44.

22. Roberts WE, Marshal KJ, Mozsary PG. Rigid endosseous implant utilized as anchorage to protract molars and close an atrophic extraction site. Angle Orthod. 1990;60(2):135-52.

23. Lee JS, Kim DH, Park YC, Kyung SH, Kim Tk, The efficient use of midpalatal miniscrew implants. Angle Othod. 2004;74(5):711-4.

24. Wehrbein H, Merz BR, Diedrich P, Glatzmaier J. The use of palatal implants for orthodontic anchorage. Design and clinical application of the orthosystem. Clin Oral Implants Res. 1996;7(4):410-6.

25. Joseph S. Petrey, Marnie M. Saunders, G. Thomas Kluemper, Larry L. Cunningham, and Cynthia S. Beeman. Temporary anchorage device insertion variables: effects on retention. Angle Orthod. 2010;80(4):634-41.

26. Lee JS, Kim DH, Park YC, Vanardall RL. Aplicação dos mini-implantes ortodônticos. São Paulo: Quintessence; 2009.

27. Joondeph DR. Mysteries of asymmetries. Am J Orthod Dentofacial Orthop. 2000;117(5):577-9.

28. Assed S. Odontopediatria: bases científicas para a prática clínica. São Paulo: Artes Médicas; 2005.

29. Tanaka OM, Amorin LH, Shintcovsk RL, Hirata TM. Treatment of patient with severaly shortened maxillary central incisor roots. J Clin Orthod. 2008;42(12):729-31.

30. Ramanathan C, Hofman Z. Root resorption in relation to orthodontic tooth movement. Acta Medica (Hradec Kralove). 2006;49(2):91-5.

19

Vertical control in the Class III compensatory treatment

Márcio Costa Sobral[1], Fernando A. L. Habib[2], Ana Carla de Souza Nascimento[3]

Introduction: Compensatory orthodontic treatment, or simply orthodontic camouflage, consists in an important alternative to orthognathic surgery in the resolution of skeletal discrepancies in adult patients. It is important to point that, to be successfully performed, diagnosis must be detailed, to evaluate, specifically, dental and facial features, as well as the limitations imposed by the magnitude of the discrepancy. The main complaint, patient's treatment expectation, periodontal limits, facial pattern and vertical control are some of the items to be explored in the determination of the viability of a compensatory treatment. Hyperdivergent patients who carry a Class III skeletal discrepancy, associated with a vertical facial pattern, with the presence or tendency to anterior open bite, deserve special attention. In these cases, an efficient strategy of vertical control must be planned and executed. **Objective:** The present article aims at illustrating the evolution of efficient alternatives of vertical control in hiperdivergent patients, from the use, in the recent past, of extra-oral appliances on the lower dental arch (J-hook), until nowadays, with the advent of skeletal anchorage. But for patients with a more balanced facial pattern, the conventional mechanics with Class III intermaxillary elastics, associated to an accentuated curve of Spee in the upper arch and a reverse Curve of Spee in the lower arch, and vertical elastics in the anterior region, continues to be an excellent alternative, if there is extreme collaboration in using the elastics.

Keywords: Orthodontics. Class III malocclusion. Camouflage.

[1] MSc in Orthodontics, Federal University of Rio de Janeiro (UFRJ). Professor, Specialization Program of Orthodontics, Federal University of Bahia (UFBA). Diplomate by the Brazilian Board of Orthodontics and Facial Orthopedics (BBO).
[2] PhD in Dentistry, Federal University of Bahia (UFBA). Specialist in Orthodontics, Federal University of Rio de Janeiro (UFRJ). Associate Professor of Orthodontics, Federal University of Bahia (UFBA).
[3] Specialist in Orthodontics, Federal University of Bahia (UFBA).

» The author reports no commercial, proprietary or financial interest in the products or companies described in this article.

Márcio Costa Sobral
Av. Anita Garibaldi, 1815, sala 315-B, C.M.E. - Ondina, Brazil
CEP: 41.170-130, Salvador / BA - E-mail: marciosobral@gmail.com

INTRODUCTION

The universe of eventual patients liable to orthodontic treatment can be divided into two large groups: With or without skeletal discrepancies. The latter, in turn, is subdivided into the presence or absence of facial growth potential, a relevant fact for the elaboration of the treatment plan, as well as to the prognosis estimate.

The interceptive treatment of important skeletal discrepancies on young patients with growth potential, together with corrective orthodontic procedures, in a subsequent step, can, in theory, redirect facial growth. Such an intervention can minimize and even correct those discrepancies, promoting good occlusion, balance between the jaws, and adequate facial esthetics.

On the other hand, for those who have already finished the outbreak of puberal growth, there are only two alternatives: Compensatory orthodontic treatment, also known as orthodontic camouflage, or orthodontic treatment associated to orthognathic surgery. The decision on what to be performed must be made together with the patient, taking into account the following aspects: Main complaint and yearnings about the treatment results, severity degree of maxillary-mandibular discrepancy, periodontal limits for orthodontic movement, clinical condition of present teeth and the impossibility of growth modification.

ORTHODONTIC CAMOUFLAGE

Orthodontic camouflage consists on the displacement of teeth in relation to the supporting bone, to compensate the discrepancy between the jaws. It can be accomplished by dental inclination. Depending on the desired level of compensation and the magnitude of orthodontic movement, some times extractions are needed.

As suggested by Proffit et al,[1] there is a limit for incisor orthodontic movement, that is, in some cases, orthodontic treatment has to be associated with the movement of the basal bones by facial orthopedics or orthognathic surgery. However, dental movement can camouflage a broad variety of skeletal discrepancies, without deleterious effects on the periodontal structures. Nevertheless, correct diagnosis and a realistic treatment plan are necessary to avoid undesirable sequelae.[5]

Orthodontic camouflage is well fit for patients that carry small skeletal Class III, with no growth potential, with a relative fine facial balance and without severe crowding. Almost always, the compensatory orthodontic treatment is followed by the patient fear of facing surgical procedure, and by his relative satisfaction with his facial aspect, generating a small demand for great changes on this feature.

In relation to Class III, when the skeletal problem is small, the facial aspect is improved after camouflage; however, in moderate and severe cases, orthodontic treatment produces considerable worsening on facial esthetics, because the slightest retraction of lower incisors increases the chin prominence.[1]

When asymmetry is added to the skeletal discrepancy, it is imperative to pay attention in the patients' expectations concerning treatment, because orthodontic camouflage is not going to correct it. Yet, facial asymmetry may not cause great impact on esthetics or, even if it is noticed, the patient may reject surgical treatment.

CLASS III CAMOUFLAGE – CLINICAL AND MECHANICAL ASPECTS

Early intervention on skeletal Class III discrepancies, in the mixed dentition and even in the deciduous dentition, is more and more attracting orthodontist's attention. However, the skeletal Class III pattern worsens with age, that is, the deformity, apparently corrected during childhood, presents relapse during adolescence. This brings great difficulties to treatment success of the problem.[2,7] Nevertheless, patients with light or moderate skeletal Class III malocclusion and with acceptable facial esthetics can benefit from a compensatory orthodontic treatment.[4]

The strategy to camouflage a Class III malocclusion usually involves buccal inclination of upper incisors and retroinclination of lower incisors to improve dental occlusion, but it does not correct the skeletal problem or modify facial profile in a meaningful way.[5,6]

It is important to notice the cases in which the facial type of the patient is characterized as vertical and/ or with a hiperdivergent tendency, or with anterior open bite. In those cases it is necessary to associate vertical control strategies during tooth movement, with the goal of avoiding undesirable opening of the mandibular plane, which would meaningfully worsen the vertical relation on the anterior region, hampering or even stopping the achievement of a satisfactory occlusion at the end of the treatment. One of the effective ways to accomplish vertical control remounts to the mechanical principles of Tweed-Merrifield technique, that nowadays, associated with skeletal anchorage devices, are extremely predictable and easily used by patients.[12]

Orthodontic camouflage treatment must be indicated for young patients, only if, before starting treatment, cephalometry shows that residual growth is not going to aggravate the deformity after treatment.[6] Besides, most of the patients that have a serious Class III skeletal deformity are liable to orthognathic surgery as the only option to obtain both normal occlusion and a pleasant profile, concerning esthetics.[2]

The goal of the present article is to illustrate the evolution of efficient strategies of vertical control in hyperdivergent patients, since the use, in the recent past, of extraoral devices on the lower arch (J-hook), until nowadays, with the advent of skeletal anchorage. But, for patients with a more balanced facial pattern, the conventional mechanics with intermaxillary elastics in Class III direction associated to an accentuated curve of Spee on the upper arch, and a reverse Curve of Spee in the lower arch, and vertical elastics in the anterior region, continues to be an excellent alternative, if there is extreme collaboration on the use of the prescribed mechanics.

PATIENTS WITH A BALANCED FACIAL PATTERN

Case 1 – Class III with anterior open bite and posterior bilateral crossbite, treated with extractions (#38, #48)

» **Vertical control**: Accentuated curve of Spee on the upper arch, reverse on lower arch and vertical elastics on anterior region.

History and etiology

The patient, 27 years old, presented for the initial exam in a good general state of health. His main complaint reported functional problems related to mastication. Facial esthetics did not seem to be a concern (Fig 1). With more detailed examination of the occlusion, a disharmony between the maxilla and the mandible, in the anteroposterior direction was noticed. There was no reference to Class III in his family medical history.

Diagnosis

Regarding facial features, he presented a mesocephalic facial type, with a straight profile, proportional and harmonious facial third, lip competence at rest, and absence of evident asymmetries. The smile was unbalanced, with exposure of lower incisors (Fig 1).

In the dental aspect, he presented an Angle Class III malocclusion, with anterior open bite (2 mm), posterior bilateral crossbite, edge to edge relationship of incisors. Also, a 2 mm anteroinferior crowding was noticed, with rotations of central incisors and canines with mesial angulation; coincident midlines (Fig 1); good oral hygiene and healthy periodontium.

The panoramic radiograph analysis did not show any significant alteration that could contraindicate the performance of orthodontic treatment (Fig 2) Cephalometric evaluation indicated important skeletal disharmony, with ANB angle equal to -1° (SNA=86° and SNB=87°), with good mandibular growth in the vertical direction (SN-GoGn=32°), highlighting the balanced facial aspect. Upper and lower incisors were slightly tipped buccally (these observations can be better evaluated on Figure 3 and Table 1).

Treatment objectives and alternatives

It is possible to present, as the main objectives for treatment of the reported patient, by its order of importance: Expansion of the upper arch, eliminating premature contacts and correcting the posterior crossbite; by extracting lower third molars, to allow for the distalization of lower teeth, with the objective of correcting Class III malocclusion and establish adequate intercuspation. Since he showed a slight anterior open bite, precautions with vertical control were set during the distalization of the lower teeth.

The possibility of surgical treatment was not considered, because of the reduced magnitude of skeletal discrepancy, as well as because of the absence of adverse features on facial esthetics that could justify such an approach.

Treatment

Despite skeletal discrepancy (ANB = -1°), the case presented treatment feasibility to be just orthodontic. By examining him in detail, it was noticed that the presence of anterior open bite was conditioned to premature contacts on the posterior region, due to the crossbite.

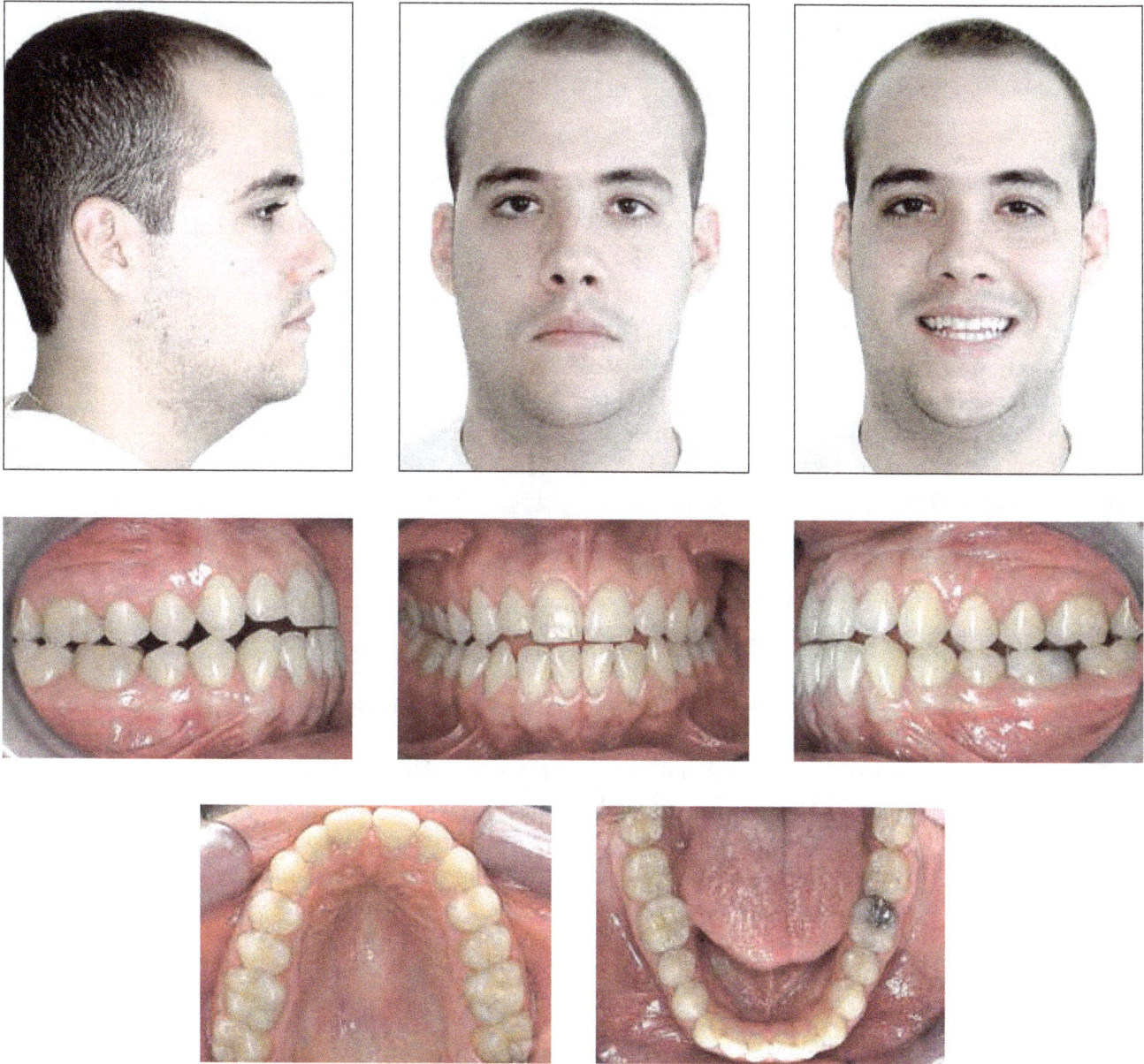

Figure 1 - Facial and intraoral initial photographs.

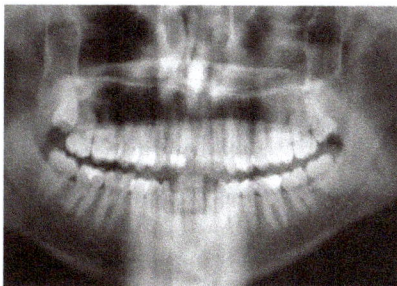

Figure 2 - Initial panoramic radiograph.

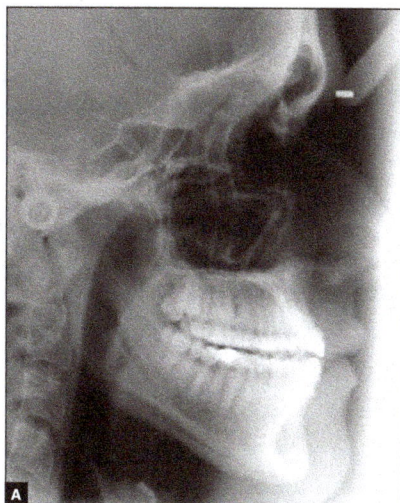

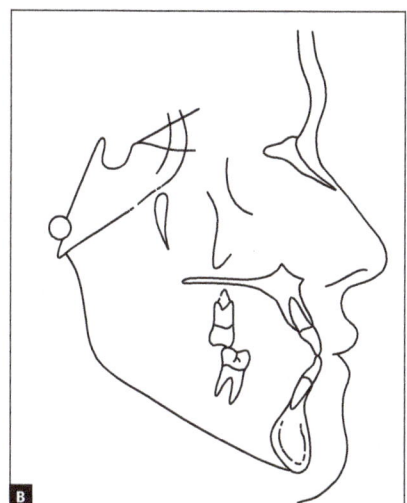

Figure 3 - Initial lateral cephalometric radiograph (**A**) and tracing (**B**).

So, the first treatment step would be to expand the upper arch, to eliminate transverse discrepancy, in order to obtain a more adequate evaluation on the real magnitude of the Class III, because it was believed that, in part, the latter was due to functional accommodation of the mandible.

The treatment itself was started with slow expansion of the upper arch (1/4 turn in alternate days, during 30 days) with a Hyrax type expander, with the objective to improving arch form, making it compatible, in the transverse dimension, with the lower arch. Three months after the correction of the posterior crossbite, the Hyrax expander was removed and then standard Edgewise 0.022 x 0.028-in slot metal brackets, with no torque or angulations, were installed.

In the lower arch, extractions of #38 and #48 were requested, with posterior appliance placement, with the exception of canines and incisors — because if they were included, it would cause undesirable projection of these teeth, due to the presence of crowding.

Once alignment and levelling of upper and lower arches (with exception of teeth #31, #32, #33, #41, #42, #43), was concluded, the improvement of coordination was beginning to be noticed on the anterior region, with the reduction of open bite (Fig 5). At this moment, 0.018 x 0.025-in steel arches were placed on both arches.

Class III mechanics (150 g/side) was started, attached to teeth #17, #27 and on long sliding jigs on the lower arch, extending from the tubes of teeth #37 and #47 to the mesial of lower canines (Figs 5 and 6). With that, the objective of this step was to use all the anchorage of the upper arch to distalize, tooth by tooth, the lower arch, by the means of light forces, in order to minimize collateral effects — such as the counterclockwise rotation of the upper occlusal plane. Thus the treatment was conducted until the correction of molar relation and the attainment of space on anteroinferior region. Then the canines and incisors were included, performing once more the alignment and levelling of the lower arch.

» **Vertical control:** At the moment the arches were found stable with rectangular 0.018 x 0.025-in wires, a specific intermaxillary Class III mechanics was started, with the objective of promoting refinement on the intermaxillary correction obtained before with the sliding jigs. Now, with heavier forces (150 g/ side), and the curve of Spee accentuated on the upper arch, reverse on the lower arch, and vertical elastics in the anterior region (150 g), the ideal conditions for adequate finishing were established (Fig 4). At this moment, the only limitation was restricted to the patient's agreement on using the elastics. The accentuated and reverse curves of Spee, respectively on the upper and lower arches, along with anterior vertical elastics, had the function of promoting efficient vertical control, with the closing of the anterior open bite due to the rotation of the upper occlusal plane with a clockwise direction and of the lower occlusal plane with a counterclockwise direction, which happened as expected (Fig 5).

The option for this kind of mechanics was because of the favorable dental and facial features presented by the patient. That would not be a good Indication for patients with excessive vertical pattern, once that, if the patient does not collaborate with the use of elastics, the effects on the occlusion may be disastrous and of harder resolution. Then, upper and lower 0.019 x 0.026-in stainless steel arches, were made with individualized bends, for proper finishing. The retention on the upper arch was accomplished with a wraparound and, on the lower one, with an intercanine fixed retainer (0,032-in).

Analysis of results

The main objectives of the treatment were accomplished, establishing an adequate dental relationship, with direct repercussion on the esthetics of the smile (Fig 7). As expected, no alteration on facial esthetics was not found. The patient was extremely cooperative, concerning the use of the proposed mechanics. With the dental alterations, the ANB angle was maintained, and there was a buccal inclination of upper incisors and retroinclination of lower ones, as well as efficient vertical control, with maintenance of the mandibular plane (Figs 8, 9, 10 and Table 1).

At the end of treatment, it was possible to observe the achievement of a Class I occlusion on canines and molars, and correction of anterior open bite, as well as adequate alignment and levelling (Fig 7).

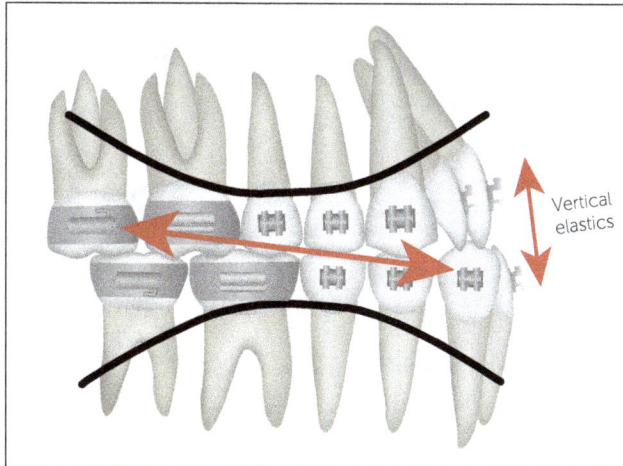

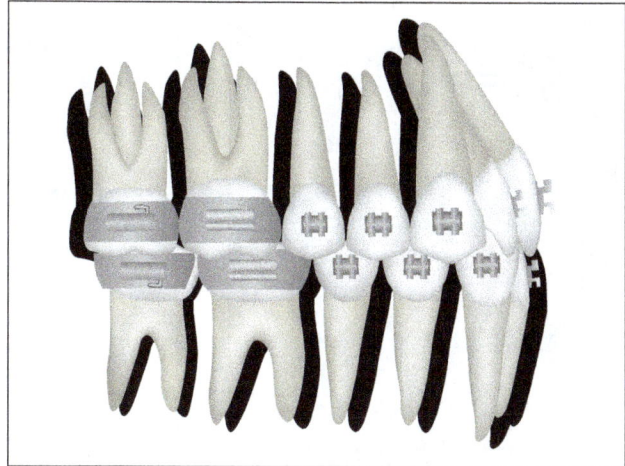

Figure 4 - Illustration of Class III mechanics use of intermaxillary elastics, reverse curve of Spee on the lower arch and accentuated Curve of Spee on the upper arch, associated to vertical elastics in the anterior region.

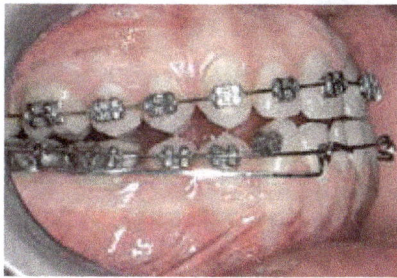

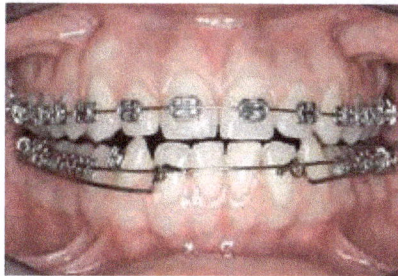

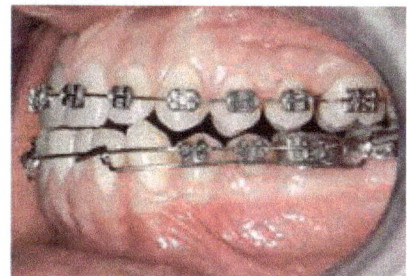

Figure 5 - Initial step of treatment. Class III mechanics with long sliding jigs (lower arch).

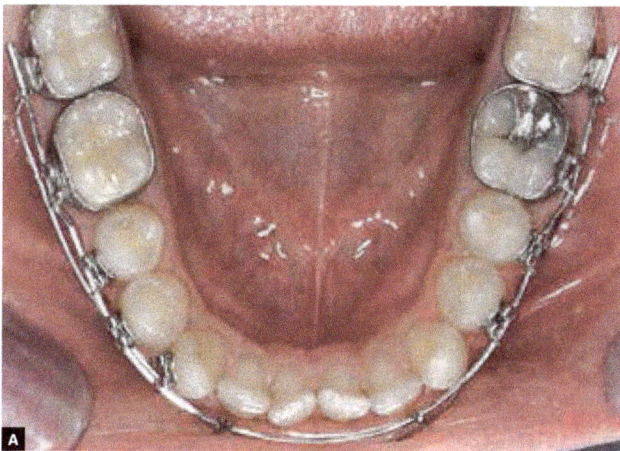

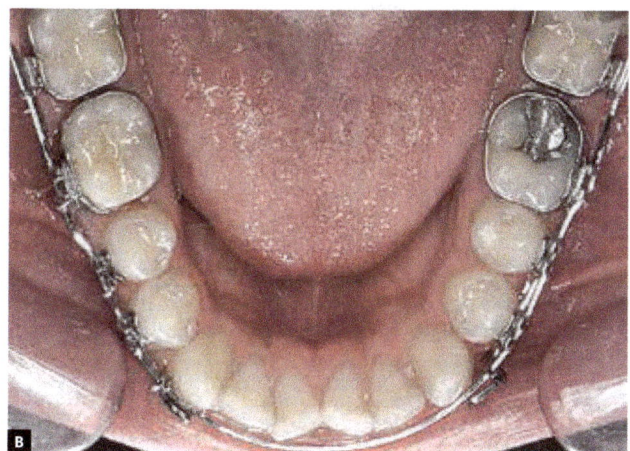

Figure 6 - A) Beginning of Class III mechanics. **B)** After 40 days, spaces between the upper teeth can be noticed.

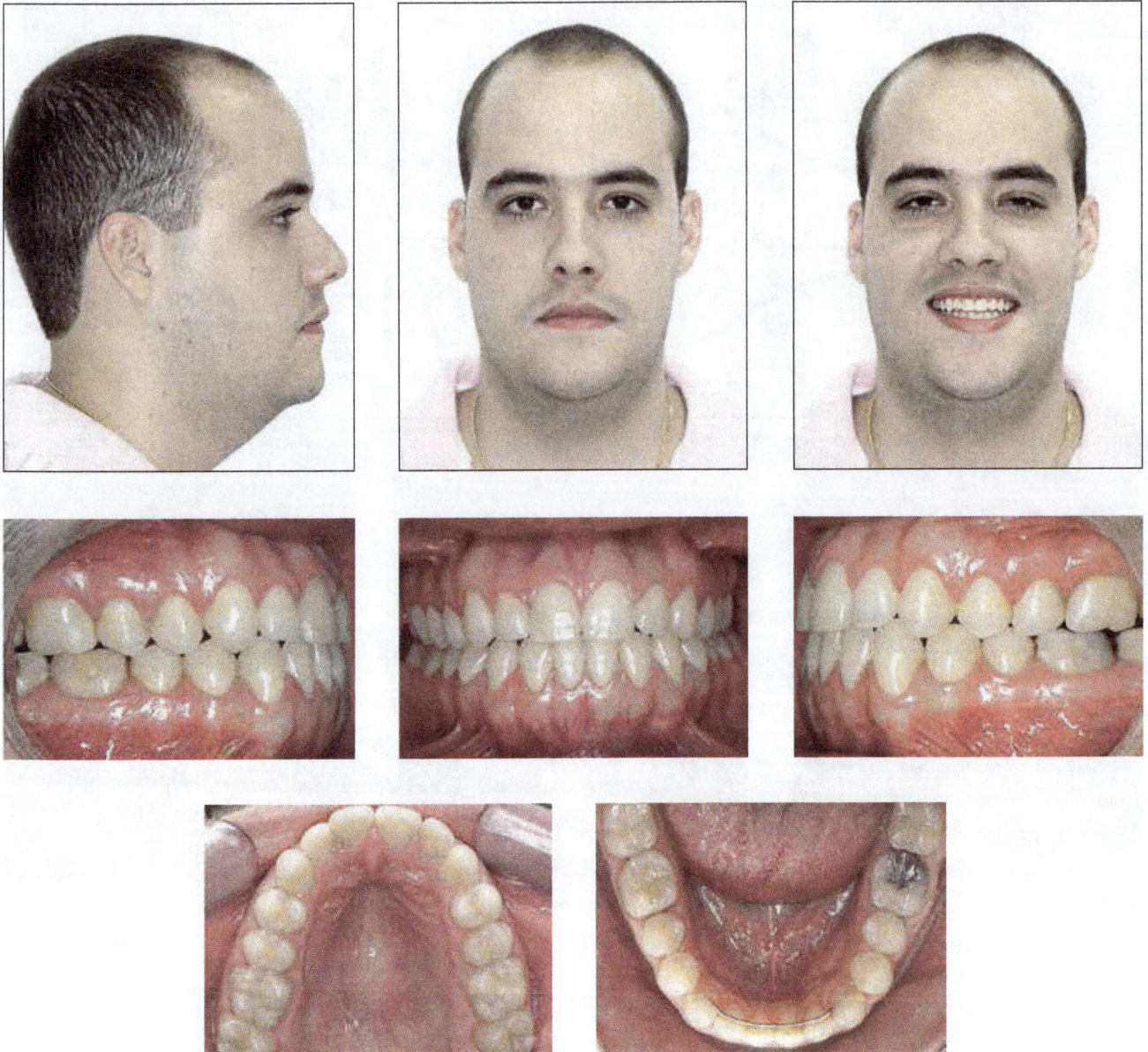

Figure 7 - Final facial and intraoral photographs.

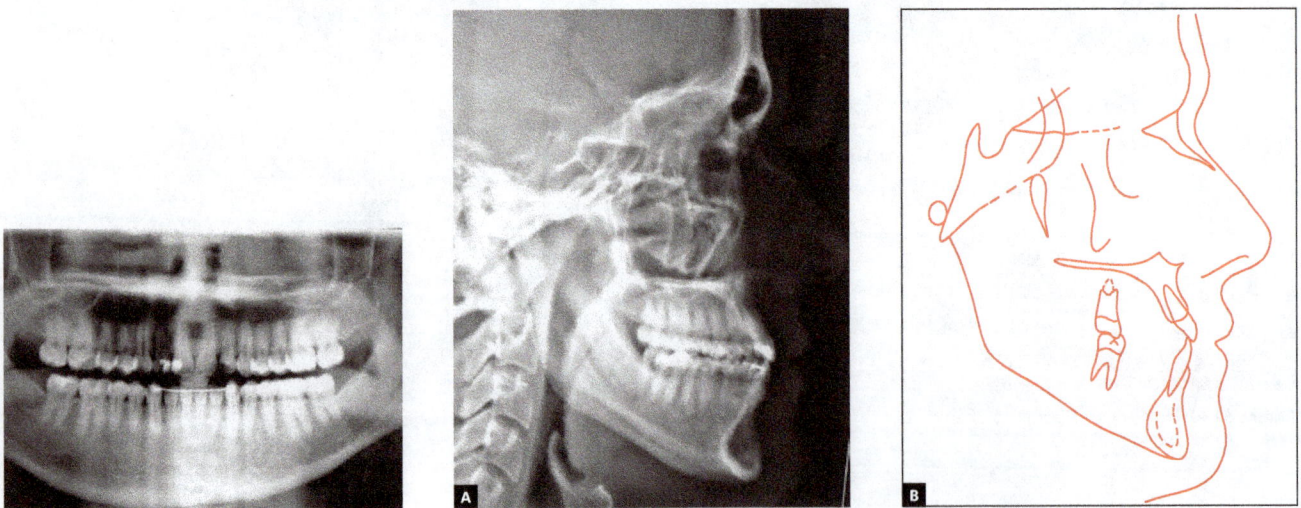

Figure 8 - Final panoramic radiograph.

Figure 9 - Final lateral cephalometric radiograph (**A**), and cephalometric tracing (**B**).

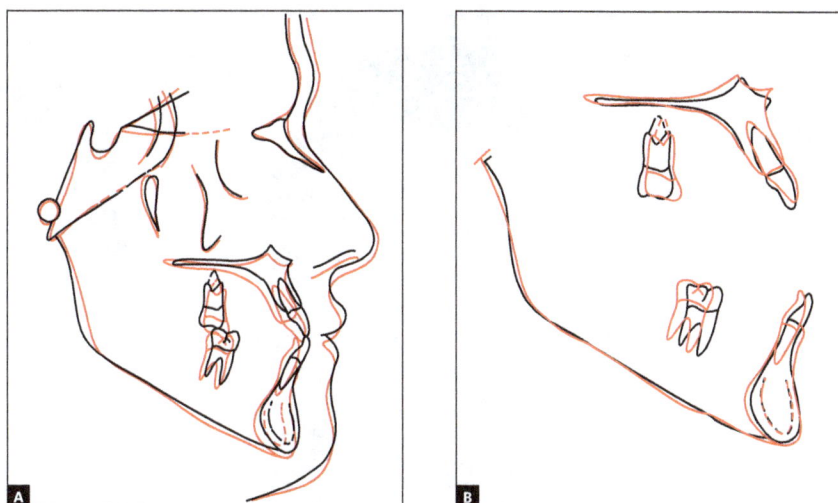

Figure 10 - Total (**A**) and partial (**B**) superimpositions of initial (black) and final (red) cephalometric tracings.

Table 1 - Summary of cephalometric measurements.

	Measures		Normal	A	B	A/B diff.
Skeletal pattern	SNA	(Steiner)	82°	86°	84°	2
	SNB	(Steiner)	80°	87°	85°	2
	ANB	(Steiner)	2°	-1°	-1°	0
	Convexity angle	(Downs)	0°	-5°	-5°	0
	Y axis	(Downs)	59°	58°	58°	0
	Facial angle	(Downs)	87°	86°	86°	0
	SN-GoGn	(Steiner)	32°	32°	33°	1
	FMA	(Tweed)	25°	27°	28°	1
Dental pattern	IMPA	(Tweed)	90°	92°	85°	7
	1.NA (degrees)	(Steiner)	22°	24°	28°	4
	1-NA (mm)	(Steiner)	4 mm	11 mm	9 mm	2
	1.NB (degrees)	(Steiner)	25°	30°	22°	8
	1-NB (mm)	(Steiner)	4 mm	9 mm	6 mm	3
	1/1 –Interincisal angle	(Downs)	130°	126°	130°	4
Profile	Upper Lip – S Line	(Steiner)	0 mm	-1 mm	-3 mm	2
	Lower Lip – S Line	(Steiner)	0 mm	-3.5 mm	-3.5 mm	0

PATIENTS WITH ADVERSE VERTICAL FACIAL PATTERN

Case 2 – Class III with anterior open bite and mandibular asymmetry, treated with extractions (#15, #25, #34, #44).

» **Vertical control**: Extraoral forces with high pull headgear (J-hooks).

History and etiology

The patient, 20 years old, presented for initial exam in a good general state of health. Her main complaint was related to the presence of anterior open bite and facial asymmetry, with mandibular deviation to the left side. Facial esthetics seemed to be a concern to the patient, due to the asymmetry caused by laterognathism (Fig 11). With more detailed examination of the occlusion, a real mandibular deviation to the left side was noticed, generated, probably, by asymmetric growth, and not by a purely functional deviation. Although, according to the mother, there was no reference to Class III on her family medical history, the peculiarities involved pointed to a multifactorial etiology.

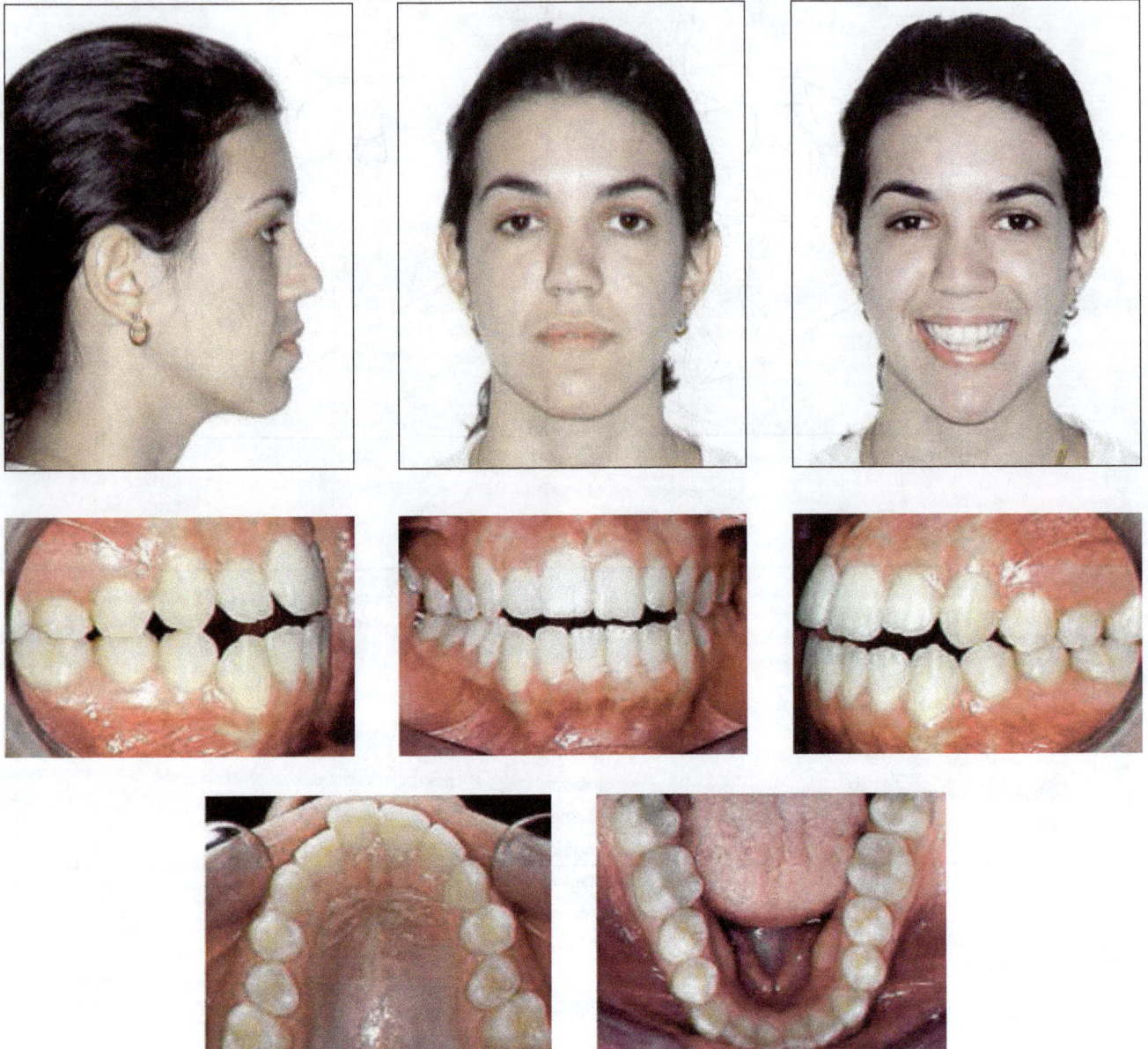

Figure 11 - Initial facial and intraoral photographs.

Diagnosis

Regarding facial features, she presented a dolichocephalic facial type, with a convex profile, inferior facial third slightly increased, lip competence, and presence of asymmetry due to mandibular deviation to the left. The lips were protruded, the lower one being slightly on front of the upper one (Fig 11).

In the dental aspect, she presented an Angle Class III malocclusion, with anterior open bite, 1 mm overjet, with buccal tipping of upper and lower incisors, characterizing a dentoalveolar double protrusion. Yet, an atresic upper arch was noticed, with a slight antero-superior crowding and rotation of teeth #15 and #25.

The lower midline was deviated 2,5 mm to the left, but was coincident with the center of the chin, characterizing a skeletal deviation, but not a dental one (Fig 11).

The panoramic radiograph analysis did not show any significative alteration that could contraindicate the performance of orthodontic treatment (Fig 12). Cephalometric evaluation indicated important skeletal disharmony, with ANB = -2° (SNA = 78° and SNB = 80°), with a poor mandible with a vertical growth direction (SN-GoGn = 39°), aggravating the vertical facial aspect. The maxilla and the mandible were slightly retruded in relation to the cranial base (this can be better evaluated on Fig 13 and Table 2).

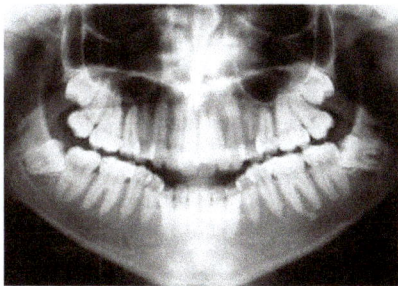

Figure 12 - Initial panoramic radiograph.

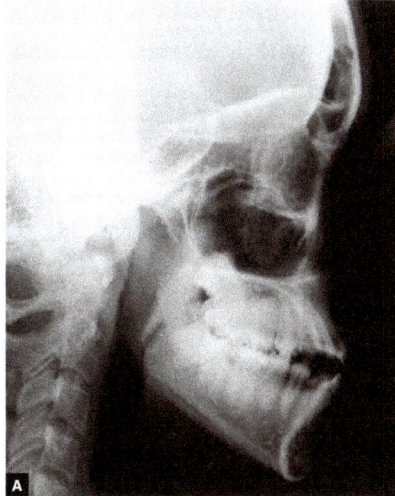

Figure 13 - Initial lateral cephalometric radiograph (**A**) and cephalometric tracing (**B**).

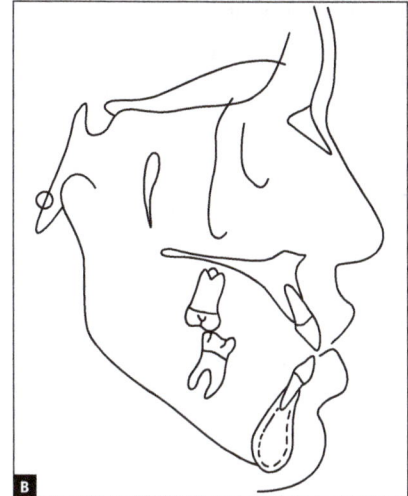

Treatment objectives and alternatives

With no doubt, the best treatment option included a surgical approach with asymmetric mandibular setback; however, this alternative was completely discarded by the patient and her parents. It was also proposed as treatment alternative a compensatory orthodontic treatment, with extraction of the second upper premolars and the first lower premolars, and the use of extraoral headgear (high-pull J-hook) on the lower arch during the retraction of canines and incisors. The achievement of this resource was pointed as indispensable for treatment success. With its use an efficient vertical control and maintenance of lower occlusal plane would be achieved, promoting a counterclockwise rotation, fundamental for the correction

of the anterior open bite. At the end of treatment, an adequate occlusion was expected, with absence of the exposure of lower incisors in the smile, which would contribute to camouflage the mandibular asymmetry and to give the smile a pleasant esthetics.

Treatment

Facing the refusal of performing a combined orthodontic and surgical treatment, a compensatory orthodontic treatment was done, with second upper premolars and first lower premolars extracted. Associated with that, the use of extraoral high-pull headgear (J-hook) on the lower arch, in order to promote efficient vertical control during treatment, specifically during canine and incisor retraction (Fig 14).

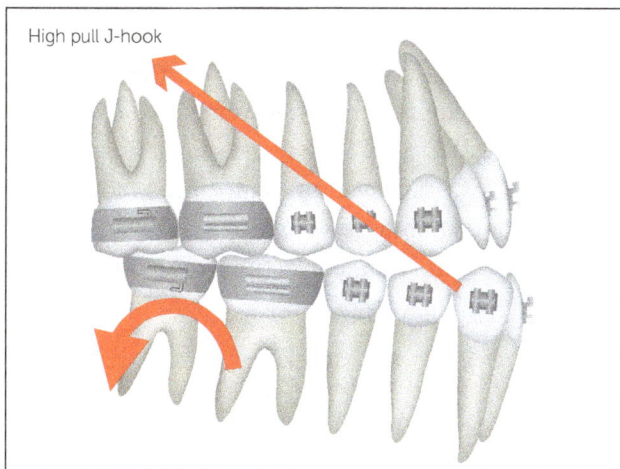

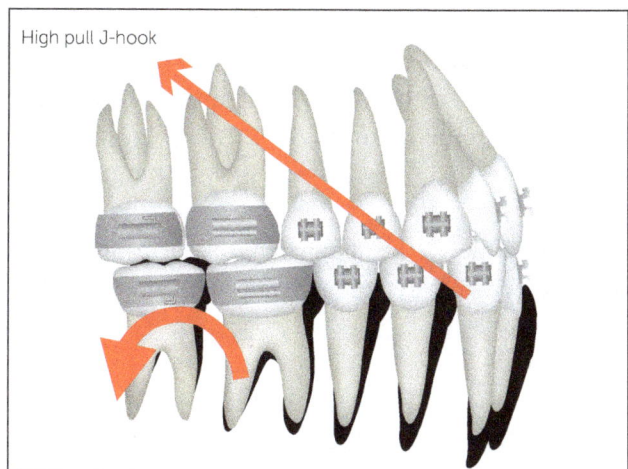

Figure 14 - Illustration of Class III mechanics employed for vertical control, anchored on J-hooks in the lower arch.

In the upper arch a slow expansion was performed (1/4 turn on alternate days, during 30 days) with a Hyrax expander, with the objective of improving arch form, making it compatible in the transverse direction with the lower arch. Then, standard metal brackets, with no torque or angulations, slot 0.022 x 0.028-in, Edgewise system were placed.

In the lower arch, apart from the fixed appliances, a high pull headgear (J-hook) was used.

After the removal of the Hyrax device, extractions of teeth #15 and #25 were requested, and then the alignment and leveling was performed, with 0.014-in, 0.016-in, 0.018-in and 0.020-in stainless steel arches, respectively. In the lower arch, initially the extractions of teeth #34 and #44 were requested and then the alignment and leveling was performed, with 0.014-in, 0.016-in, 0.018-in and 0.020-in sequential stainless steel wires. With the 0.018 x 0.025-in rectangular wire, the J-hook headgear was adapted on the lower arch, with high pull direction (150 g/side). The patient was instructed to use it for at least 12h/day. It was directly anchored on the arch, hooked to the canines, working as jigs, with the objective of distalizing the lower canines and, at the same time, due to the high pull, promote efficient vertical control, generating a rotation of the lower occlusal plane in the counterclockwise direction – which was favorable for the closure of the open bite (Fig 14). Due to the asymmetry and the greater need for distal movement of tooth #43, after distalization of tooth #33, the J-hook was anchored to a hook welded to the arch between teeth #32 and #33, while the right side would continue to play the role of a jig, moving tooth #43.

Meanwhile, in the upper arch, space closure would be executed in a reciprocal way, with the objective of enabling posterior anchorage loss, together with retraction and uprighting of the incisors, and consequent closure of the open bite.

Then, upper and lower 0.019 x 0.026-in stainless steel arches, with bends and torques were made, individualized, as needed for adequate finishing (Fig 15). The retention on the upper and lower arches, was done with wraparound type removable appliances.

Analysis of results

The main objectives of the treatment were accomplished, establishing an adequate dental relationship, with important repercussion on the general esthetics of the face, and, in a specific way, significative improvement on the smile, with the absence of exposure lower teeth (Fig 15), collaborating for mandibular asymmetry camouflage. It is worth to highlight that a preponderant factor for the success of the treatment was patient collaboration, with the use of extraoral mechanics, resulting in excellent vertical control. With the dental alterations, there was a significative change on the ANB angle, from -2° to 3° (Figs 17, 18 and Table 2).

That fact can be attributed to remodeling of the alveolar processes on lower and upper anterior regions, as response to the retraction mechanics employed. There was also significative improvement on the inclination on lower and upper incisors, with a decrease of 1-NA from 30° to 20°, and from 1-NB from 32° to 24°, effecting directly on the closure of the open bite and on the improvement of facial profile (Figs 17, 18, and Table 2). A Class I occlusion relationship was achieved on canines and molars, and the anterior open bite was corrected. Alignment, leveling, and inclination correction were successfully achieved (Fig 7).

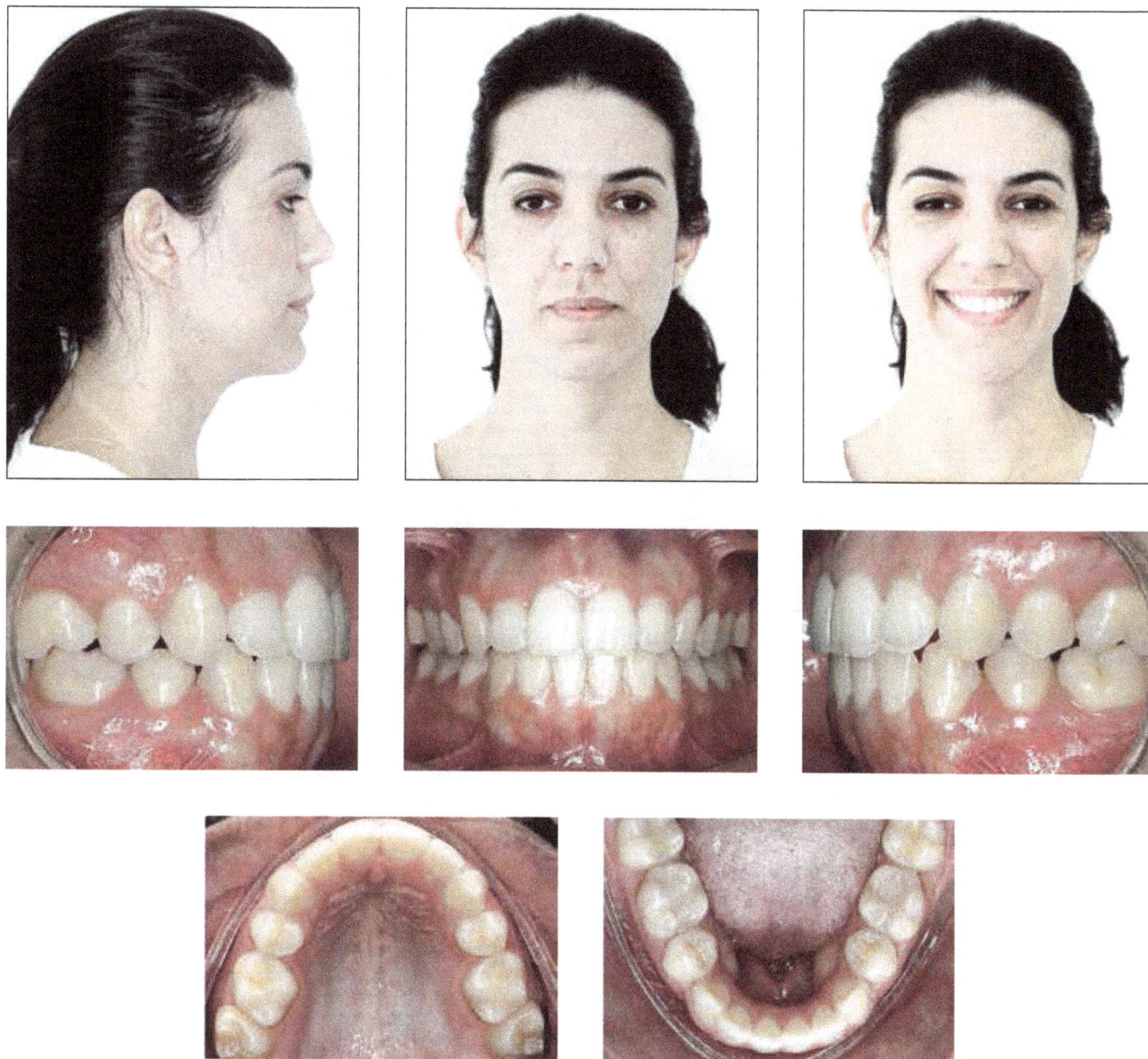

Figure 15 - Final facial and intraoral photographs.

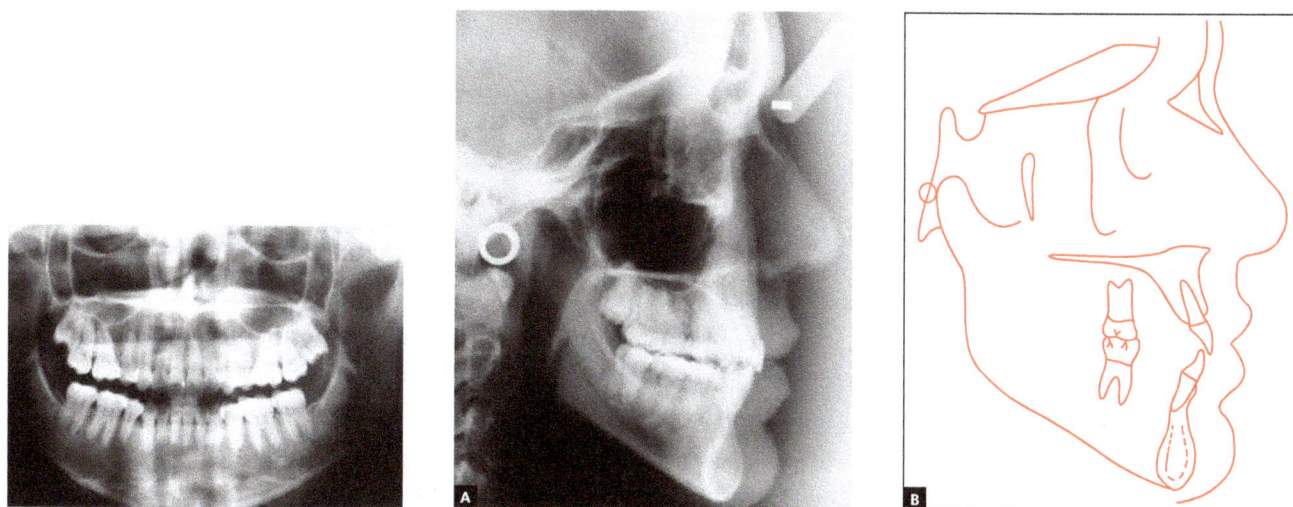

Figure 16 - Final panoramic radiograph.

Figure 17 - Final lateral cephalometric radiograph (**A**) and cephalometric tracing (**B**).

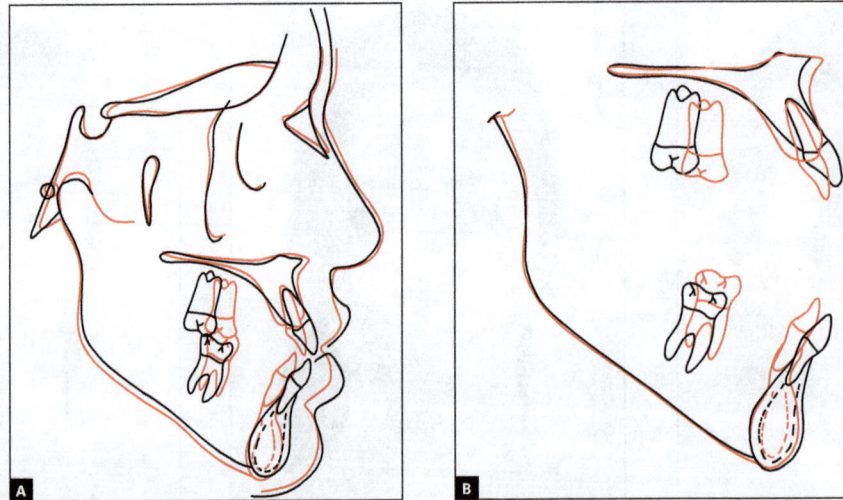

Figure 18 - Total (**A**) and partial (**B**) superimpositions of initial (black) and final (red) cephalometric tracings.

Table 2 - Summary of cephalometric measurements.

	Measures		Normal	A	B	A/B diff.
Skeletal pattern	SNA	(Steiner)	82°	78°	79°	1
	SNB	(Steiner)	80°	80°	76°	4
	ANB	(Steiner)	2°	-2°	3°	5
	Convexity angle	(Downs)	0°	-3°	2°	5
	Y axis	(Downs)	59°	66°	69°	3
	Facial angle	(Downs)	87°	82°	80°	2
	SN-GoGn	(Steiner)	32°	39°	40°	1
	FMA	(Tweed)	25°	37°	40°	3
Dental pattern	IMPA	(Tweed)	90°	93°	86°	7
	1.NA (degrees)	(Steiner)	22°	34°	18°	16
	1-NA (mm)	(Steiner)	4 mm	9 mm	5 mm	4
	I.NB (degrees)	(Steiner)	25°	32°	24°	8
	I-NB (mm)	(Steiner)	4 mm	7 mm	6 mm	1
	$\frac{1}{1}$ – Interincisal Angle	(Downs)	130°	116°	137°	21
	I – APO (mm)	(Downs)	1 mm	7 mm	2 mm	5
Profile	Upper Lip – S Line	(Steiner)	0 mm	1 mm	-1 mm	2
	Lower Lip – S Line	(Steiner)	0 mm	3 mm	-0.5 mm	3.5

Case 3 – Class III with anterior open bite treated with extractions (#38, #48)

» **Vertical control:** Skeletal anchorage

History and etiology

The patient, 29 years old, presented for initial exam in a good general state of health. His main complaint was related to the presence of anterior open bite, associated with masticatory difficulty. Facial esthetics did not seem to be a concern (Fig 19). With more detailed examination of the occlusion, a disharmony was noticed between the maxilla and the mandible, on the anteroposterior direction. There was reference to Class III on his family medical history.

Diagnosis

Regarding facial features, he presented a dolichocephalic facial type, with a convex profile, lower facial

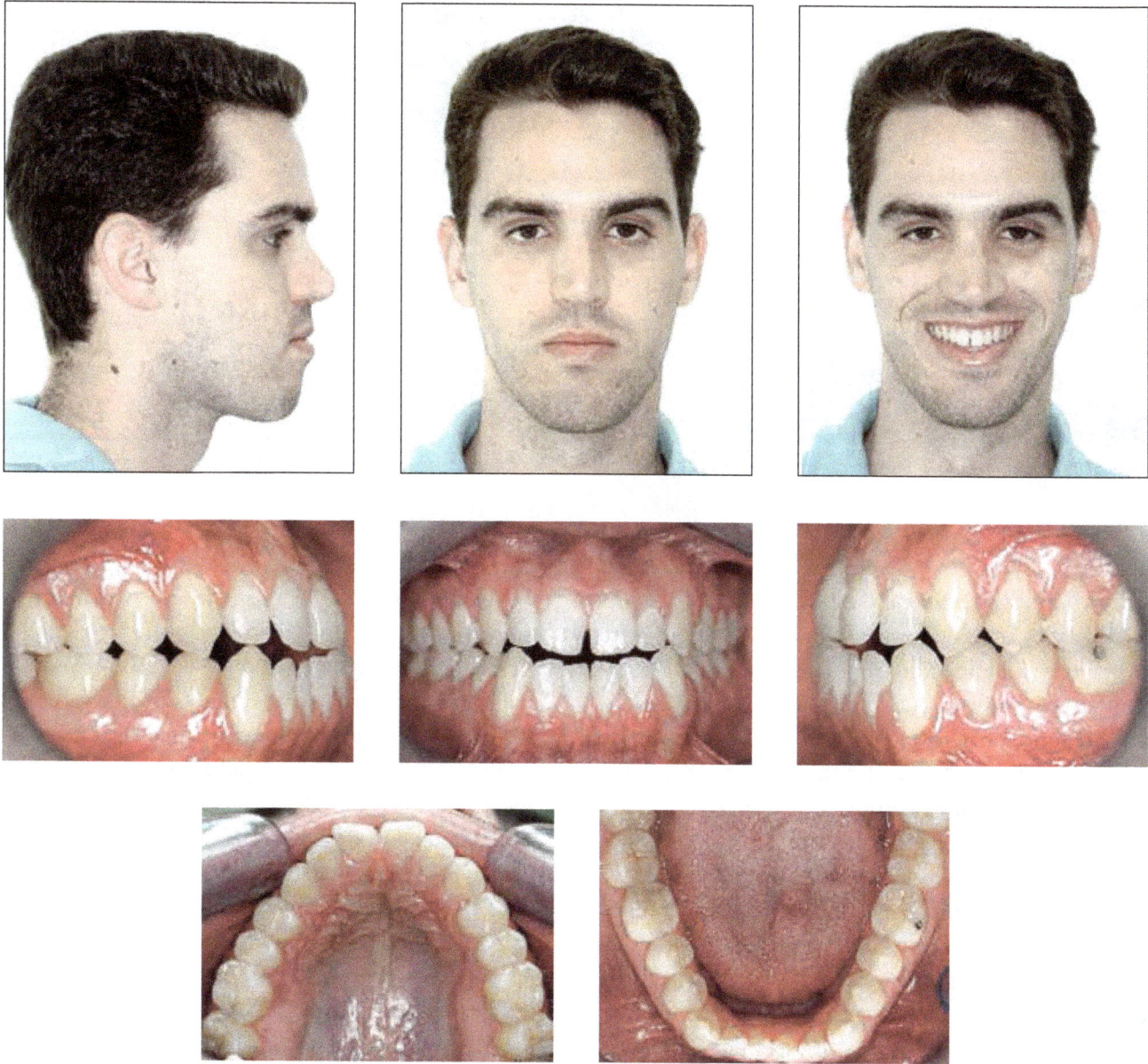

Figure 19 - Initial facial and intraoral photographs.

third largely increased and lip incompetence at rest. The lips presented a unbalanced relation, the lower being in front of the upper. He presented adequate exposure of upper incisors, when smiling (Fig 19).

Regarding the dental aspect, he had an Angle Class III malocclusion, with anterior open bite (2 mm), and a -2 mm overjet. Also, an ample upper arch was noticed, with rotations of central incisors and interincisal diastema. There was a reverse curve of Spee on the lower arch, with significative unevenness between posterior and anterior segments of the arch; upper and lower occlusal planes were divergent, and midlines were coincident (Fig 19). The presence of countless gingival recessions was, probably, related to the inad-

equate and traumatic form with which the patient performed brushing, conjugated to extremely fine periodontal profile, especially on the lower incisor region.

The panoramic radiograph analysis did not show any significant alteration that could contraindicate the performance of orthodontic treatment (Fig 20). Cephalometric evaluation indicated important skeletal disharmony, with ANB = -1° (SNA = 79° and SNB = 80°), with poor mandibular growth in the vertical direction (SN-GoGn=34°), highlighting the vertical hyperdivergent facial aspect. Upper incisors were tipped buccally and lower ones were vertical, in relation to the basal bone (those observations can be better evaluated on Fig 21 and Table 3).

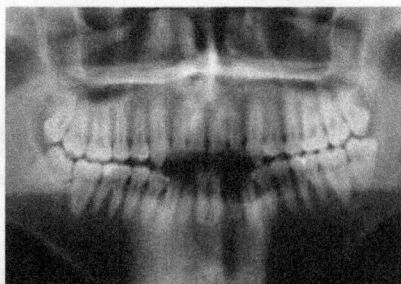

Figure 20 - Initial panoramic radiograph.

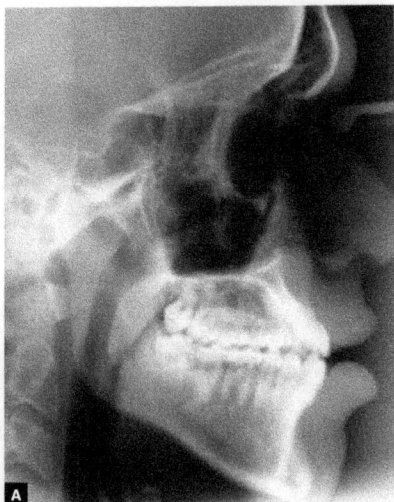

Figure 21 - Initial lateral cephalometric radiograph (**A**) and tracing (**B**).

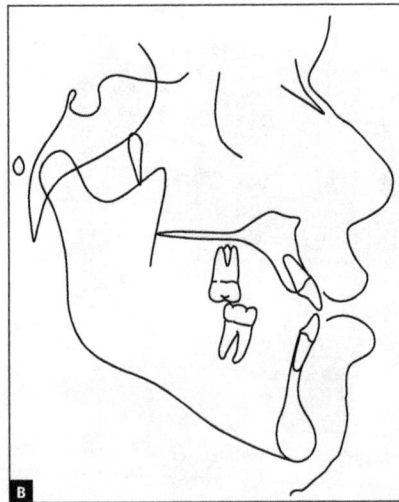

Treatment objectives and alternatives

Initially, orthosurgical treatment, probably with need of maxillomandibular manipulation, was presented as the only option to establish adequate esthetic and functional patterns. The surgical alternative was completely discarded by the patient. As another alternative, a compensatory orthodontic treatment was suggested with extraction of lower third molars, the use of skeletal anchorage on the upper arch (mini-implants) to support Class III intermaxillary mechanics, in order to reproduce the system of directional forces presented by Tweed-Merrifield, during distal lower tooth movement.[12] The achievement of this mechanic was pointed as indispensable for treatment success. With its use, efficient vertical control and maintenance of inferior occlusion plane would be achieved, promoting its rotation in a counterclockwise direction, fundamental for the correction of the anterior open bite. At the end of the treatment, an adequate occlusion was expected to be found, with counterclockwise rotation of the lower occlusal plane and decrease of lower incisor exposure in the smile. Periodontal control, associated with adequate brushing technique, was fit to minimize progression of recession, which was also part of the objectives.

Treatment

Even with the absence of complaint about facial esthetics, it was clear that the best option for the treatment would be the combination of orthodontics with orthognathic surgery. The patient readily manifested his aversion to surgery, questioning the alternatives. After careful analysis of the case, a compensatory orthodontic treatment was proposed, with the purpose of offering satisfactory occlusion with no worries about changes in the facial aspect. The greatest concern on the elaboration of the treatment plan was due to the need of efficient vertical control, because of the hyperdivergent pattern of the patient. The control of the lower occlusal plane, as well as its rotation in a counterclockwise direction, was made necessary to promote closure of the anterior open bite. This aspect was obtained with the use of specific mechanics, with origin in points of skeletal anchorage on the upper arch (mini-implants) (Fig 22). The mechanic described followed the directional force principles of Tweed-Merrifield technique.[12]

The treatment itself had its start with the extraction of the lower third molars, the installation of mini-implants between teeth #15-#16 and #25-#26, and the setting of 0.022 x 0.028-in Edgewise standard metal brackets in both arches, except on the lower incisors that were included only in a posterior step of the treatment.

The superior arch had its normal sequence of alignment and leveling with 0.014-in NiTi wire, as well as 0.016-in; 0.018-in and 0.020-in, and finally with a 0.018 x 0.025-in, stainless steel archwire. In the lower arch a specific mechanic was applied to perform vertical control and distalization of the lower teeth after the removal of the third molars. The mini-implants on the posterior region of the upper arch worked as points of skeletal anchorage, in order to apply intermaxillary mechanics with Class III direction. The presence of those devices resulted on several advantages, such as: 1) It completely eliminated the undesirable effects of intermaxillary mechanics on the upper arch, which would provide an even bigger projection of upper incisors. 2) The direction of the high-pull on the anterior region of the lower arch gave a vigorous vertical control, promoting counterclockwise rotation of the lower occlusal plane, so important for the evolution of the treatment during distalization of the lower teeth and closure of the open bite, quite similar to the high pull J-hook extraoral device on the lower arch, as described and applied on the technique by Tweed-Merrifield[12] (Figs 22 to 25).

As the posterior region of the lower arch presented a relative degree of alignment and leveling, the treatment started with a 0.017 x 0.022-in rectangular stainless steel archwire, passively adapted, highlighting only the presence of tip back bends with intensity of about 30° on teeth #37 and #47.

Molar correction was performed with the help of long sliding jigs that received elastics from mini-implants on the upper arch (Fig 23). Those jigs were near the tubes on teeth #37 and #47, extending anteriorly

until the canine distal surface. The force exerted by the elastics (150 g) on the high pull potentiated the distal inclination bends of teeth #37 and #47, distalizing them, at the same time in which promoted efficient control of the lower occlusal plane (Figs 22 and 23). As the second molars were distalized and reached their proper place, the jigs were being transferred to the next molar, and so on.

When posteroinferior teeth had already been considerably distalized, so that some diastemas appeared between the canines and the lateral incisors, the incisors were included in the treatment. A 0.018-in archwire with "T" loops, to allow for the correct alignment and leveling of these teeth, replaced the rectangular arch. However, the intermaxillary mechanics continued.

After alignment and leveling of incisors, a new 0.018 x 0.025-in rectangular lower archwire was made. Intermaxillary mechanics persisted until the achievement of the molar and canine Class I occlusion, and the establishment of adequate overbite and overjet.

Then, upper and lower 0.019 x 0.026-in stainless steel archwires, in an ideal form were made, individualized as needed for adequate finishing. The retention on the upper arch was done with a wraparound type plate, and on the lower arch with intercanine fixed retainer made with 0,032-in wire.

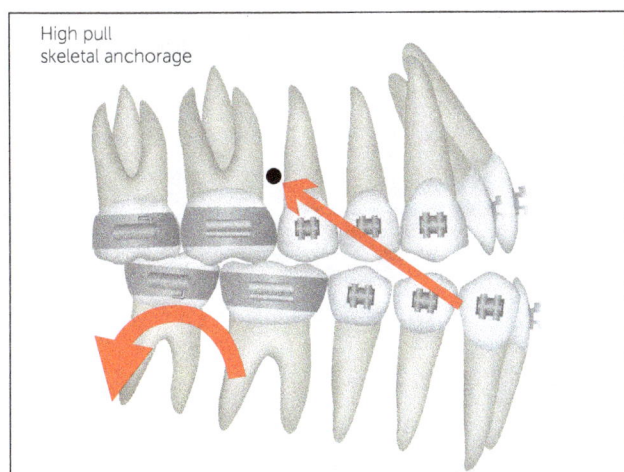

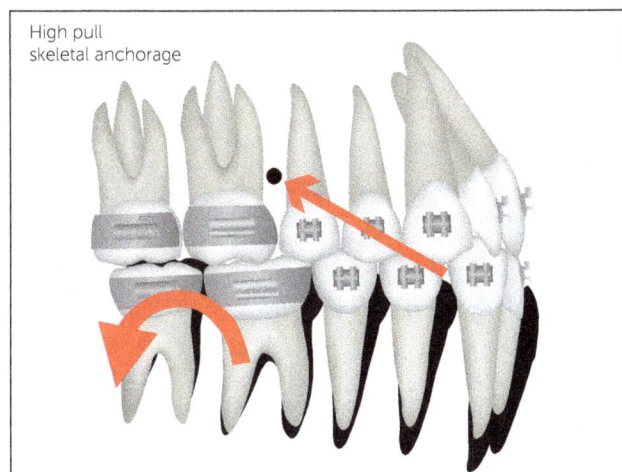

Figure 22 - Illustration of the Class III mechanics employed in the vertical control, anchored in mini-implants on the upper arch, between the first molars and second premolars.

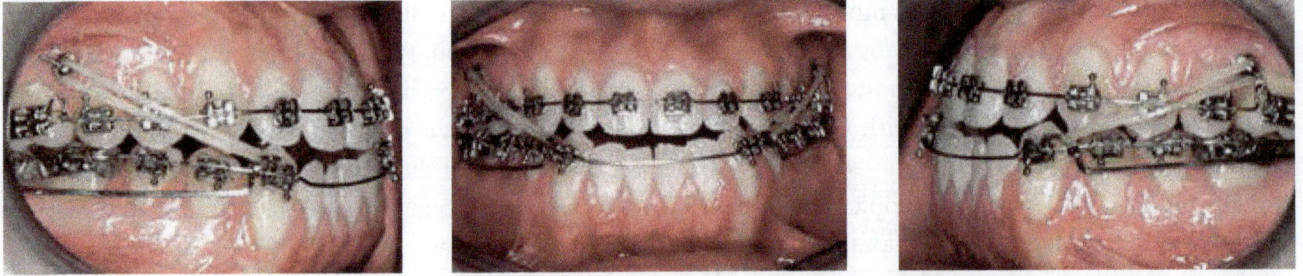

Figure 23 - Initial step of treatment. Class III mechanics supported by mini-implants (upper arch) and with sliding jigs (lower arch).

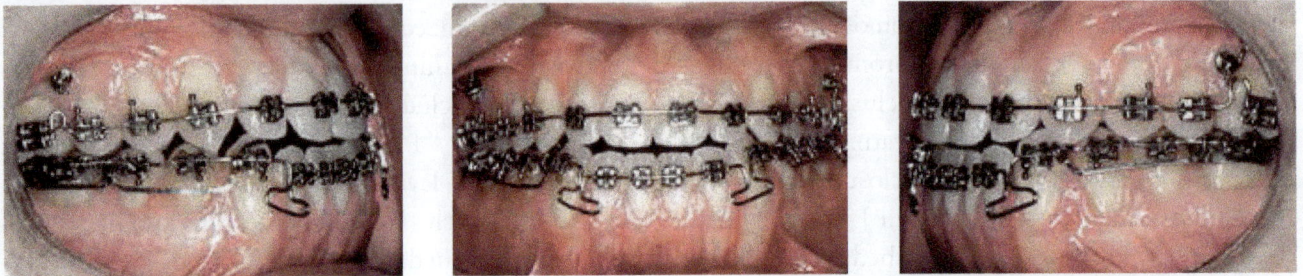

Figure 24 - Intermediate treatment step. Lower incisors were included after reasonable distalization of the other teeth in this arch. Observe the control of the lower occlusal plane, as well as the closure of the bite, produced by Class III mechanics supported by mini-implants.

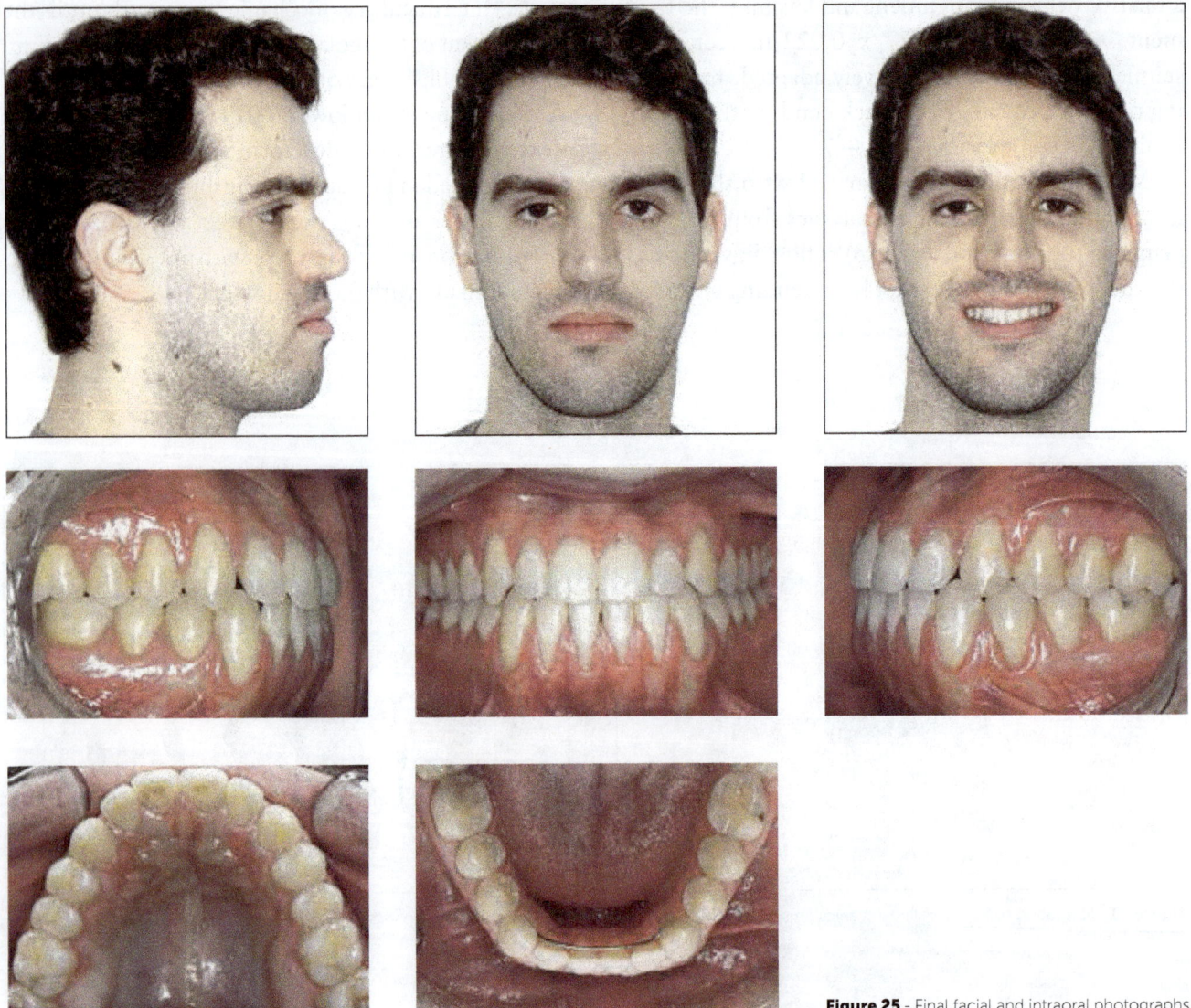

Figure 25 - Final facial and intraoral photographs.

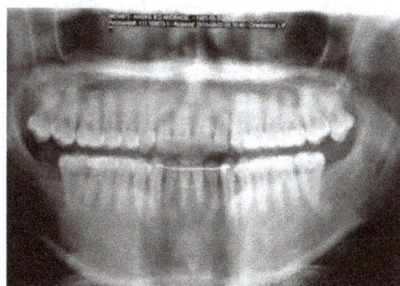

Figure 26 - Final panoramic radiograph.

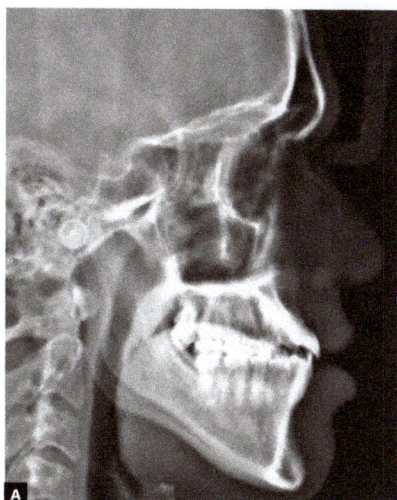

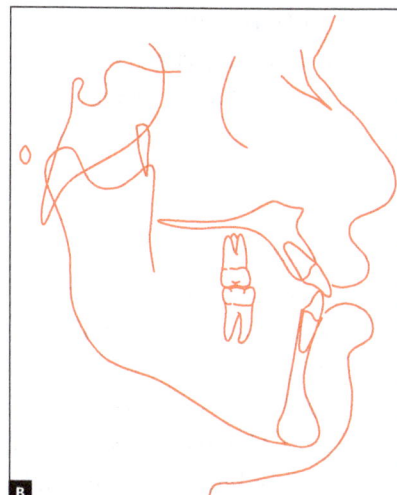

Figure 27 - Final lateral cephalometric radiograph (**A**), and cephalometric tracing (**B**).

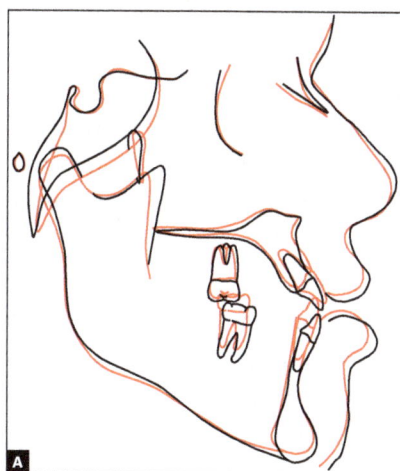

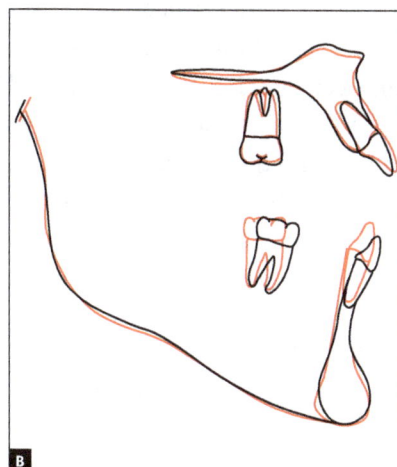

Figure 28 - Total (**A**) and partial (**B**) superimpositions of initial (black) and final (red) cephalometric tracings.

Table 3 - Summary of cephalometric measurements.

	Measures		Normal	A	B	A/B diff.
Skeletal pattern	SNA	(Steiner)	82°	79°	78°	1
	SNB	(Steiner)	80°	80°	79°	1
	ANB	(Steiner)	2°	-1°	-1°	0
	Convexity angle	(Downs)	0°	-6°	-7°	1
	Y axis	(Downs)	59°	57°	57°	0
	Facial angle	(Downs)	87°	94°	93°	1
	SN-GoGn	(Steiner)	32°	34°	32°	2
	FMA	(Tweed)	25°	27°	24°	3
Dental pattern	IMPA	(Tweed)	90°	85°	83°	2
	1.NA (degrees)	(Steiner)	22°	33°	42°	9
	1-NA (mm)	(Steiner)	4 mm	8 mm	11 mm	3
	1.NB (degrees)	(Steiner)	25°	23°	18°	5
	1-NB (mm)	(Steiner)	4 mm	7 mm	6 mm	1
	$\frac{1}{1}$ –Interincisal Angle	(Downs)	130°	124°	122°	2
Profile	Upper Lip – S Line	(Steiner)	0 mm	0.5 mm	0 mm	0.5
	Lower Lip – S Line	(Steiner)	0 mm	6 mm	4 mm	2

Analysis of results

The main objectives of the treatment were accomplished, establishing an adequate dental relationship, with significative improvement on esthetics of the smile, with the minimization of lower incisor exposure (Fig 25). No important repercussion was noticed on general facial esthetics, since that was not an original objective. It is worthy to highlight that a preponderant factor for the success of the treatment was patient collaboration on the use of intermaxillary elastics. Skeletal alterations can be summarized on mandibular counterclockwise rotation, with decrease of 2°, at SN-GoGn (from 34° to 32°), proving the efficient control of used mechanics (Figs 27 and 28, and Table 3). From the dental point of view, there was and increase of upper incisor inclination, with 1-NA from 33° to 42°, and slight retroinclination and extrusion of lower incisors, 1-NB from 23° to 18°, effecting directly on the closure of the open bite (Fig 27 and 28, and Table 3).

A Class I relationship on canines and molars was obtained, and the anterior open bite was corrected. Alignment, leveling, and inclination and rotation correction were successfully achieved (Fig 17). There was a slight increase of gingival recessions on the region of lower incisors, but not in a single moment that fact could be attributed to dental movement, since those movements were slowly accomplished, with lingual inclination. The patient admitted to persist with inadequate brushing, which surely contributed to this situation. He was referred to evaluation by a periodontist, regarding the need for performing free gingival grafts.

CONCLUSION

On the importance of vertical control on Class III orthodontic compensatory treatment (camouflage), we understand that:

1. The control of the occlusal plane and of the mandibular plane provided by efficient and easily applied mechanics can bring benefits that characterize Class III compensatory treatment as a great alternative for the resolution of those problems. It is important to highlight that there are limitations, and that not every case can be treated in a compensatory manner.

2. Orthodontic camouflage is not able to produce great changes on the face, neither to correct asymmetry, that is, it should not be used on patients who yearn for great facial esthetics alteration, who, therefore, are candidates to orthognathic surgery.

3. It is important to highlight that, in cases treated with orthodontic camouflage, skeletal discrepancy remains. Therefore, it is most important to verify in detail the patient's complaint before beginning any kind of treatment. That prevents future frustration regarding the result achieved at the end of the treatment.[3]

4. Orthodontics is not a exact science, therefore, it is the clinical experience of the professional that will dictate treatment planning, always paying attention to the limitations and particularities of each patient, in order to raise the possibilities of treatment success.

REFERENCES

1. Proffit WR. Ortodontia contemporânea. 3ª ed. Rio de Janeiro: Guanabara Koogan; 2002.

2. Jiuxiang L, Yan G. Preliminary investigation of nonsurgical treatment of severe skeletal Class III malocclusion in the permanent dentition. Angle Orthod. 2003;73(4):401-10.

3. Silva AAF, Manganello-Souza LC, Freitas SLA. Tratamento das deformidades maxilofaciais. Rev Bras Cir Craniomaxilofac. 2009;2(3):129-32.

4. Troy BA, Shanker S, Fields HW, Vig K, Johnston W. Comparison of incisor inclination in patients with Class III malocclusion treated with orthognathic surgery or orthodontic camouflage. Am J Orthod Dentofacial Orthop. 2009;135(2):146.e1-9; discussion 146-7.

5. Burns NR, Musich DR, Martin C, Razmus T, Gunel E, Ngan P. Class III camouflage treatment: what are the limits? Am J Orthod Dentofacial Orthop. 2010 Jan;137(1):9.e1-9.e13; discussion 9-11.

6. Sakai A, Haraguchi S, Takada K. Orthodontic camouflage of a late adolescent patient with Class III malocclusion. Orthod Waves. 2006;65(3):127-33.

7. Ning F, Duan Y, Huo N. Camouflage treatment in skeletal Class III cases combined with severe crowding by extraction of four premolars. Orthod Waves. 2009;68(2):80-7.

8. Mihalik CA, Proffit WR, Phillips C. Long-term follow-up of Class II adults treated with orthodontic camouflage: A comparison with orthognathic surgery outcomes. Am J Orthod Dentofacial Orthop. 2003;123(3):266-78.

9. Bishara SE. Class II malocclusions: diagnostic and clinical considerations with and without treatment. Semin Orthod. 2006;12(1):11-24.

10. Araújo TM. Cefalometria, conceitos e análises [tese]. Rio de Janeiro (RJ): Universidade Federal do Rio de Janeiro; 1983.

11. Arnett W, Bergman RT. Facial keys to orthodontic diagnosis and treatment planning—part II. Am J Orthod Dentofacial Orthop. 1993;103(5):395-411.

12. Merrifield L. Edgewise sequential directional force technology. J Charles H. Tweed Int Found. 1986;14:22-37.

20

Sagittal and vertical aspects of Class II division 1 subjects according to the respiratory pattern

Laura de Castro Cabrera[1], Luciana Borges Retamoso[2], Raul Magnoler Sampaio Mei[3], Orlando Tanaka[4]

Introduction: The teeth position, specially maxillary and mandibular incisors, in relation to basal bone and surrounding soft tissues must be considered in the elaboration of diagnosis, treatment planning and execution to obtain alignment, leveling, intercuspation, facial balance and harmony with stability of results. **Objectives:** To evaluate the modifications in the positioning of incisors in individuals with Angle Class II, division 1 malocclusion in two distinct moments of dentocraniofacial development, with mean interval of 2 years and 5 months. **Methods:** The measures were obtained by means of lateral cephalograms of 40 individuals, being 23 nasal breathers (NB) and 17 mouth breathers (MB). The analyzed measures were overjet, overbite, UCI-NA, LCI-NB, UCI.NA, LCI.NB, UCI.SN, LCI.GoGn, UCI.LCI, ANB, GoGn.SN, and OccPl.SN. Statistical analysis (2-way repeated-measures ANOVA) was applied to verify intergroups differences. **Results:** Overjet, UCI-NA, LCI-NB, ANB, GoGn.SN, and OccPl.SN demonstrated statistically significant difference ($p < 0.05$) when observed the moment or the respiratory method. **Conclusion:** There is alteration in the positioning of incisors during growth with interference of the respiratory pattern.

Keywords: Angle Class II malocclusion. Mouth breathing. Breathing. Vertical dimension.

[1] MSc Student in Dentistry.
[2] PhD Student in Dental Materials, PUCPR.
[3] MSc in Orthodontics, PUCPR.
[4] Responsible for the area of concentration in Orthodontics of PPGO-PUCPR.

» The authors report no commercial, proprietary or financial interest in the products or companies described in this article.

Orlando Tanaka
Rua Imaculada Conceição, 1155
CEP: 80.215-901 – Curitiba / PR, Brazil
Email: tanakaom@gmail.com

INTRODUCTION

Overbite is the vertical trespass and overjet is the horizontal trespass, which suffer significant alterations during development of dentition, from initial mixed dentition to permanent occlusion.[16] Overbite is correlated to other measures that indicate facial dimensions, such as mandibular plane and occlusal plane angles. Overjet usually is a reflex of the anteroposterior skeletal relation,[8] and it is sensible to the atypical function of lips and tongue. On the development of Class II and III malocclusions, these dental measurements tend to adapt to abnormal skeletal relations. The position of maxillary and mandibular incisors, the relation between both and to the surrounding tissues, are important characteristics in the diagnosis, execution and stability of the treatment. The measures related to positioning of incisors affect the balance and harmony of facial profile. Due to its importance, since the introduction of craniometry, the position of mandibular incisor on sagittal plane became a precious tool to assess a malocclusion.[3,7] The determination of positioning of maxillary and mandibular incisor is part of most cephalometric analysis.[4] Downs[6] and Riedel[19] advocated specific values for the position of mandibular incisor, however, other values were suggested and used to predict the stability of the treatment results.[22,25,26] The maxillary incisors perform an important role because they provide the inclination for protrusive mandibular movement.[20] Also, the position and specially the axial inclination of maxillary and mandibular incisors, are determinative on facial esthetics, as incisors with increased axial inclinations, create protruded lips and, many times, absence of passive lip seal. The orthodontic treatment is frequently performed during adolescence, between 10 and 16 years of age.[17] Consequently, the evaluation of incisors positioning, its relation to adjacent structures, overjet and overbite during this period may provide information and contribute to the elaboration of diagnosis, planning, treatment and assessment of the post treatment stability. Thus, this work aims to assess the alterations on the position of maxillary and mandibular incisors in individuals with Angle Class II malocclusion, division 1, in two distinct moments of the dentocraniofacial development, with mean interval of 2 years and 5 months according to respiratory pattern.

MATERIAL AND METHODS

To perform this research it was used lateral cephalograms of 40 individuals with Angle Class II division 1 malocclusion, where 23 were nasal breathers (NB) and 17 mouth breathers (MB), aged between 10 years and 9 months and 14 years (T_1), and between 13 years and 4 months and 16 years and 6 months (T_2). The classification of respiratory pattern was done according to protocol described by Wieler et al,[27] which includes clinical evaluation of lip seal performed by dental surgeon, survey answered by the parents regarding respiratory habits, otorhinolaryngological assessment and speech evaluation. From these evaluations it was assigned scores and weighting for each evaluation, creating an index to classify the individual's predominant respiratory pattern. On each cephalogram it was fixed a sheet of acetate paper, 50 μm thick and 18 cm high x 17 cm wide. The cephalograms were traced with mechanical pencil Pentel P203 and graphite 2B, 0,3 mm of diameter, considering the interesting anatomic structures, and only on the left side, by a single operator, in a darkened room, being the only source of light the one from the negatoscope. The linear measures were performed with a single ruler with precision of 0.5 mm, and the angular measures with a protractor, precision of 0.5 degrees. The used angular and linear measures were the following, showed in Figure 1:

1. Overjet: Distance from vestibular surface of mandibular central incisor to palatine surface of maxillary central incisor, in millimeters.
2. Overbite: Distance, in millimeters, that the maxillary central incisor trespass the mandibular central incisor.
3. UCI-NA: Distance, in millimeters, from the vestibular surface of maxillary central incisor to the NA line.
4. LCI-NB: Distance, in millimeters, from the vestibular surface of mandibular central incisor to the NB line.
5. UCI.NA: Angle, measured in degrees, formed by the intersection of the long axis of maxillary central incisor and the NA line.
6. LCI.NB: Angle, measured in degrees, formed by the intersection of the long axis of mandibular central incisor and the NB line.
7. UCI.SN: Angle, measured in degrees, formed by the intersection of the long axis of maxillary central incisor and the SN line.

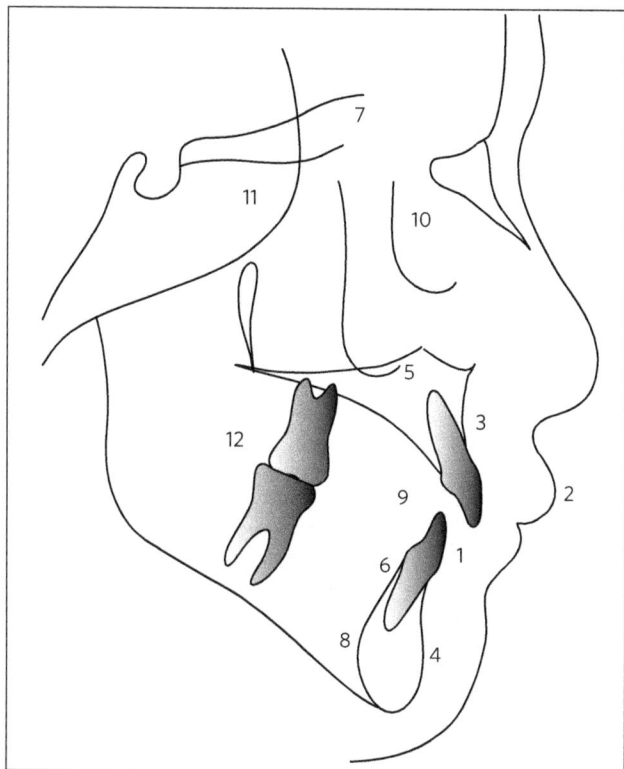

Figure 1 - Linear and angular measurements used.

8. LCI.GoGn: Angle, measured in degrees, formed by the intersection of the long axis of mandibular central incisor and the mandibular plane.

9. UCI.LCI: Angle, measured in degrees, formed by the intersection of the long axis of maxillary central incisor and the long axis of mandibular central incisor.

10. ANB: Difference, measured in degrees, between the angles SNA and SNB, determines the position of the maxilla and mandible in the anteroposterior direction.

11. GoGn.SN: Angle, measured in degrees, that determines the facial pattern in vertical direction.

12. OccPl.SN: Angle, measured in degrees, that determines the inclination of occlusal plane in relation to SN line.

STUDY'S REPRODUCIBILITY ERROR

To evaluate the reproducibility error, it was randomly selected 30 teleradiographs and a single operator performed the cephalometric evaluation for the second time, with interval of 30 days. It was calculated the systematic error[5] between the two evaluations

and it was observed that, for all the studied measures, this did not exceed 3%, thus obtaining reliability for all obtained data.

RESULTS

The statistical analysis was performed using the Statistical Package for the Social Science 15.0 for Windows (SPSS, Inc., Chicago, IL, USA). The verification of normality was performed through Kolmogorov-Smirnov test, at significance level of 0.05. Once it was found the normal distribution, the verification of existence or absence of difference between the means (Table 1) of the two types of breathers for each one of the two moments, was performed with the aid of ANOVA with two criteria for classification, with repeated measures.

When ANOVA demonstrated that there was a statistically significant difference ($p < 0.05$) between the mean values of overjet, UCI-NA, LCI-NB, ANB, GoGn.SN and OccPl.SN according to moment or respiratory pattern, it was used Tukey's HSD test of multiple comparison to identify which groups were different from one another (Table 2).

DISCUSSION

The results of the present work showed that there were alterations on the measures related to positioning of incisors according to moments and respiratory pattern, agreeing with Ceylan et al.[4] It was observed reduction of the overjet from T_1 to T_2 in both analyzed groups of individuals (nasal and mouth breathers). This behavior occurs because of the mandibular growth that tends to reduce the facial convexity and the overjet, according to proved studies by Ceylan et al.[4] Besides, the modification in the positioning of incisors may also have caused the reduction of overjet, for the measure LCI-NB increased in larger proportion than the UCI-NA. Another factor to be considered, is the reduction of the occlusal plane, probably caused by the counterclockwise rotation of the mandible, and consequently reduction of overjet. It is emphasized that the respiratory pattern affected this measure, since mouth breathers present greater overjet than nasal breathers, according to Mocellin[15] and Ricketts,[18] who point the respiratory pattern as an etiologic factor for malocclusions. Generally, mouth breathing patients tend to present a protruded maxilla and maxillary atresia, consequence of the alteration on the tongue position, which becomes lower, breaking the

Table 1 - Mean and standard deviation of linear and angular measures.

MEASURE	GROUP	n	MEAN	S.D.	MEASURE	GROUP	n	MEAN	S.D.
Overjet	NB T$_1$	23	4.21	2.14	UCI.SN	NB T$_1$	23	75.96	5.18
	NB T$_2$	23	3.74	1.77		NB T$_2$	23	74.96	5.53
	MB T$_1$	17	5.35	1.86		MB T$_1$	17	75.71	5.82
	MB T$_2$	17	5	1.7		MB T$_2$	17	74.59	5.29
Overbite	NB T$_1$	23	3.26	2.18	LCI.GoGn	NB T$_1$	23	98.78	4.23
	NB T$_2$	23	3.35	1.7		NB T$_2$	23	99.09	4.33
	MB T$_1$	17	3.15	2.26		MB T$_1$	17	99.29	4.81
	MB T$_2$	17	3.38	1.98		MB T$_2$	17	99.53	5.52
UCI-NA	NB T$_1$	23	5.28	1.66	UCI.LCI	NB T$_1$	23	125.7	7.5
	NB T$_2$	23	5.85	1.84		NB T$_2$	23	124.61	7.59
	MB T$_1$	17	5.56	1.69		MB T$_1$	17	121.41	6.44
	MB T$_2$	17	5.71	1.93		MB T$_2$	17	120.82	7.35
LCI-NB	NB T$_1$	23	5.61	1.8	ANB	NB T$_1$	23	4.48	2.19
	NB T$_2$	23	6.13	1.53		NB T$_2$	23	4	2.15
	MB T$_1$	17	6.97	1.75		MB T$_1$	17	5.94	1.68
	MB T$_2$	17	7.15	1.82		MB T$_2$	17	5.24	1.56
UCI.NA	NB T$_1$	23	22.22	4.78	GoGn.SN	NB T$_1$	23	31.83	5.1
	NB T$_2$	23	22.83	5.27		NB T$_2$	23	30.7	5.09
	MB T$_1$	17	22.88	6.5		MB T$_1$	17	34.71	4.04
	MB T$_2$	17	23.82	6.43		MB T$_2$	17	33.71	4.57
LCI.NB	NB T$_1$	23	28.09	4.94	OccPl.SN	NB T$_1$	23	16.48	4.83
	NB T$_2$	23	27.87	4.88		NB T$_2$	23	14.83	5.21
	MB T$_1$	17	29.59	4.09		MB T$_1$	17	19.12	2.26
	MB T$_2$	17	29.76	5.52		MB T$_2$	17	17.53	2.21

Table 2 - Mean, standard deviation and p value for the variables.

MEASURE	GROUP	n	MEAN	S.D.	intra and intergroups difference
Overjet	NB T$_1$	23	4.21	2.14	NS
	NB T$_2$	23	3.74	1.77	*NB T$_2$ X MB T$_1$
	MB T$_1$	17	5.35	1.86	*NB T$_2$ X MB T$_1$
	MB T$_2$	17	5	1.7	NS
UCI-NA	NB T$_1$	23	5.28	1.66	*NB T$_1$ X NB T$_2$
	NB T$_2$	23	5.85	1.84	*NB T$_1$ X NB T$_2$
	MB T$_1$	17	5.56	1.69	NS
	MB T$_2$	17	5.71	1.93	NS
LCI-NB	NB T$_1$	23	5.61	1.8	*NB T$_1$ X NB T$_2$, *NB T$_1$ X MB T$_2$
	NB T$_2$	23	6.13	1.53	*NB T$_1$ X NB T$_2$
	MB T$_1$	17	6.97	1.75	NS
	MB T$_2$	17	7.15	1.82	*NB T$_1$ X MB T$_2$
ANB	NB T$_1$	23	4.48	2.19	NS
	NB T$_2$	23	4	2.15	**NB T$_2$ X MB T$_1$
	MB T$_1$	17	5.94	1.68	**NB T$_2$ X MB T$_1$
	MB T$_2$	17	5.24	1.56	NS
GoGn.SN	NB T$_1$	23	31.83	5.1	**NB T$_1$ X NB T$_2$
	NB T$_2$	23	30.7	5.09	**NB T$_1$ X NB T$_2$
	MB T$_1$	17	34.71	4.04	NS
	MB T$_2$	17	33.71	4.57	NS
OccPl.SN	NB T$_1$	23	16.48	4.83	***NB T$_1$ X NB T$_2$
	NB T$_2$	23	14.83	5.21	***NB T$_1$ X NB T$_2$, ***NB T$_2$ X MB T$_1$
	MB T$_1$	17	19.12	2.26	***NB T$_2$ X MB T$_1$
	MB T$_2$	17	17.53	2.21	NS

NOTE: Significance level for Tukey HSD multiple comparisons *p < 0.05; **p < 0.03; ***p < 0.01.

balance with the buccinator muscle. It was verified an increase of the linear measures UCI-NA and LCI-NB from 10 to 16 years of age, which may be related to projection of maxillary and mandibular incisors, agreeing with Bishara.[2] On the other hand, Forsberg[9] observed verticalization of the incisors with facial growth. In this research, the measurement LCI-NB presented an increase proportionally larger than UCI-NA, explained as a way to camouflage the Class II skeletal relation. It is suggested that the alteration observed in the positioning of incisors can also be explained by the action of tongue muscles. However, Baydas et al[1] did not observe statistically significant difference in the positioning of these teeth during growth. From analysis of the ANB angle it was verified that there was a reduction on the difference between maxillary and mandibular bone bases in the sagittal plane, which seems to be directly related to mandibular growth and overjet alterations. The fact that the linear measurements related to the positioning of the mandibular incisor increases in larger proportion than the maxillary incisor may have caused the reduction on ANB. The respiratory pattern affected this result, where mouth breathers presented a larger ANB, disagreeing with the results of Frasson et al.[10] It is suggested that the decline on the tongue rest position, affected the maxillary growth, according to Subtelny[23] nasal breathing is essential for a correct growth and development of the craniofacial complex. However, Jakobsone et al[12] advocate that the respiratory pattern does not affect the soft tissue profile, and that such changes depend of the craniocervical posture and age of the patients. The angular measurement GoGn.SN presented a reduction from initial to final moment. It is concluded that this reduction can be related to counterclockwise mandibular rotation, as consequent reduction of overjet and ANB, as occurred in this work. The facial growth pattern is also responsible for alterations in this measure, for individuals with tendency to horizontal growth, will present a reduced GoGn.SN, and individuals with vertical growth, an increased GoGn.SN. As all patients were in growth

stage, the difference can be explained by a genetic horizontal growth pattern disagreeing with results of Lessa et al,[14] which did not observe significant differences on these measures. Likewise, the measure OccPl.SN also reduced, due to reduction on the inclination of occlusal plane, consequence of the change on positioning of maxillary and mandibular incisors and the mandibular rotation. This measurement was affected by the respiratory pattern, according to Lessa et al,[14] mouth breathers present greater mandibular inclination and vertical growth pattern. This work obtained statistically significant differences in the positioning of incisors in individuals with distinct respiratory patterns, agreeing with results by Spinelli.[21] Thus, the mouth breathing affected growth of some facial structures, causing a mandibular rotation down and backwards, in relation to the palate; and reduction of angle formed by intersection of mandibular plane with nasal plane.[13] According to literature, there is correlation between alterations caused by mouth breathing and the occlusion,[13] fact also verified in this work. It is assumed that alterations occurred on measures were consequence of genetic growth pattern, for with aging there is a tendency of the facial profile to become relatively more straight[28] associated to environmental factors, especially the respiratory method. However, this result disagree with Gwynne-Evans and Ballard;[11] Tomer and Harvold,[24] which indicated that muscle patterns and skeletal growth are genetically defined and, therefore, the individual characteristics, favorable or not, are inherited and little influenced by the alterations on respiratory pattern. Therefore, the alterations in positioning of incisors and the individual's respiratory pattern must be considered on the diagnosis, elaboration of treatment plan and execution of treatment in individuals in growth stage.

CONCLUSION

It is concluded that there was alteration in the positioning of incisors and overjet, during growth and with interference on the respiratory pattern.

REFERENCES

1.   Baydas B, Yavuz I, Atasaral N, Ceylan I, Dagsuyu I. Investigation of the changes in the positions of upper and lower incisors, overjet, overbite, and irregularity index in subjects with different depths of curve of Spee. Angle Orthod. 2004;74(3):349-55.

2.   Bishara SE. Longitudinal cephalometric standards from 5 years of age to adulthood. Am J Orthod. 1981;79(1):35-44.

3.   Broadbent BH. A new X-ray technique and its application in Orthodontics. Angle Orthod. 1931;1(2):45-6.

4.   Ceylan I, Baydas B, Bolukbasi B. Longitudinal cephalometric changes in incisor position, overjet, and overbite between 10 and 14 years of age. Angle Orthod. 2002;72(3):246-50.

5. Dahlberg G. Statistical methods for medical and biological students. New York: Interscience; 1940.

6. Downs WB. Variation of facial relationships: their significance in treatment and prognosis. Am J Orthod. 1948;34(10):812-40.

7. Ellis EE, McNamara JA. Cephalometric evaluation of incisor position. Angle Orthod. 1986;56(4):324-44.

8. Fleming H. An investigation of the vertical overbite during the eruption of the permanent dentition. Am J Orthod. 1961;31(1):53-62.

9. Forsberg CM. Facial morphology and ageing: a longitudinal cephalometric investigation of young adults. Eur J Orthod. 1979;1(1):15-23.

10. Frasson JMD, Magnani MBBA, Nouer DF, Siqueira VCV, Lunardi NC. Cephalometric study between nasal and predominantly mouth breathers. Braz J Otorhinolar. 2006;72(1):72-81.

11. Gwynne-Evans E, Ballard CF. The mouth-breather. Am J Orthod. 1958;44(7):559.

12. Jakobsone G, Urtane I, Terauds I. Soft tissue profile of children with impaired nasal breathing. Stomatol. 2006;8(2):39-43.

13. Kerr WJS, McWilliam JS, Linder-Aronson S. Mandibular form and position related to changed mode of breathing — a five-year longitudinal study. Angle Orthod. 1989;59(2):91-6.

14. Lessa FCR, Enoki C, Feres MFN, Valera FCP, Lima WTA, Matsumoto MAN. Influência do padrão respiratório na morfologia craniofacial. Rev Bras Otorrinolaringol. 2005;71(2):156-60.

15. Mocellin M. Respirador bucal. In: Petrelli, E. Ortodontia para Fonoaudiologia. São Paulo: Lovise; 1992. p. 131-43.

16. Moyers RE. Ortodontia. 4ª ed. Rio de Janeiro: Guanabara Koogan; 1991. 786 p.

17. Prahl-Andersen B, Ligthelm-Bakker AS, Wattel E, Nanda R. Adolescent growth changes in soft tissue profile. Am J Orthod Dentofacial Orthop. 1995;107(5):476-83.

18. Ricketts RM. Perspectives in the clinical application of cephalometrics. Angle Orthod. 1981;51(2):115-50.

19. Riedel RA. The relation of maxillary structures to cranium in malocclusion and in normal occlusion. Angle Orthod. 1952;22(3):142-5.

20. Russouw PE, Preston CB, Lombard CJ, Truter JW. A longitudinal evaluation of the anterior border of the dentition. Am J Orthod Dentofacial Orthop. 1993;104(2):146-152.

21. Spinelli MLM, Casanova PC. Respiração bucal. [acesso em 2002 Fev 2] Disponível em: www.odontologia.com.br/artigos.

22. Steiner CC. Cephalometrics for you and me. Am J Orthod. 1953;39(10):729-55.

23. Subtelny JD. Oral respiration: facial mal development and corrective dentofacial orthopedics. Angle Orthod. 1980;50(3):147-64.

24. Tomer BS, Harvold EP. Primate experiments on mandibular growth direction. Am J Orthod. 1982;82(2):114-9.

25. Tweed CH. The Frankfurt-mandibular incisor angle (FMIA) in orthodontic diagnosis, treatment planning and prognosis. Angle Orthod. 1954;24(3):121-69.

26. Tweed CH. Clinical orthodontics. St. Louis: CV Mosby; 1966. v. 1.

27. Wieler WJ, Barros AM, Barros LA, Camargo EL, Ignácio SA, Maruo H, et al. Combined protocol to aid diagnosis of breathing mode. Rev Clín Pesq Odontol. 2007;3(2):101-11.

28. Zylinski CG, Nanda RS, Kapila S. Analysis of soft tissue facial profile in white males. Am J Orthod Dentofacial Orthop. 1992;101(6):514-8.

Permissions

List of Contributors

Helder Baldi Jacob
Post doc student in Orthodontics, Texas A&M Baylor College of Dentistry

Ary dos Santos-Pinto
Full professor in Orthodontics, School of Dentistry — State University of São Paulo/Araraquara

Peter H. Buschang
Professor, Department of Orthodontics, Texas A&M Baylor College of Dentistry

Aristeu Corrêa de Bittencourt Neto
MSc in Dentistry, Orthodontics, Uningá, Maringá, Paraná, Brazil

Armando Yukio Saga
Professor at the Specialization course in Orthodontics, Pontifícia Universidade Católica do Paraná (PUCPR) and ABO-PR, Curitiba, Paraná, Brazil

Ariel Adriano Reyes Pacheco
PhD resident in Dentistry, Orthodontics, Pontifícia Universidade Católica do Paraná (PUCPR), Curitiba, Paraná, Brazil

Orlando Tanaka
Full professor of Dentistry, Orthodontics, Pontifícia Universidade Católica do Paraná (PUCPR), School of Health and Biosicences, Curitiba, Paraná, Brazil

José Valladares Neto
Adjunct Professor, Department of Orthodontics, Federal University of Goiás. Certified by the Brazilian Board of Orthodontics and Facial Orthopedics

Adriano Porto Peixoto
PhD resident in Oral and Maxillofacial Surgery, School of Dentistry – State University of São Paulo/Araraquara

Daniela Gamba Garib
Full Professor, Department of Orthodontics. Hospital of Rehabilitation of Craniofacial Anomalies, School of Dentistry — University of São Paulo/Bauru

João Roberto Gonçalves
Assistant Professor, Department of Orthodontics, School of Dentistry-State University of São Paulo/Araraquara

Davidson Fróis Madureira
PhD resident, Biological Sciences Institute of UFMG

Viviane Elisângela Gomes and Ana Cristina Borges de Oliveira
Professor, School of Dentistry — UFMG

Luís Fernando Castaldi Tocci
MSc in Orthodontics, UNIMAR

Omar Gabriel da Silva Filho
MSc in Orthodontics, UNESP

Acácio Fuziy
Post-Doc in Dentistry, FOB-USP

José Roberto Pereira Lauris
Full Professor, USP. PhD in Human Communication Disturb, University of São Paulo

Marcel Marchiori Farret
Professor, post-graduation courses, Specialization in Orthodontics, Centro de Estudos Odontológicos Meridional (CEOM), Passo Fundo, Rio Grande do Sul, Brazil; and Fundação para Reabilitação das Deformidades Crânio-Faciais (FUNDEF), Lajeado, Rio Grande do Sul, Brazil

Daniella Borges Machado and Valéria Silva Cândido Brizon
MSc in Dentistry, Federal University of Minas Gerais (UFMG)

Gláucia Maria Bovi Ambrosano
Professor, School of Dentistry — State University of Campinas (UNICAMP)

Milton M. Benitez Farret
Professor, Universidade Federal de Santa Maria (UFSM), Santa Maria, Rio Grande do Sul, Brazil

Aparecida Fernanda Meloti and Renata de Cássia Gonçalves
PhD in Orthodontics and Facial Orthopedics, School of Dentistry — State University of São Paulo (UNESP)/Araraquara

Ertty Silva
Specialist in Orthodontics and Facial Orthopedics, PUC-RJ

Milton M. Benitez Farret
Professor, Universidade Federal de Santa Maria (UFSM), Santa Maria/RS, Brazil

Alessandro Marchiori Farret
Private practice, Santa Maria/RS, Brazil

Melissa Proença Nogueira Fialho
Professor, School of Dentistry, CEUMA Univeristy, UNICEUMA

Célia Regina Maio Pinzan-Vercelino
Assistant professor, Department of Orthodontics, School of Dentistry, CEUMA Univeristy, UNICEUMA

Rodrigo Proença Nogueira
Assistant professor, Brazilian Dental Association/ Maranhão

Júlio de Araújo Gurgel
Assistant professor, Department of Orthodontics, CEUMA University, UNICEUMA

Bruno Boaventura Vieira, Ana Carolina Meng Sanguino and Marilia Rodrigues Moreira
Post-Graduation Student, FORP-USP

Elizabeth Norie Morizono
Professor at the Specialization Course in Orthodontics, FORP-USP

Mírian Aiko Nakane Matsumoto
Associated Professor at the Department of Pediatric Clinic, Preventive and Social Dentistry, FORP-USP

Francyle Simões Herrera-Sanches
MSc in Orthodontics, FOB-USP

José Fernando Castanha Henriques and Guilherme Janson
Full Professor, Department of Orthodontics, FOB-USP
Full professor, School of Dentistry — USP/Bauru

Leniana Santos Neves
Professor of the Specialization Course in Orthodontics, Federal University of Vale do Jequitinhonha and Mucuri

Karina Jerônimo Rodrigues Santiago de Lima
Adjunct Professor, Federal University of Paraíba

Rafael Pinelli Henriques and Lucelma Vilela Pieri
PhD in Orthodontics, FOB-USP

Ruben Leon-Salazar
Masters student in Orthodontics, School of Dentistry — USP/Bauru

Vladimir Leon-Salazar
PhD resident in TMD and Orofacial Pain, School of Dentistry — University of Minnesota

Susiane Allgayer
PhD student of Orthodontics and Facial Orthopedics, PUC-RS

Deborah Platcheck
PhD and Professor of Orthodontics, ABO/RS

Ivana Ardenghi Vargas
PhD in Dentistry, ULBRA

Raphael Carlos Drumond Loro
PhD in Oral and Maxillofacial Surgery and Professor at Graduation and Postgraduation courses, PUCRS

Mariana Roennau Lemos Rinaldi and Susana Maria Deon Rizzatto
PhD resident in Orthodontics, Pontifícia Universidade Católica do Rio Grande do Sul (PUCRS), Porto Alegre, Rio Grande do Sul, Brazil

Lídia Parsekian Martins and Ary dos Santos-Pinto
Adjunct professor, Department of Pediatric Dentistry and Orthodontics, School of Dentistry — State University of São Paulo (UNESP)/Araraquara

Luciane Macedo de Menezes and Waldemar Daudt Polido
PhD in Oral and Maxillofacial Surgery, Pontifícia Universidade Católica do Rio Grande do Sul (PUCRS), Porto Alegre, Rio Grande do Sul, Brazil

Eduardo Martinelli Santayanna de Lima
Adjunct professor of Orthodontics, Pontifícia Universidade Católica do Rio Grande do Sul (PUCRS), Porto Alegre, Rio Grande do Sul, Brazil

Milena Peixoto Nogueira de Sá
MSc in Integrated Dentistry, State University of Maringá (UEM)

Jacqueline Nelisis Zanoni
PhD in Cell Biology and Associate professor at the Department of Morphological Sciences, UEM

Carlos Luiz Fernandes de Salles
PhD in Pediatric Dentistry, University of São Paulo (USP). Adjunct professor at the Department of Dentistry, UEM

Fabrício Dias de Souza
PhD in Endodontics, College of Dentistry — Pernambuco

Uhana Seifert Guimarães Suga
Masters student in Integrated Dentistry, UEM

Raquel Sano Suga Terada
PhD in Dentistry, USP. Associate professor at the Department of Dentistry, UEM

Márcio Costa Sobral
MSc in Orthodontics, Federal University of Rio de Janeiro (UFRJ). Professor, Specialization Program of Orthodontics, Federal University of Bahia (UFBA) Diplomate by the Brazilian Board of Orthodontics and Facial Orthopedics (BBO)

Fernando A. L. Habib
PhD in Dentistry, Federal University of Bahia (UFBA) Specialist in Orthodontics, Federal University of Rio de Janeiro (UFRJ)
Associate Professor of Orthodontics, Federal University of Bahia (UFBA)

Ana Carla de Souza Nascimento
Specialist in Orthodontics, Federal University of Bahia (UFBA)

Osama Hasan Alali
MDS in Orthodontics, Teaching Assistant, Graduate-PhD

André da Costa Monini
Specialist and Master in Orthodontics UNESP-Araraquara

Luiz Gonzaga Gandini Júnior
Professor, School of Dentistry of Araraquara, UNESP Assistant Professor, Baylor College of Dentistry, Dallas, Texas, USA

Luiz Guilherme Martins Maia
Master and Doctorate student in Orthodontics UNESP-Araraquara

Ary dos Santos-Pinto
Professor, School of Dentistry of Araraquara, UNESP

Laura de Castro Cabrera
MSc Student in Dentistry

Luciana Borges Retamoso
PhD Student in Dental Materials, PUCPR

Raul Magnoler Sampaio Mei
MSc in Orthodontics, PUCPR

Orlando Tanaka
Responsible for the area of concentration in Orthodontics of PPGO-PUCPR

Index